Tackling the World's Fastest-Growing HIV Epidemic

HUMAN DEVELOPMENT PERSPECTIVES

Tackling the World's Fastest-Growing HIV Epidemic

More Efficient HIV Responses in Eastern Europe and Central Asia

Feng Zhao, Clemens Benedikt, and David Wilson, Editors

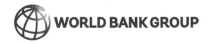 WORLD BANK GROUP

Human Development Perspectives

The books in this series address main and emerging development issues of a global/regional nature through original research and findings in the areas of education, gender, health, nutrition, population, and social protection and jobs. The series is aimed at policy makers and area experts and is overseen by the Human Development Practice Group Chief Economist.

Previous titles in this series

Meera Shekar and Barry Popkin, *Obesity: Health and Economic Consequences of an Impending Global Challenge* (2020).

Truman Packard, Ugo Gentilini, Margaret Grosh, Philip O'Keefe, Robert Palacios, David Robalino, and Indhira Santos, *Protecting All: Risk Sharing for a Diverse and Diversifying World of Work* (2019).

Damien de Walque, *Risking Your Health: Causes, Consequences, and Interventions to Prevent Risky Behaviors* (2014).

Rita Almeida, Jere Behrman, and David Robalino, *The Right Skills for the Job? Rethinking Training Policies for Workers* (2012).

Barbara Bruns, Deon Filmer, and Harry Anthony Patrinos, *Making Schools Work: New Evidence on Accountability Reforms* (2011).

Harold Alderman, *No Small Matter: The Impact of Poverty, Shocks, and Human Capital Investments in Early Childhood Development* (2011).

All books in the Human Development Perspectives series are available at https://openknowledge.worldbank.org/handle/10986/2161.

Contents

Chapter 12: Uzbekistan 273

*Toward Effective Prevention and Treatment
for Key Populations*

*Predrag Duric, Christoph Hamelmann,
and John Macauley*

Chapter 13: Optima HIV Methodology and Approach 291

*Cliff C. Kerr, Robyn M. Stuart, David J. Kedziora,
Amber Brown, Romesh Abeysuriya,
George L. Chadderdon, Anna Nachesa,
and David P. Wilson*

Boxes

Figures

Maps

Tables

Acknowledgments

The country studies presented in this book were carried out within the HIV allocative efficiency program managed by the World Bank and supported by the Global Fund to Fight AIDS, Tuberculosis and Malaria (Global Fund); the Joint United Nations Programme on HIV/AIDS (UNAIDS); and the United Nations Development Programme (UNDP).

The Steering Committee of the program—composed of Committee Chair Feng Zhao (World Bank), Christoph Hamelmann (UNDP), Manoela Manova (UNAIDS), Emiko Masaki (World Bank), and Shufang Zhang (Global Fund)—provided overall guidance to the country studies. The four agencies also cosponsored the various study activities. Michael Borowitz and Nicolas Cantau (Global Fund), Jean-Elie Malkin and Vinay P. Saldanha (UNAIDS), Christoph Hamelmann (UNDP), and David Wilson (World Bank) conceptualized the regional initiative on HIV allocative efficiency.

The Optima model, which was applied in the study, was developed by the University of New South Wales (UNSW), the Burnet Institute, and the World Bank. Data collation involved inputs from various national experts and was financially supported by UNAIDS, UNDP, and the World Bank, and in specific country studies also by the US Agency for International Development (USAID)/US President's Emergency Plan for AIDS Relief (PEPFAR) and the government of Germany.

Substantial technical inputs across various country studies were provided by Feng Zhao (World Bank Task Team Leader), Marelize Görgens, Clemens Benedikt, Son Nam Nguyen, Nejma Cheikh, Nicole Fraser-Hurt, Emiko Masaki, and Michael Obst (World Bank); David Kokiashvili and Shufang Zhang (Global Fund); Roman Hailevich and Manoela Manova (UNAIDS);

Predrag Duric, Christoph Hamelmann, Boyan Konstantinov, and John Macauley (UNDP); Cliff C. Kerr, Robyn M. Stuart, Iyanoosh Reporter, and Azfar Syed Hussain (UNSW); David P. Wilson (Burnet Institute); and Hassan Haghparast-Bidgoli, Laura Grobicki, Jolene Skordis-Worrall, and Jasmina Panovska-Griffiths (University College London).

Valeria Grishechkina, Sandra Irbe, Giedrius Likatavicius, Dejan Loncar, Corina Maxim, Nino Mdivani, Tsovinar Sakanyan, George Sakvarelidze, and Tatyana Vinichenko (all Global Fund); Otilia Scutelniciuc and Jacek Tyszko (UNAIDS); Nešad Seremet (UNDP); Rajeev Patel (USAID); Ulrich Laukamm-Josten (consultant); and Paolo Belli, Olena Doroshenko, Marcelo Bortman, Rosalia Rodriguez Garcia, Zara Shubber, and Baktybek Zhumadil (World Bank) provided inputs in the review of specific initial country analyses.

Feng Zhao, Clemens Benedikt, and David Wilson (all World Bank) developed the overall concept and structure of this book and supported the countries in compiling priority content and developing the country chapters. All book chapters were technically reviewed and edited by Katherine Ward. Theo Hawkins designed the figures in the book and the art on the cover of the book. Initial analytical country reports benefitted from editing by Alicia Hetzner. Marjia Jannati (World Bank) also provided important support for the overview chapter.

Armenia
The core analysis and report-writing team for the Armenia study included Samvel Grigoryan, Trdat Grigoryan, Ruben Hovhannisyan, and Arshak Papoyan (all National AIDS Center); Sherrie L. Kelly (Burnet Institute); and Clemens Benedikt, Diego Cuadros, Wendy Heard, and Emiko Masaki (all World Bank).

Belarus
The core analysis and report-writing team for the Belarus study included Olga Atroshchanka (UNDP), Alena Fisenka (AIDS Prevention Department at the Republican Centre of Hygiene, Epidemiology and Public Health), Vera Ilyenkova (UNAIDS); Predrag Duric (UNDP); Richard T. Gray (UNSW); and Clemens Benedikt and Emiko Masaki (both World Bank).

Bulgaria
The core analysis and report-writing team for the Bulgaria study included Tonka Varleva, Bahtiyar Karaahmed, Mariya Zamfirova, Mariya Tyufekchieva, Emilia Naseva, Veselina Tiholova, Desislava Mitova, Kristiyan Hristov, Velimira Sergieva, Elena Kabakchieva, Tsveta Raycheva, Stefka Boneva, and Petar Tsintsarski (Bulgarian Directorate of Management of Specialized Donor-Funded Programmes of the Ministry of Health); Hristo Taskov (National Center for Infectious and Parasitic Diseases);

Hassan Haghparast-Bidgoli, Laura Grobicki, and Jolene Skordis-Worrall (University College London); Clemens Benedikt and Feng Zhao (World Bank); and David J. Kedziora and Robyn M. Stuart (UNSW).

Georgia
The core analysis and report-writing team for the Georgia study included Alexander Asatiani, David Baliashvili, Irma Khonelidze, Ekaterine Ruadze, Ketevan Stvilia, and Maia Tsereteli (National Center for Disease Control and Public Health); Otar Chokoshvili (Infectious Diseases, AIDS and Clinical Immunology Research Center); Hassan Haghparast-Bidgoli, Laura Grobicki, Jasmina Panovska-Griffiths, and Jolene Skordis-Worrall (University College London); Clemens Benedikt and Feng Zhao (World Bank); and Cliff C. Kerr (UNSW).

Kazakhstan
The core analysis and report-writing team for the Kazakhstan study included Baurzhan S. Baiserkin (Republican AIDS Center); Aliya Bokazhanova (UNAIDS Kazakhstan); Lolita U. Ganina, N. F. Kalinich, Assem A. Kazimova, Irina I. Petrenko, and Alla V. Yelizarieva (national experts); Predrag Duric (UNDP), Andrew J. Shattock (UNSW); and Clemens Benedikt and Emiko Masaki (World Bank).

Kyrgyz Republic
The core analysis and report-writing team for the Kyrgyz Republic study comprised Venera Maitieva (Ministry of Health, Kyrgyz Republic); Liutsiia Ianbukhtina and Talgat Mambetov (National AIDS Center); Larisa Bashmakova and Meerim Sarybaeva (both UNAIDS); Predrag Duric (UNDP); Andrew J. Shattock (UNSW); and Clemens Benedikt and Emiko Masaki (World Bank). Substantial technical inputs also were provided by Dinara Soorombaeva (National Statistic Committee of the Kyrgyz Republic), as well as Aida Abarbekova and Meerim Kazizova (Ministry of Finance, Kyrgyz Republic).

Moldova
The core analysis and report-writing team for the Moldova study included Tatiana Alexeenco (HIV regional program, Eastern region); Liliana Caraulan (Center of Health Policies and Studies); Tatiana Costin and Valeriu Plesca (both National Center of Health Management); Lilia Gantea (Ministry of Health); Stefan Gheorghita (National Center of Public Health); Lucia Pirtina and Svetlana Popovici (both Hospital of Dermatology and Communicable Diseases); Svetlana Plamadeala (UNAIDS); Richard T. Gray (UNSW); and Clemens Benedikt, Alona Goroshko, and Emiko Masaki (all World Bank).

North Macedonia
The core analysis and report-writing team for the North Macedonia study included Vladimir Mikik (Institute for Public Health of the Republic of

North Macedonia); Natasha Nikolovska Stankovikj and Lidija Kirandjiska (GFATM-HIV Program Implementation Unit at the Ministry of Health, Republic of North Macedonia); Hassan Haghparast-Bidgoli, Laura Grobicki, Jasmina Panovska-Griffiths, and Jolene Skordis-Worrall (University College London); Clemens Benedikt and Feng Zhao (World Bank); and Iyanoosh Reporter and Azfar Syed Hussain (UNSW).

Tajikistan
Christoph Hamelmann and Predrag Duric developed the original Tajikistan country study and report. David P. Wilson and Cliff C. Kerr developed and ran the mathematical model. The original analysis built on the inputs and reviews of the Tajikistan country team working on the development of an HIV investment case for Tajikistan: Tatjana Majitova, Zuhra Nurlyaminova, Murodali Mehmondustovich Ruziev, Safarhon Sattorov, and Alijon Soliev (Republican AIDS Center); Muratboki Beknazarovich Beknazarov (Country Coordinating Mechanism Secretariat); Ulugbek Aminov (UNAIDS Tajikistan); and Mavzuna Burkhanova, Saodat Kasymova, Zarina Iskhanova, and Tedla Mezemir (UNDP Tajikistan).

Ukraine
The core analysis and report writing team for the Ukraine study included Igor Kuzin (Ukrainian Center for Socially Dangerous Disease Control [UCDC]); Eleonora Hvazdziova and Katerina Sharapka (UNAIDS); Cliff C. Kerr and Robyn M. Stuart (UNSW); and Clemens Benedikt, Alona Goroshko, Emiko Masaki, and Feng Zhao (all World Bank). Substantial technical inputs were also provided by Natalia Nizova (UCDC) and Jana Boyko (International HIV/AIDS Alliance in Ukraine).

Uzbekistan
Christoph Hamelmann and Predrag Duric developed the original Uzbekistan country study and report. David P. Wilson and Cliff C. Kerr developed and ran the mathematical model. The original analysis built on the inputs and reviews of the Uzbekistan country team working on the development of an HIV investment case for Uzbekistan: Nurmat Satiniyazovich Atabekov (Republican AIDS Center); Umida Islamova (Centre for Economic Research); Zakir Kadirov and Liya Perepada (UNDP); and Flora Sallikhova.

Production of the volume was managed by Susan Mandel of the World Bank's formal publishing program; Jewel McFadden, of the Development Economics unit, was the acquisitions editor. Deborah Appel-Barker, also with the World Bank publishing program, was the print coordinator.

Abbreviations

AA	Association Agreement
ABC-MCMC	approximate Bayesian computation Markov chain Monte Carlo
AEM	AIDS Epidemic Model
AIDS	acquired immune deficiency syndrome
API	application programming interface
ART	antiretroviral therapy
ARV	antiretroviral
ASD	adaptive stochastic descent
ASEAN	Association of Southeast Asian Nations
BCC	behavior change communication
BOC	budget-outcome curve
CCM	Country Coordinating Mechanism
CDC	Centers for Disease Control and Prevention (United States)
CEA	cost-effectiveness analysis
CHEM	Cambodian HIV Epidemic Model
CI	confidence interval
CIS	Commonwealth of Independent States
CSW	client of female sex worker
DALY	disability-adjusted life year
DCFTA	Deep and Comprehensive Free Trade Area
DFAT	Department of Foreign Affairs and Trade (Australia)

EACS	European AIDS Clinical Society
ECDC	European Center for Disease Prevention and Control
ECEA	extended cost-effectiveness analysis
EECA	Eastern Europe and Central Asia
EIMC	early infant male circumcision
ELISA	enzyme-linked immunosorbent assay
EU	European Union
FSW	female sex worker
GA	geospatial analysis
GARPR	Global AIDS Response Progress Reporting
GDP	gross domestic product
Global Fund	Global Fund to Fight AIDS, Tuberculosis and Malaria
GUI	graphical user interface
HBP	health benefits package
HCV	hepatitis C virus
HIM	HIV in Indonesia Model
HIV	human immunodeficiency virus
HR	human resources
HTA	health technology assessment
HTC	HIV testing and counseling
HTS	HIV testing services
IBBS	integrated biobehavioral surveillance
IBBSS	integrated biobehavioral surveillance survey
ICER	incremental cost-effectiveness ratio
iDSI	international Decision Support Initiative
IDU	injecting drug use
IEID	Institute of Epidemiology and Infectious Diseases of the Academy of Science of Ukraine
INSERM	l'Institut national de la santé et de la recherche médicale
IPH	Institute of Public Health of the Republic of North Macedonia
JSON	JavaScript Object Notation
KP	key population
LGBT	lesbian, gay, bisexual, and transgender
M&E	monitoring and evaluation
MC	Monte Carlo
MDG	Millennium Development Goal
MHSP	Ministry of Health and Social Protection of the Population (Tajikistan)
mm^3	cubic millimeter
MMC	medical male circumcision
MSM	men who have sex with men
MSP	multiple sexual partners

MSW	male sex worker
MTCT	mother-to-child transmission
NAP	National HIV/AIDS Prevention Program (Belarus)
NAP	National HIV/AIDS/STI Prophylaxis Program (Moldova)
NASA	National AIDS Spending Assessment
NCC	National Coordination Committee (Tajikistan)
NCD	noncommunicable disease
NCDC	National Center for Disease Control and Public Health (Georgia)
NFM	new funding model
NGO	nongovernmental organization
NHIF	National Health Insurance Fund (Bulgaria)
NICE	National Institute for Health and Care Excellence
NSP	needle and syringe exchange program
odict	ordered dictionary
OECD	Organisation for Economic Co-operation and Development
OI	opportunistic infections
OST	opioid substitution therapy
OVC	orphans and vulnerable children
PEP	post-exposure prophylaxis
PEPFAR	US President's Emergency Plan for AIDS Relief
PLHIV	people living with HIV
PMTCT	prevention of mother-to-child transmission
PrEP	pre-exposure prophylaxis
PSI	Population Services International
PWID	people who inject drugs
PY	person-year
QALY	quality-adjusted life year
RAC	Republican AIDS Center
RPC	remote procedure call
SBCC	social and behavior change communication
SDG	Sustainable Development Goal
SIR	susceptible–infected–recovered
STI	sexually transmitted infection
SW	sex workers
TB	tuberculosis
TDF	tenofovir disoproxil fumarate
UCDC	Ukrainian Center for Socially Dangerous Disease Control
UHC	universal health coverage
UID	unique identifier
UNAIDS	Joint United Nations Programme on HIV/AIDS
UNDP	United Nations Development Programme

UNFPA	United Nations Population Fund
UNGASS	United Nations General Assembly Special Session
UNICEF	United Nations Children's Fund
UNODC	United Nations Office on Drugs and Crime
UNSW	University of New South Wales
USAID	US Agency for International Development
WHO	World Health Organization
YLL	years of life lost
µL	microliter

Introduction

HIV and Allocative Efficiency in Eastern Europe and Central Asia

Feng Zhao, Clemens Benedikt, and Katherine Ward

Part I
The Growing Challenge

Although only a relatively small proportion of all new human immunodeficiency virus (HIV) infections globally occurs in the Eastern Europe and Central Asia (EECA) region, the trends are a cause for concern. The region saw an estimated 30 percent increase in new infections between 2010 and 2017, and acquired immune deficiency syndrome (AIDS)-related mortality also increased steadily between 2010 and 2016, before dropping in 2017. Moreover, the epidemic, although still concentrated, has now diversified, affecting more key populations in many countries in the region. This diversification has increased the number of people in need, the ways the epidemic can further spread to sexual partners of key populations, and the complexity of formulating an effective strategy.

While the epidemic in the region is on the rise, international funding for the response in many countries in the region is decreasing rapidly, with funding from the Global Fund to Fight AIDS, Tuberculosis and Malaria (the Global Fund) in the process of ending entirely for many nations. Domestic plans to cover the funding losses are, in many cases, far from complete. Moreover, other long-standing challenges have yet to be adequately addressed in many instances: barriers to access to treatment remain too widespread, as does the weight of social discrimination due to stigmatization of some of the most vulnerable communities, which are also in greatest need of support.

This section briefly reviews each of these key components, helping readers better understand why the region is reaching a critical inflection point in the course of the epidemic and efforts to respond to it. Unless otherwise noted, this chapter refers to the situation in 2017, the most recent year for which data from the Joint United Nations Programme on HIV/AIDs (UNAIDS) were available at the time of writing.

The Fastest-Growing HIV Epidemic in the World

Whereas the absolute numbers for the HIV epidemic in the EECA region are still comparatively small, the trends are a cause for real concern. Thus, although the UNAIDS statistics for 2017 make clear that the region accounts for only a small proportion of global totals—1.4 million of 36.9 million (3.79 percent of the total) people living with HIV (PLHIV), and 7.22 percent of all the new cases globally (130,000 of 1.8 million)[1]—the trends paint a different picture. While HIV prevalence and incidence in general have decreased in almost every other region of the world, they are increasing in the EECA region. In 2017, the region saw an estimated 130,000 new infections—30,000 more than the annual total in 2010. This rising rate of new infections (30 percent over that period) represents a worrisome increase and stands in clear contrast to the trends in other regions. During that same time period, new HIV infections declined by 33.3 percent in Eastern and Southern Africa, 9.75 percent in Western and Central Africa, 12.5 percent in Asia and the Pacific, 21.0 percent in the Caribbean, and no change in Latin America; the rate in the Middle East and North Africa increased by 11.1 percent (rising from 16,000 new cases in 2010 to 18,000 in 2017).

From 2010 through 2016, AIDS-related deaths globally decreased by 29.3 percent. At the same time, AIDS-related mortality in the EECA region increased by 15 percent before experiencing a drop in 2017, which returned the 2017 mortality number to the 2010 level of 34,000 individuals. In 2016, AIDS-related mortality claimed 30,550 lives in the Russian Federation, accounting for most of the increase in AIDS-related mortality in the EECA region (UNAIDS 2017c). As demonstrated in figure I.1,

Figure I.1   Global AIDS-Related Death Change, 2010–16

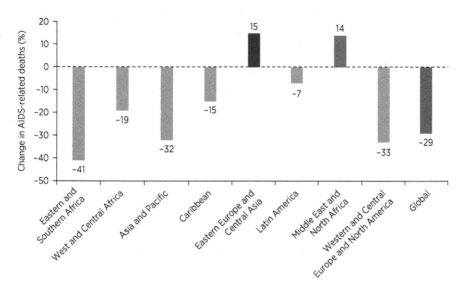

Source: AIDSinfo, http://aidsinfo.unaids.org (UNAIDS 2017 estimates).
Note: AIDS = acquired immune deficiency syndrome.

between 2010 and 2016 AIDS-related deaths decreased in every region—with the exception of EECA (which saw an increase of 15 percent) and the Middle East and North Africa (increase of 14 percent). The increase in AIDS-related mortality in the EECA region between 2010 and 2016 could be due to low coverage of HIV testing and treatment programs combined with a rise in new infections.

In the EECA region, the number of PLHIV increased from 890,000 people in 2010 to 1.4 million in 2017. As figure I.2 shows, the number of PLHIV increased continuously among all ages in the EECA region not only since 2010 but also stretching back to 1990.

Globally, the number of new HIV infections dropped from 2.2 million in 2010 to 1.8 million in 2017—primarily driven by reductions in Sub-Saharan Africa and the region encompassing Asia and the Pacific.[2] During the same time period, the annual rates of new adult HIV infections remained relatively constant in Latin America, declined somewhat in the Caribbean and in the combined regions of Western and Central Europe and North America, and rose by 2,000 in the Middle East and North Africa (increasing from 16,000 to 18,000). In the EECA region, however, the number of new HIV infections increased from 100,000 in 2010 to 130,000 in 2017, reflecting an

Figure I.2 People Living with HIV in Eastern Europe and Central Asia, 1990–2017

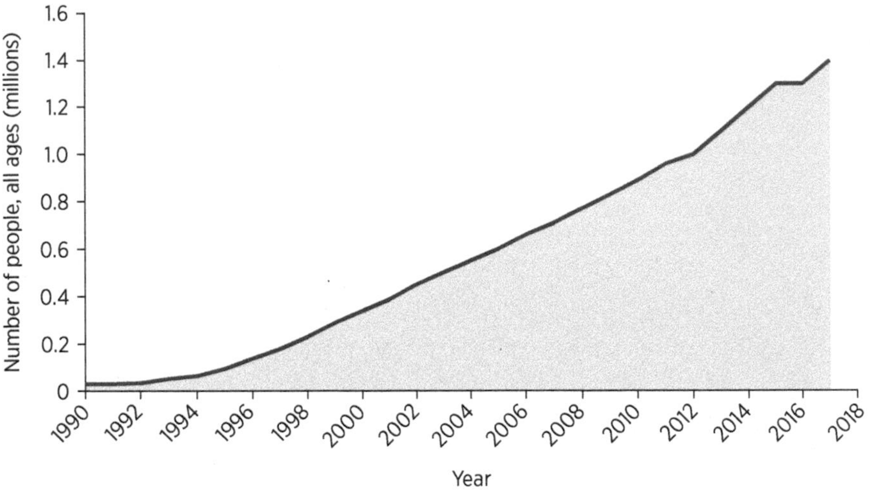

Source: AIDSinfo, http://aidsinfo.unaids.org (UNAIDS 2018 estimates).
Note: HIV = human immunodeficiency virus.

estimated 30 percent increase in new HIV infections in the EECA region in that time period, as noted previously.[3] In the EECA region the annual number of new HIV infections has approximately doubled since 2000 (UNAIDS 2018a). To provide a longer-term picture of the trends, figure I.3 and figure I.4 present the trend lines not only for 2010 through 2017 but also extending back to 1990.

During the same time period, progress on antiretroviral coverage was a bright spot, both globally and in the EECA region. Globally, the number of PLHIV who were on antiretroviral treatment rose by more than 270 percent between 2010 and 2017, increasing from 8 million to 21.7 million. In EECA, the number of people living with HIV on antiretroviral treatment rose by over 460 percent, increasing from 103,000 in 2010 to almost 520,000 in 2017.[4]

A Concentrated but Diversifying Epidemic

Available data suggest that approximately 47 percent of new HIV infections globally in 2017 were among key populations and their sexual partners (UNAIDS 2018a). In 2017, members of key populations and their sexual

Figure I.3   New HIV Infections—Global Trend, 1990–2017

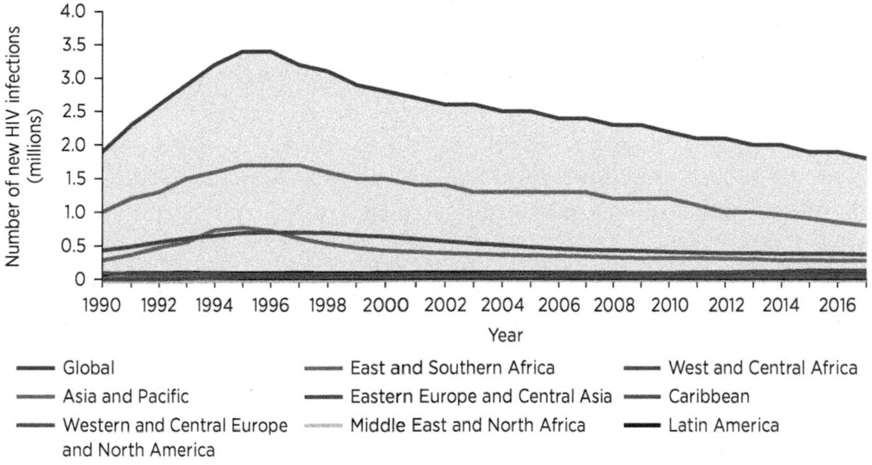

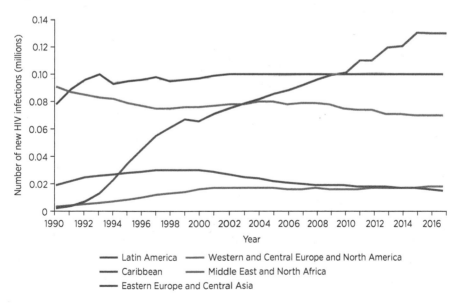

Source: AIDSinfo, http://aidsinfo.unaids.org (UNAIDS 2018 estimates).
Note: HIV = human immunodeficiency virus.

Figure I.4   New HIV Infections—Regional Trends, 1990–2017

Source: AIDSinfo, http://aidsinfo.unaids.org (UNAIDS 2018 estimates).
Note: HIV = human immunodeficiency virus.

partners accounted for over 95 percent of new infections in the EECA region (UNAIDS 2018c). In the past, people who inject drugs (PWID) were the focus of a concentrated epidemic in the region. Despite its concentration, however, the epidemic has now also diversified to other high-risk populations as well—particularly men who have sex with men (MSM), female sex workers (FSWs), and prisoners. In 2017, the distribution of new HIV infections among population groups in the EECA region was as follows: PWID accounted for 39 percent of all new infections in the region, clients of sex workers and other sexual partners of key populations 28 percent, MSM 21 percent, and sex workers 9 percent; the rest of the population accounted for 3 percent (UNAIDS 2018c). This spread to a wider set of high-risk populations can increase the number of people in need, the ways the epidemic can further spread to the general population, and the complexity of formulating an effective strategy.

PWID are the key population group most affected by HIV infections in the EECA region, although unprotected sex is also becoming a leading factor in transmission. Moreover, PWID are at a higher risk of HIV transmission because of needle sharing, criminalization and marginalization, poverty, sex work, and imprisonment and detention. In 2016, one in eight PWID was reported to be living with HIV (UNODC 2018). An estimated 3.1 million PWID reside in EECA (Harm Reduction International 2016), constituting 2.3 percent of the adult population in Russia, 1.1 percent in Belarus, 1 percent in Moldova, and between 0.8 percent and 1.2 percent in Ukraine (UNODC 2016). HIV prevalence among PWID in the region is notably higher than the global average; it is also higher than the prevalence for this population in neighboring regions—including Asia and Western and Central Europe. Globally, 12 million people inject drugs and one in seven PWID lives with HIV, accounting for 1.6 million people. In the EECA region, an estimated 2.86 million people inject drugs, and 22.9 percent of them are HIV-positive; this proportion is in contrast to the region of Western and Central Europe where 11.2 percent of its 700,000 PWID are HIV-positive and Asia where 12.5 percent of its 4.67 million injecting drug users are HIV-positive (UNODC 2016). In 2017, globally 8 percent of new HIV infections were found among PWID, compared to a much higher rate of 39 percent in EECA (UNAIDS 2018a). In the EECA region, examples of national HIV prevalence in 2017 among PWID were as high as 30.8 percent in Belarus and 25.6 percent in Russia, and include 14.3 percent in the Kyrgyz Republic, 13.9 percent in Moldova, and 2.3 percent in Georgia.[5]

In 2017, 3 percent of new HIV infections globally were among sex workers and 18 percent were among clients of sex workers and other sexual partners of key populations. In contrast, 9 percent of new HIV infections in the EECA region were among sex workers and 28 percent were among clients of sex workers and other sexual partners of key populations (UNAIDS 2018a). Most sex workers in the EECA region are female. Among sex workers, examples of national HIV prevalence range from 0.1 percent in Armenia to 7 percent in Belarus.[6] Sex workers who also inject drugs or have been in prison are at an increased risk of living with HIV (ECUO 2016). In Central Asia, FSWs who inject drugs had 20 times higher HIV prevalence compared to sex workers who did not (Baral et al. 2013). In 2017, globally, FSWs had 13 times higher relative risk of HIV acquisition than adult women aged 15–49 (UNAIDS 2018a). Women face multiple risk factors for HIV including economic vulnerability, fearing or experiencing violence, and difficulties in negotiating safe sex. In Ukraine, women aged 15–24 have over three times the HIV prevalence of men of the same age group; among 15-to-24-year-olds in 2017, the number of women living with HIV was 10,000, whereas the number of men living with AIDS was 3,200.[7]

In many EECA countries, HIV data concerning MSM are inconclusive or largely underreported in official epidemiological data. According to survey results, HIV prevalence among gay men or MSM was estimated to be 6 percent in Ukraine and 7 percent in Georgia in 2011 and 9.2 percent in Moscow in 2010. The rate of new infections among MSM in 2014, which was 6 percent in EECA, was much lower compared to the rate of 49 percent in Western Europe (UNAIDS 2016a). In 2017, 18 percent of new HIV infections globally were among MSM, compared to 21 percent of new HIV infections for the same key population group in the EECA region (UNAIDS 2018a). Of the countries with available reported data, the rate was highest in Georgia (20.7 percent) and lowest in Armenia (0.8 percent).[8]

In EECA, prisoners are at high risk for HIV. Harsh criminalization of drug use has led to high incarceration rates, which subsequently has led to HIV transmission among PWID. In short, incarcerating drug users increases HIV transmission, especially in overcrowded prisons where syringe sharing and unprotected sex are very common (Global Commission on HIV and the Law 2012). Altice et al. (2016) reported an HIV prevalence among prisoners of 19.4 percent in Ukraine and 10.3 percent in the Kyrgyz Republic. Results from surveillance studies in the region found that HIV prevalence in prisons was 22 times, 19 times, and 34 times higher compared to its prevalence in the general population in Ukraine, Azerbaijan, and the Kyrgyz Republic, respectively (Azbel et al. 2013). A 2016 Lancet study estimates that between 28 percent and 55 percent of all new HIV infections in the EECA region are due to heightened HIV transmission risk among current or previously incarcerated people who were injecting drug users (Altice et al. 2016).

Ongoing Barriers to Treatment

The EECA region has seen high rates of HIV/AIDS cases due to late diagnosis, low treatment coverage, and delayed initiation of HIV treatment. In fact, coverage of key HIV interventions in the EECA region has not been on par with the global level in recent years. The effective prevention and treatment measures against HIV/AIDS implemented elsewhere, which have significantly helped control the HIV epidemic, have unfortunately not been consistently implemented in the EECA region. As UNAIDS (2018c, 272) has noted, "Political, legal and technical barriers in many national HIV programmes are delaying the use of new, innovative approaches and tools, such as self-testing and pre-exposure prophylaxis (PrEP)."

In the EECA region, 73 percent of all PLHIV know their HIV status.[9] The rates vary significantly across countries in region—as high as 84 percent in Montenegro and as low as 41 percent in Uzbekistan. Trends in testing also diverge when comparing testing overall versus testing in key populations, and late diagnosis also remains an issue. In the analysis of its 2017 data, UNAIDS (2018c, 277) explained:

> While the overall number of annual HIV tests in the region continues to increase, the proportion of tests among key populations—including people who use drugs, gay men and other men who have sex with men, and patients with sexually transmitted infections—is shrinking, declining from 4.5 percent of all HIV tests conducted annually in 2010 to 3.2 percent in 2016. Late HIV diagnosis also remains a major challenge in the region: in the Russian Federation, almost 69 percent of patients who started treatment in 2016 had CD4 cell counts below 350 cells per mm^3.[10, 11]

In the region, 36 percent of all PLHIV are receiving antiretroviral therapy (ART), a rate significantly lower than the global figure of 59 percent. That rate is as low as 29 percent in Uzbekistan and as high as 59 percent in Montenegro.[12] In the EECA region, 50 percent of PLHIV who know their status are on treatment, which is significantly lower than the global figure of 79 percent.

UNAIDS data[13] show that coverage of viral load testing in the EECA region was 77 percent as of 2015 for countries in the region with available data (11 out of 17) (UNAIDS 2016a). Viral suppression for those on ART has been one of the more successful stories in tackling HIV in the region, with 72 percent of those on ART having achieved viral suppression. Montenegro has the highest viral suppression rate among people on ART at 91 percent, followed by Georgia at 89 percent and Armenia at 85 percent, whereas the rate in Albania is the lowest at 33 percent. Overall, however, only 26 percent of the total number of PLHIV in the region are virally suppressed; therefore, the risk of passing on the virus remains high among those not on treatment.

The region is also not on track to reach the Fast Track 90-90-90 targets for 2020 set by UNAIDS (2017a). The targets are that 90 percent of all PLHIV know their status (the EECA region is at 73 percent), 90 percent of all PLHIV who know their status are on treatment (the EECA region is at 50 percent), and 90 percent of people on treatment are virally suppressed (the EECA region is at 72 percent).[14]

In short, although knowledge of HIV status is not bad overall, ART coverage and viral suppression among all PLHIV in the EECA region are poor. Moreover, adequate availability of community-based testing and counseling or lay provider testing is lacking in most countries in the region, as is ART provision in community settings. The fact that most countries in the region now have national policies on routine viral load testing for adults and adolescents offers some cause for optimism (UNAIDS 2017c). Most countries in EECA, however, largely ignored the World Health Organization's 2013 treatment guidelines for HIV until recently (WHO 2013). With other competing needs, policy makers and also the general public in the EECA region have not paid enough attention to HIV/AIDS programs, and global resources against HIV have largely been allocated to Africa and elsewhere. This lack of attention has consequences. The recent trends have been alarming and deserve global attention.

Treatment has been shown to be effective in the EECA region; however, coverage is low (only 36 percent in 2017) because of barriers to accessing treatment. Barriers to HIV prevention in EECA include economic, social, legal, and other barriers. Lack of funding for HIV is a major economic barrier for scaling up HIV prevention programs. When the funds are available, they are put toward programs for the general population instead of key populations. In addition, prevention programs are under threat in the region because of reduced international support and often inadequate domestic funding (UNAIDS 2016b).

Social barriers include stigma and discrimination against PLHIV such as denying health or dental services and refusing employment. Stigma and discrimination against key populations prevent them from accessing HIV services (UNAIDS 2018c), and women experiencing gender-based violence and marginalization due to injecting drug use have difficulty accessing HIV prevention services. In Kazakhstan and the Kyrgyz Republic, Stigma Index surveys found that notably high numbers of PLHIV reported being denied health services: at least 18 percent and 20 percent, respectively. In addition, disclosure by health care workers of patient HIV status without consent remains too common. Discrimination and misunderstanding in the wider society also remain a concern, with 50 percent or more of adults in eight surveyed countries stating that they would not buy vegetables from a merchant living with HIV (UNAIDS 2018c). Some places, however, have made progress. For example, in Ukrainian medical facilities, discrimination against PLHIV dropped from 22 percent in 2010 to 8 percent in 2016 (UNAIDS 2018c).

Legal barriers include the criminalization of same-sex sexual acts and drug use, police corruption, and administrative barriers to accessing HIV reduction programs. Conservative legislators have placed restrictions on same-sex relationships, sex work, and drug use, which have made accessing HIV services more difficult. Laws prohibiting same-sex relationships are still enforced in Turkmenistan and Uzbekistan. Age-restrictive access to harm reduction services exists. Registration for opioid substitution therapy (OST) services can lead to employment restriction, loss of privileges, and targeting by police in Belarus, Latvia, Lithuania, Moldova, Russia, Ukraine, and Uzbekistan (Altice et al. 2016).

Other barriers include poor HIV epidemic surveillance, unemployment, and health care costs. Because of discrepancies among prevalence studies between nongovernmental organizations and government statistics, the true data and need for HIV services are hidden. In addition, organizational barriers include hours of operation, inconvenient locations, and transportation costs.[15]

The Rising Importance of Domestic Financing

Lack of funding for HIV has been a major economic barrier to scaling up HIV prevention programs. Although global resources to fight HIV have long been largely allocated to Sub-Saharan Africa and other regions, the EECA region was still able to access fairly significant international funding. But that access is no longer so clear. Epidemiological indicators suggest the need for strengthened responses, but many countries in the region face rapidly declining access to long-relied-upon international funding as 14 countries in the region have moved up into lower-middle-income status and Russia has moved into the high-income category (UNAIDS 2016b). A clear and important case in point is financing from the Global Fund. With many countries in the region moving up economically, the Global Fund is phasing out or has already ended its grants for HIV programming. For example, the Global Fund provided Ukraine with US$51 million in 2014 and 2015; however, with Ukraine's new middle-income status, the Global Fund announced it would cut its funding by half (Cook et al. 2014).

Unfortunately, the domestic funds allocated to HIV have failed to meet the funding gap. With a decrease in external financing, domestic financing is urgently needed to sustain the high-impact programs. Because of other competing needs, policy makers and also the general public in the EECA region have not paid enough attention to HIV/AIDS programs. For example, for many countries in the region (Armenia, Azerbaijan, Belarus, Georgia, Kazakhstan, the Kyrgyz Republic, and Ukraine), general government health expenditures as a percentage of gross domestic product in 2014 were below the global average of 4.2 percent.[16]

This is not to say that the picture is uniform across the EECA region. Countries are in different phases of the transition in financing the HIV response. Figure I.5 shows the 2016 and 2017 HIV expenditures for selected countries in the region by funding source. In 2016, the total HIV resource availability for low- and middle-income EECA countries was US$639 million. Of this amount, most came from domestic sources (75 percent), followed by the Global Fund (9.9 percent), other international sources (8.0 percent), and the United States (7.5 percent) (UNAIDS 2017c). The total resource availability for HIV responses in the

Figure I.5   HIV Expenditure in Selected Eastern European and Central Asian Countries, 2016 versus 2017

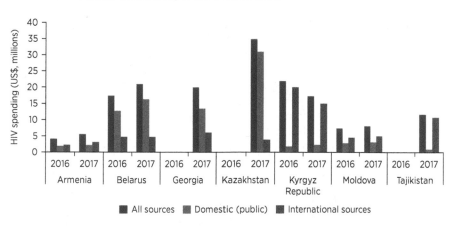

Source: AIDSinfo, http://aidsinfo.unaids.org (UNAIDS 2017 estimates).
Note: HIV = human immunodeficiency virus; US$ = US dollar.

EECA region decreased between 2012 and 2016, followed by a notable increase in domestic spending in 2017 to reach US$739 million (UNAIDS 2018c).

The bottom line is that, despite its increase in domestic funding, the region still relies significantly on external financing, especially for the highest-impact interventions. As the funding from the Global Fund in the region continues to drop, ensuring domestic spending from national budgets for key populations has been and will likely continue to be difficult.[17] In 2017, approximately 3 percent of total HIV spending in the region went toward programs focused on key populations (UNAIDS 2018b). In 2016, allocation of HIV resources for key populations in Ukraine was 6 percent (UNAIDS 2018a). In addition, large gaps in per capita resource availability exist in the region (UNAIDS 2018a).

Part II
Using Allocative Efficiency Analysis to Chart the Way Forward

Against the background described in part I, the World Bank and partner agencies jointly conducted HIV allocative efficiency studies in 11 countries in the EECA region: Armenia, Belarus, Bulgaria, Georgia, Kazakhstan, the Kyrgyz Republic, Moldova, North Macedonia, Tajikistan, Ukraine, and Uzbekistan. The countries were selected on the basis of both demand by the countries and regional considerations, to address different needs, and particularly to

- Better inform the next round of country strategies;
- Generate evidence for improving the impact of the HIV spending, often requested by the relevant ministry of finance;
- Provide inputs to Global Fund proposals;
- Support the formulation of the transitional plans during the phasing-out of international resources; and
- Address specific policy issues for high-risk populations (for example, migration-related issues in Armenia).

This book includes country-specific chapters that provide detailed analysis of the findings from the allocative efficiency studies for each country. This section summarizes the general findings among the 11 countries.

Scaling Up Treatment and Prevention

HIV programs in the EECA region need simultaneously to scale up treatment to a larger number of PLHIV than ever before and also to provide prevention at scale. HIV testing among key populations, such as PWID and MSM, remains low. In fact, in 2017, even as the overall number of HIV tests was increasing, the proportion of tests for these key populations and patients with sexually transmitted infections was in decline—dropping from 4.5 percent of all tests in 2010 to 3.2 percent in 2016 (UNAIDS 2018c).

In this context, it should be noted that, in the 2011 United Nations Political Declaration on HIV and AIDS, countries agreed to reduce sexual and injection-related HIV transmission by 50 percent by 2015 (United Nations General Assembly 2011). Globally, the estimated number of new HIV infections among PWID rose from 114,000 in 2011 to 152,000 in 2015, and the 2015 target of a 50 percent reduction was missed (UNAIDS 2016b). In 2017, 8 percent of new HIV infections globally were found among PWID, compared to a much higher rate of 39 percent in EECA (UNAIDS 2018a).

At the same time, after a decade of rapid growth, international HIV financing stabilized around 2010 (UNAIDS 2015); but it was projected to decline thereafter in middle-income countries (Cook et al. 2014). The shortfall in funding will be detrimental, especially for harm reduction programs. Comprehensive packages of services with needle and syringe exchange programs (NSP), OST, and a suitable legal and policy environment are needed to prevent HIV infections and to decrease HIV/AIDS-related illness and mortality (UNAIDS 2017b).

In this environment, two main courses of action exist for achieving HIV impact targets: (1) increased domestic financing for HIV programs, and (2) greater efficiency in program design and delivery in order to ensure that programs can do more with available resources. Given the large gaps in HIV prevention coverage and treatment programs in the EECA region during a time of limited resources, efficiency will become essential not only for impact but also for the sustainability of the response.

The concept of allocative efficiency refers to the maximization of health outcomes using the least costly mix of health interventions. HIV allocative efficiency analysis addresses the question: How can HIV funding be optimally allocated to the combination of HIV response interventions that will yield the highest impact? Technically, allocative efficiency can be accomplished either within a fixed budget envelope to achieve maximum impact with a given amount of money or within defined impact targets to achieve a given impact with minimal cost. In both cases, allocative efficiency is realized by optimizing the mix of interventions to achieve specific impact-level goals. Implementation efficiency can be defined as a set of measures to ensure that programs are delivered in a way that achieves outputs with the lowest input of resources.

HIV allocative efficiency analyses were conducted, using a similar analytical framework, in 11 EECA countries with significant HIV epidemics. Figure I.6 summarizes allocations of HIV resources to different HIV response programs for the 11 countries covered in this book. The first bar for each country represents the total annual HIV spending from the latest year with reported data at the time of the analysis (either 2013 or 2014 for all countries). The second bar for each country represents optimized allocations for the same amount of funding to minimize cumulative HIV incidence and AIDS-related deaths by 2020 according to the Optima HIV model, which was used to conduct the analysis. The HIV programs analyzed in this book vary substantially in size, ranging from Ukraine's HIV program with a spending volume of US$80 million in 2013–14 to programs in Armenia and North Macedonia with less than US$5 million in annual spending at the time of analysis.

Variations in HIV Spending Levels

Large variations in the total population size of countries make it important to understand HIV spending levels per person living with HIV (as represented in figure I.7). As figure I.7 shows, a large variation exists between countries in HIV spending per person living with HIV—ranging in the 2013–14 budget year from US$300 in Ukraine to more than US$18,000 in North Macedonia.

As subsequent chapters of this book illustrate, many reasons account for the differences. One factor is economies of scale, which allow for achieving lower unit costs in countries with larger numbers of PLHIV such as Ukraine and Uzbekistan. Ukraine's low spending per person living with HIV reflects its already relatively efficient resource allocation and low-cost models in place for reaching key populations at scale. At the same time, Ukraine's low spending per person living with HIV reflects a substantial HIV treatment gap. In contrast, North Macedonia's exceptionally high spending per person living with HIV reflects its very small number of PLHIV—only about 400. A relatively wide range of services funded from HIV budgets—which, because of low HIV incidence among certain populations such as PWID in North Macedonia—mainly have no HIV benefits. In Bulgaria, high spending per person living with HIV reflects particularly high unit costs of treatment. Relatively higher spending per person living with HIV in other countries reflects factors such as high unit cost of programs for key

Figure I.6 HIV Spending in 11 Countries, Eastern Europe and Central Asia, 2013 and 2014

Actual and optimized allocations

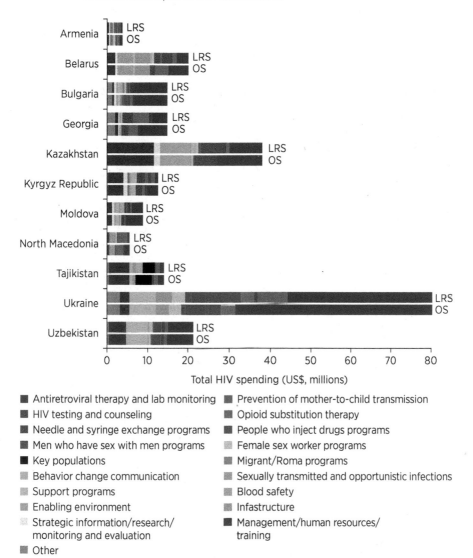

Total HIV spending (US$, millions)

- Antiretroviral therapy and lab monitoring
- Prevention of mother-to-child transmission
- HIV testing and counseling
- Opioid substitution therapy
- Needle and syringe exchange programs
- People who inject drugs programs
- Men who have sex with men programs
- Female sex worker programs
- Key populations
- Migrant/Roma programs
- Behavior change communication
- Sexually transmitted and opportunistic infections
- Support programs
- Blood safety
- Enabling environment
- Infastructure
- Strategic information/research/ monitoring and evaluation
- Management/human resources/ training
- Other

Source: Optima HIV model results.

Note: HIV = human immunodeficiency virus; LRS = the total annual HIV spending from the latest year with reported data at the time of the analysis (either 2013 or 2014 for all countries); OS = optimized allocations for the same amount of funding to minimize cumulative HIV incidence and AIDS-related deaths by 2020, according to analysis using the Optima HIV model. HIV = human immunodeficiency virus; US$ = US dollar.

Figure I.7 HIV Spending Levels per Person Living with HIV in 11 Countries, Eastern Europe and Central Asia

Actual and optimized allocations

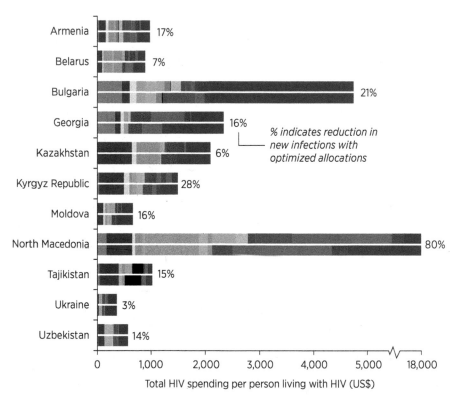

Source: Optima HIV model results.

Note: The top bar for each country represents HIV spending per person living with HIV in 2013–14; the bottom bar represents optimized allocations to minimize HIV incidence and deaths for 2016–20. HIV = human immunodeficiency virus; US$ = US dollar.

populations (the Kyrgyz Republic), high costs for procurement of antiretroviral medicines (Kazakhstan), or combinations of coverage and above-average unit cost in specific programs (Georgia). Across most countries, coverage of ART was relatively low, with less than 40 percent of PLHIV on ART at the time of analysis; hence, ART coverage was not the major factor in explaining differences in spending per PLHIV.

Countries also varied substantially in relation to the size of efficiency gains that can be achieved. The percentage values in figure I.7 show the proportion of new HIV infections that could be averted by optimally allocating the same amount of money that was available in 2013–14. With the given level of available resources and unit costs, the analyses found only limited efficiency gains through reallocations for Belarus, Kazakhstan, and Ukraine. In Ukraine, limited potential for reallocation pointed to already strong prioritization, but Belarus's HIV response required an increase in resource allocation in order to be able to reallocate. In Kazakhstan, the largest efficiency gain was found to be not reallocation, but reduction of drug prices, which would in turn allow for ART scale-up and programs for key populations. In North Macedonia, particularly large allocative efficiency gains of 80 percent—the highest potential for allocative efficiency gains found in Optima HIV studies globally—were found to be possible through increasing coverage of ART and other programs for MSM, while also sustaining programs for PWID for multiple health benefits. The scale of these gains was largely due to the concentration of North Macedonia's epidemic among MSM, whereas spending was focused on PWID and general populations. Relatively large efficiency gains in Bulgaria were found to be possible through focusing on key populations; in the Kyrgyz Republic increased focus on ART, which had the lowest allocation of all countries studied, was found to be critical.

Across all countries, optimized allocations also reduced the number of AIDS-related deaths by between 7 percent and 53 percent. In the Kyrgyz Republic, the reduction in deaths to be achieved through optimized allocations was the highest (53 percent), reflecting the potential effects of increasing focus on and coverage of ART.

Varying Costs per Person Reached

Costs have varied significantly across the region. As part of the regional overview, the teams involved in the allocative efficiency analyses also compared costs in five EECA countries: Armenia, Belarus, Georgia, Moldova, and Ukraine. The variations among these five EECA countries appear to be due to differences in packages, procurement, and economies of scale.

Table I.1 summarizes the cost per person reached from actual country spending/planning data collected for the allocative efficiency analyses. It therefore includes existing packages in countries, not the cost of implementing the same package of services in different countries.

A separate comparison exercise found that the costs per person reached in four EECA countries (Belarus, Georgia, Moldova, and Tajikistan) for OST also vary. The World Health Organization (WHO) recommends OST as a core component of care packages and harm reduction for PWID who have been diagnosed with HIV. Studies have shown that OST in conjunction with HIV treatment is more effective in saving the lives of drug users than ART by itself (Alcorn 2015). Since January 2014, OST has been introduced in nine countries in the region but has reached less than 1 percent of the population of PWID. Whereas some countries in the region have scaled up OST programs, others have offered them at a limited scale (Azerbaijan, Kazakhstan, Moldova, and Tajikistan), and some countries have criminalized OST (Russia and Turkmenistan) (Harm Reduction International 2018; UNAIDS Regional Support Team for Eastern Europe and Central Asia 2014).

Harm reduction program coverage has been low, but scaling up programs will lead to returns on investment. Table I.2 lists the estimated annual costs of scaling up harm reduction in the EECA region, from 2009 coverage levels, by region, to meet WHO guideline coverage targets. For ART, the

Table I.1 Costs per Person Reached in Five Countries, Eastern Europe and Central Asia

Cost per person reached (US$)	Derived from 2013 spending/coverage data				From two national strategies costed in 2014/15	
	Lowest	Highest	Average	Median		
FSW programs	41.66	166.24	102.80	107.05	29.84	112.03
MSM programs	23.67	232.35	76.87	47.79	18.87	133.99
PWID-NSP programs	40.90	129.25	76.87	66.86	35.36	79.02
OST	431.41	1,645.24	838.16	935.15	248.07	1,835.18
PMTCT	738.08	8,905.27	3,808.05	4,068.39	649.94	7,147.23
ART	576.48	1,464.71	987.86	1,127.29	696.23	1,410.97
HTC	0.55	34.72	11.22	3.05	0.76	15.50

Source: World Health Organization Global Price Reporting Mechanism, data verified February 2016.

Note: ART = antiretroviral therapy; FSW = female sex worker; HTC = HIV testing and counseling; MSM = men who have sex with men; NSP = needle and syringe exchange program; OST = opioid substitution therapy; PMTCT = prevention of mother-to-child transmission; PWID = people who inject drugs; US$ = US dollar.

Table I.2   Estimated Annual Cost of Scaling Up Harm Reduction in Eastern Europe and Central Asia

Harm reduction strategy (2009 coverage) (Mathers et al. 2010)	Annual cost (US$) of scale-up to reach medium coverage targets (level of coverage)	Annual cost (US$) of scale-up to reach high coverage targets (level of coverage)
NSP (11.7%)	19.1 million (20% coverage)	111.5 million (60% coverage)
OST (<1.0%)	715.5 million (20% coverage)	1.5 billion (40% coverage)
ART (1.1%)	1.2 billion (25% coverage)	3.6 billion (75% coverage)

Sources: Mathers et al. 2010 and Optima HIV models populated for each country.

Note: Table shows estimates of the total annual costs of scaling up each of the harm reduction strategies from existing coverage levels, by region, to meet WHO guideline coverage targets. ART = antiretroviral therapy; NSP = needle and syringe exchange program; OST = opioid substitution therapy; US$ = US dollar.

annual cost to reach medium coverage targets (25 percent) is approximately US$1.2 million; reaching high coverage targets (75 percent) would cost approximately US$3.6 million.

Recommendations

Figure I.8 summarizes the patterns of recommended reallocations in all 11 countries. Across nearly all countries, the optimization analyses suggested that allocations to ART should increase. Only in Bulgaria, which had the highest ART unit costs, did the analysis suggest that scaling up programs for key populations was more cost-effective at then-current levels of resources and with then-current unit costs. Most prevention programs for key populations also remained cost-effective across countries, but some shifts between different groups were recommended in some countries. Prevention and HIV testing programs for low-risk populations were not found to be cost-effective across countries, and defunding was suggested. The analysis also revealed that countries were allocating a substantial proportion of HIV response funding to management and cross-cutting support costs. Although the mathematical model could not assess these costs, the considerable variation suggests potential for implementation efficiency gains in these indirect areas of spending.

For reasons of comparability, the findings summarized in figures I.6 through I.8 represent optimized allocations of resources that assume that future funding would remain stable compared to the baseline (2013–14).

Figure I.8 HIV Spending, 2013–14 Levels and Optimized Allocations for 2016–20

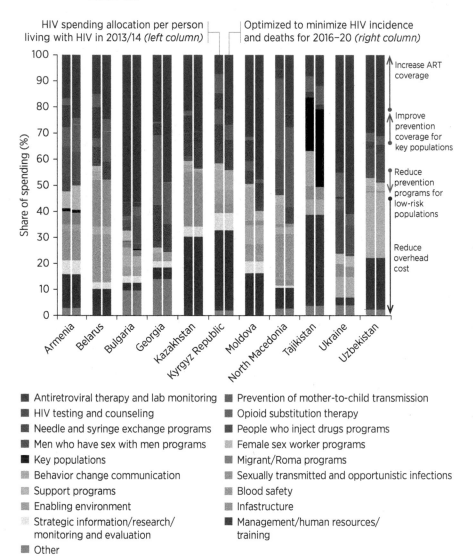

HIV spending allocation per person living with HIV in 2013/14 *(left column)*

Optimized to minimize HIV incidence and deaths for 2016–20 *(right column)*

- Increase ART coverage
- Improve prevention coverage for key populations
- Reduce prevention programs for low-risk populations
- Reduce overhead cost

■ Antiretroviral therapy and lab monitoring
■ HIV testing and counseling
■ Needle and syringe exchange programs
■ Men who have sex with men programs
■ Key populations
■ Behavior change communication
■ Support programs
■ Enabling environment
■ Strategic information/research/ monitoring and evaluation
■ Other

■ Prevention of mother-to-child transmission
■ Opioid substitution therapy
■ People who inject drugs programs
■ Female sex worker programs
■ Migrant/Roma programs
■ Sexually transmitted and opportunistic infections
■ Blood safety
■ Infastructure
■ Management/human resources/ training

Source: Optima HIV model results.

Note: The left column for each country shows HIV spending allocation per person living with HIV in 2013–14; the right column for each country shows optimized allocations to minimize HIV incidence and deaths for 2016–20. ART = antiretroviral therapy; HIV = human immunodeficiency virus.

Given that all countries in the region have a substantial gap in treatment and that ART is the only intervention directly reducing AIDS-related deaths, the optimized allocation suggests that a substantial proportion of resources be allocated to ART programs across all countries. In the analyses using constant budgets, this priority reduced the remaining resources available for reallocation to the next most effective programs. For example, in optimized allocations in Kazakhstan, funding for programs for PWID did not increase, because 56.4 percent of the total budget was already being absorbed by fixed costs and another 29.3 percent by ART—leaving only 14.3 percent of the budget for reallocation. Additional optimization analyses were conducted assuming a 67 percent reduction in prices of antiretroviral (ARV) medicines—in line with benchmarks of unit costs from other countries in the EECA region and a 20 percent reduction in management costs. When applying the reduced unit costs, allocations to programs for PWID would increase to 15.5 percent and new injection-related HIV infections would decline from an estimated 570 per year to only 210 (Shattock et al. 2017; World Bank 2015). The competing needs for ART and prevention for key populations imply that, at then-current levels of spending and at then-current unit costs, most programs would not be universal in optimized allocations.

Coverage rates refer to annual coverage rates of public sector and nongovernmental organization programs. Data from several countries suggest that behavioral outcomes (use of clean needles and condoms) among key populations tend to be higher than the annual reach of public programs, because some PWID, sex workers, and MSM buy condoms and needles from the private sector. For example, additional analysis for five countries (Armenia, Belarus, Kazakhstan, the Kyrgyz Republic, and Moldova) established that, after optimization, coverage of NSP increased from a range of 14 percent to 60 percent with then-current allocations rising to 30–70 percent with optimized allocations using the same amount of money. With full funding required to achieve national HIV incidence and mortality targets (in most countries 50 percent reductions by 2020), the coverage of NSP would need to increase further in some countries to levels between 56 percent and 70 percent.

The analyses also revealed important differences in costs per person reached, although those differences were not the central focus of the country studies and, because of different methods of recording, were not systematically comparable. Table I.1 earlier in this section illustrates costs per person reached for a selected group of countries. Figure I.9 shows that significant differences were also found for ARV medicine prices, presenting

Figure I.9 Cost of Antiretroviral Products in Eastern European and Central Asian Countries, 2014–15

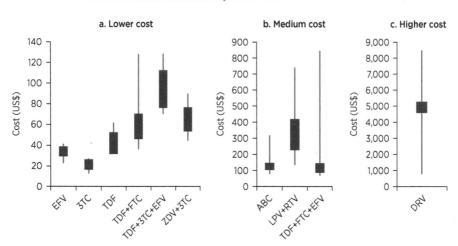

Source: World Bank based on data from World Health Organization Global Price Reporting Mechanism for HIV, Tuberculosis and Malaria, http://apps.who.int/hiv/amds/price/hdd/, accessed May 13, 2016.

Note: The endpoints of vertical lines represent maximum and minimum cost. The solid column represents the interquartile range; 3TC = lamivudine; ABC = abacavir; DRV = darunavir; EFV = efavirenz; FTC = emtricitabine; LPV = lopinavir/ritonavir; RTV = ritonavir; TDF = tenofovir; US$ = US dollar; ZDV = zidovudine.

prices from highest, lowest, using interquartile ranges for a 365-day supply of the drug components, and combinations, which account for more than 80 percent of the purchases.

Although domestic funding has been increasing, a large resource gap is still prominent in the region. Analysis has found a need for funding to more than double in low- and middle-income countries in order for them to reach Fast Track targets (UNAIDS 2017a). If a country can allocate resources properly, it can achieve significant gains. Resource allocations at the time of the analyses discussed in this book, although not off-track, were not optimal; and the impact of optimized resource allocation can be significant. The analyses identified a need for stronger links between targets and the right interventions as well as resource allocation. Nonhealth decision-makers in resource allocation need to be informed.

The region saw some progress in 2017, reflected in a notable increase in domestic HIV investment in the region: reaching a total of US$739 million and 81 percent of all HIV spending in the EECA region in that year. Total domestic spending, however, accounted for only 46 percent of the total

US$1.6 billion per year needed to meet the 2020 Fast Track Targets for the EECA region (UNAIDS 2018c). Moreover, the fact remains that, as support from the Global Fund decreases, ensuring that money from national budgets is used for key populations has been difficult (UNAIDS 2018c).

Advanced Concentrated HIV Epidemics

The subsequent country chapters explore in more detail the actual allocation patterns at the time of analysis and optimized allocation patterns including their interactions with unit costs and implementation contexts. Regional comparison has shown important similarities and differences. Despite some universal major trends—such as the need to scale up ART and enhance focus on key populations and their sexual partners—heterogeneity of contexts persists as epidemics progress. The term "advanced concentrated HIV epidemics" is proposed to describe the situation for the EECA region. This term reflects a shift in transmission pattern with increases of sexual transmission. It is not a shift in the sense of a generalization of the epidemic; instead it represents a shift in the sense of the increasing roles of sexual partners of drug users and emerging and growing epidemics among MSM. This pattern varies among countries. Although HIV prevalence remains high among injecting drug users in some contexts, HIV prevalence among MSM exceeds HIV prevalence among PWID in other contexts now such as Georgia. The country chapters work out these nuances in epidemic trends, describe optimized allocations, and outline actions taken by countries to enhance outcomes of national HIV responses.

Notes

1. Data from the UNAIDS (Joint United Nations Programme on HIV/AIDS) AIDSinfo page, http://aidsinfo.unaids.org.
2. AIDSinfo.
3. AIDSinfo.
4. AIDSinfo.
5. AIDSinfo.
6. AIDSinfo.
7. AIDSinfo.
8. AIDSinfo.
9. AIDSinfo.
10. UNAIDS (Joint United Nations Programme on HIV/AIDS) special 2017 analysis of national program data from 11 countries.

11. Presentation by N. Ladnaya on peculiarities in the development of the HIV epidemic in Russia.
12. AIDSinfo.
13. Data in this paragraph from AIDSinfo.
14. AIDSinfo.
15. Data from Avert's "HIV and AIDS in Eastern Europe & Central Asia Overview" web page (accessed March 22, 2018), https://www.avert.org/hiv-and-aids -eastern-europe-central-asia-overview.
16. Global Health Expenditure Database, World Health Organization, Geneva (accessed December 4, 2017), http://www.who.int/health-accounts/ghed/en/.
17. AIDSinfo.

References

Alcorn, K. 2015. "Opioid Substitution Therapy Combined with HIV Treatment Saves the Lives of More Drug Users than ART Alone." NAM AIDSmap, July 23. https:// www.aidsmap.com/Opioid-substitution-therapy-combined-with-HIV-treatmen t-saves-the-lives-of-more-drug-users-than-ART-alone/page/2987340.

Altice, F. L., L. Azbel, J. Stone, E. Brooks-Pollock, P. Smyrnov, S. Dvoriak, F. S. Taxman, N. El-Bassel, N. K. Martin, R. Booth, H. Stöver, K. Dolan, and P. Vickerman. 2016. "The Perfect Storm: Incarceration and the High-Risk Environment Perpetuating Transmission of HIV, Hepatitis C Virus, and Tuberculosis in Eastern Europe and Central Asia." *Lancet* 388 (10050): 1228–48.

Azbel, L., J. A. Wickersham, Y. Grishaev, S. Dvoryak, and F. L. Altice. 2013. "Burden of Infectious Diseases, Substance Use Disorders, and Mental Illness among Ukrainian Prisoners Transitioning to the Community." *PloS ONE* 8 (3): e59643.

Baral, S., C. S. Todd, B. Aumakhan, J. Lloyd, A. Delegchoimbol, and K. Sabin. 2013. "HIV among Female Sex Workers in the Central Asian Republics, Afghanistan, and Mongolia: Contexts and Convergence with Drug Use." *Drug and Alcohol Dependence* 132 (Supplement 1): S13–S16.

Cook, C., J. Bridge, S. McLean, M. Phelan, and D. Barrett. 2014. *The Funding Crisis for Harm Reduction, Donor Retreat, Government Neglect and the Way Forward.* London: International Harm Reduction Association.

ECUO (East Europe and Central Asia Union of People Living with HIV). 2016. "Eastern Europe and Central Asia: Let's Not Lose Track!" Report prepared for the 2016 High-Level Meeting on HIV/AIDS. ECUO. http://ecuo.org/wp -content/uploads/2016/09/eeca_position_document_hlm.pdf.

Global Commission on HIV and the Law. 2012. "Risks, Rights & Health." United Nations Development Program, HIV/AIDS Group, New York.

Harm Reduction International. 2016. *Regional Overview: 2.2 Eurasia.* Harm Reduction International. https://www.hri.global/files/2016/11/15/Eurasia.pdf.

Harm Reduction International. 2018. *The Global State of Harm Reduction 2018.* Harm Reduction International. https://www.hri.global/files/2019/02/05/global-state -harm-reduction-2018.pdf.

Mathers, B. M., L. Degenhardt, H. Ali, L. Wiessing, M. Hickman, R. P. Mattick, B. Myers, A. Ambekar, and S. A. Strathdee for the 2009 Reference Group to the

UN on HIV and Injecting Drug Use. 2010. "HIV Prevention, Treatment, and Care Services for People Who Inject Drugs: A Systematic Review of Global, Regional, and National Coverage." *Lancet* 375 (9719): 1014–28.

Shattock A. J., C. Benedikt, A. Bokazhanova, P. Duric, I. Petrenko, L. Ganina, S. L. Kelly, R. M. Stuart, C. C. Kerr, T. Vinichenko, S.-F. Zhang, C. Hamelmann, M. Manova, E. Masaki, and D. P. Wilson. 2017. "Kazakhstan Can Achieve Ambitious HIV Targets despite Expected Donor Withdrawal by Combining Improved ART Procurement Mechanisms with Allocative and Implementation Efficiencies." *PLoS One* 12 (2): e0169530.

UNAIDS (Joint United Nations Programme on HIV/AIDS). 2015. *How AIDS Changed Everything. MDG 6: 15 Years, 15 Lessons of Hope from the AIDS Response.* Geneva: UNAIDS.

UNAIDS (Joint United Nations Programme on HIV/AIDS). 2016a. "Global AIDS Update 2016." Special analysis reference report, UNAIDS, Geneva.

UNAIDS (Joint United Nations Programme on HIV/AIDS). 2016b. *Prevention Gap Report.* Geneva: UNAIDS.

UNAIDS (Joint United Nations Programme on HIV/AIDS) 2017a. "Ending AIDS: Progress towards the 90-90-90 Targets." UNAIDS, Geneva.

UNAIDS (Joint United Nations Programme on HIV/AIDS) 2017b. "Stopping the Rise of New HIV Infections among People Who Inject Drugs." Feature story, UNAIDS, March 16, 2017.

UNAIDS (Joint United Nations Programme on HIV/AIDS) 2017c. "UNAIDS Data 2017." UNAIDS, Geneva.

UNAIDS (Joint United Nations Programme on HIV/AIDS). 2018a. *Global AIDS Update: Miles to Go: Closing Gaps, Breaking Barriers, Righting Injustices.* Geneva: UNAIDS.

UNAIDS (Joint United Nations Programme on HIV/AIDS). 2018b. "Sixth Eastern Europe and Central Asia Conference on HIV/AIDS Opens in Moscow." UNAIDS Update, April 20. http://www.unaids.org/en/resources/presscentre/featurestories /2018/april/sixth-eastern-europe-and-central-asia-conference-on-hiv-aids.

UNAIDS (Joint United Nations Programme on HIV/AIDS). 2018c. "UNAIDS Data 2018." UNAIDS, Geneva.

UNAIDS (Joint United Nations Programme on HIV/AIDS) Regional Support Team for Eastern Europe and Central Asia. 2014. "Synthesis on Opioid Substitution Therapy in Eastern Europe and Central Asia." Unpublished manuscript.

United Nations General Assembly. 2011. "Political Declaration on HIV and AIDS: Intensifying Our Efforts to Eliminate HIV and AIDS." Resolution 65/277 adopted June 10, 2011. United Nations, New York.

UNODC (United Nations Office on Drugs and Crime). 2016. *World Drug Report 2016.* Vienna: UNODC.

UNODC (United Nations Office on Drugs and Crime). 2018. *World Drug Report 2018.* Vienna: UNODC.

WHO (World Health Organization). 2013. *Consolidated Guidelines on the Use of Antiretroviral Drugs for Treating and Preventing HIV Infection: Recommendations for a Public Health Approach.* Geneva: World Health Organization.

World Bank. 2015. "Optimizing Investments in Kazakhstan's HIV Response." World Bank, Washington DC.

1

Cost-Effectiveness 2.0
Improving Allocative Efficiency with Decision Science Analytics

*David P. Wilson and Marelize Görgens**

Introduction

In September 2015, the United Nations General Assembly adopted a set of goals to "end poverty, protect the planet, and ensure prosperity for all as part of a new sustainable development agenda" (United Nations General Assembly 2015). The third of the 17 Sustainable Development Goals (SDGs) is to "ensure healthy lives and promote well-being for all at all ages." Measuring progress toward achieving SDG 3 has been quantified in 13 health-related targets, including targets related to universal health coverage and to communicable diseases:

- SDG Target 3.3: By 2030, end the epidemics of acquired immune deficiency syndrome (AIDS), tuberculosis, malaria, and neglected tropical diseases and combat hepatitis, waterborne diseases, and other communicable diseases.
- SDG Target 3.8: Achieve universal health coverage (UHC), including financial risk protection, access to quality essential health care services, and access to safe, effective, quality, and affordable essential medicines and vaccines for all.

Achieving these targets would substantially reduce morbidity and mortality worldwide—from about 5 million deaths annually and 250 million disability-adjusted life years (DALYs) due to these diseases, particularly in lower-income countries that carry most of the overall and infectious disease burden (GBD 2015 DALYs and HALE Collaborators 2016; GBD 2015 Disease and Injury Incidence and Prevalence Collaborators 2016; GBD 2015 SDG Collaborators 2016). As seen in some countries, purposeful investment in interventions against these conditions leads to improved individual and population health, well-being, and equity (Jamison et al. 2013). Until two decades ago, elimination of these diseases seemed unlikely, but advances in treatments and an improved focus on primary prevention have given some cause for optimism if effective technologies are financed, scaled up, and implemented efficiently.

It is a more promising time than ever to be addressing these communicable diseases because there is now an armory of biomedical technologies that were previously unavailable. These advances and technologies have contributed to observed decreases in the major burdens of disease—that is, 37 percent, 33 percent, and 17 percent declines in deaths due to malaria, human immunodeficiency virus/acquired immune deficiency syndrome (HIV/AIDS), and tuberculosis (TB) respectively since 2005 (Wang et al. 2016). For HIV, antiretroviral therapy (ART)—itself having clinical benefit to HIV-positive individuals and population-level prevention benefits to reduce HIV incidence—combined with other, nonbiomedical primary prevention programs like harm reduction for sex workers is reducing new infections and deaths in countries that have scaled up these programs and obtain high adherence levels (Cohen et al. 2011; Fonner et al. 2016; Verguet et al. 2016). TB elimination may be possible because of improved environmental conditions and emerging innovative biomedical technologies (WHO 2015). Malaria has been successfully eliminated from several countries, and recent years have seen considerable technological, clinical, and public health strategy advances to drive the elimination agenda (WHO 2016a). For hepatitis C, the advent of new direct-acting antiviral treatments has led to a cure (Burki 2014); for hepatitis B, a highly effective vaccine combined with improving therapies, both used in combination with high-quality harm reduction, makes the viral hepatitis targets achievable (WHO 2016b). The search to use these innovations most effectively in intervention technologies has led to exciting advances in decision science analytics.

Achieving the best use of those innovations, however, will require prioritization, allocative efficiency, and a laser-like focus on effectiveness.

Governments in low- and middle-income countries are legitimizing the implementation of universal health coverage (UHC), following a United Nations General Assembly Resolution on UHC in 2014 and its reinforcement in the sustainable development goals set in 2015. UHC will differ in each country depending on country contexts and needs, as well as demand

and supply in health care. Therefore, fundamental issues such as objectives, users, and cost-effectiveness of UHC have been raised by policy makers and stakeholders. While priority-setting is done on a daily basis by health authorities—implicitly or explicitly—it has not been made clear how priority-setting for UHC should be conducted. (Chalkidou et al. 2016)

In order to prioritize, governments need to use data to make the best possible decisions about how to create client-centered health systems that deliver personalized, predictive, preemptive, and participative health care that is delivered efficiently. To help governments be as data-driven as possible when prioritizing health service delivery, a suite of quantitative approaches exists—ranging from more straightforward static cost-effectiveness analyses (CEAs), to mathematical modeling using optimization algorithms, to the use of big data, predictive analytics, and artificial intelligence.

Along this continuum of quantitative approaches, the lowest-hanging fruit is CEA. When considering only health gains and noninteracting interventions, CEA is a widely accepted analytical method used in choosing interventions that offer good value for money. The "value" of a health outcome is expressed by a single measure encompassing mortality and morbidity aspects, either DALYs or quality-adjusted life years (QALYs). Because these measures capture both life span and quality of life, either can assess the outcome of a wide range of health interventions and their individual impact on such health outcomes, but generally not a package of interventions and its impact on one health outcome. Although it has been a good start, CEA also has other weaknesses—such as its inability to look at dynamic population-level outcomes beyond the life span of the intervention and beyond the population targeted through an individual intervention.

To address the limits of CEA and consider broader factors in decision systems, packages of services and technologies should be considered together rather than in isolation and analyses should incorporate overall health, financial, and equity objectives and relevant constraints. Optimization tools have recently emerged for this purpose and can help to optimize a health benefits package tailored to specific objectives and time horizons within available budget envelopes, local and changing epidemiology, dynamic costs, and variable, nonlinear benefits on different populations (Görgens et al. 2017). This chapter describes the evolution of the next-generation analytical approach and how it may be expanded beyond current applications to further the international goals of improved health outcomes for all.

The aspiration of health systems includes providing quality health services with equitable access for all who need them and ensuring that no one who receives these services suffers negative financial shocks as a result of doing so—in other words, the aspiration is UHC. All health systems work within a limited budget, however, which means priority setting in health is both inevitable and essential.

Resource allocation decisions are often influenced by competing criteria—including socioeconomic, political factors, and historical precedent—rather than by rational calculations based on scientific evidence of effectiveness and best practice. It is now generally accepted that resource allocation decisions should be informed by, or grounded in, explicit criteria based on cost-effectiveness to maximize health benefits with the resources available. A challenge faced by decision-makers is how to use their limited funds optimally across the large set of health conditions, technologies, health care programs, and patient groups to target the right people, in the right locations, at the right time, and in the right way to achieve the greatest population health gains while also addressing issues of equity, access, and protection against financial catastrophe.

This introduction describes the rationale for and history of the design, development, and use of the Optima approach, an innovative framework for decision-making designed to assist in prioritizing health spending in specific areas, and the analytic tools that have been developed to implement the Optima approach for specific problems. Analytic tools such as these— together with big data, predictive analytics, and artificial intelligence—are at the cutting edge of methods to improve health-financing efficiency and effectiveness. This introduction (1) demonstrates that it is possible to achieve greater allocative and implementation efficiency in health; (2) argues that traditional CEAs on their own are inadequate for priority setting in health; (3) presents how the Optima approach addresses many of the limitations of traditional CEAs; (4) describes how tools to implement the Optima approach have evolved over time, including its foundations in HIV in the Eastern Europe and Central Asia region; (5) explains how countries have used the results of Optima analyses to improve priority setting in health; and (6) outlines planned future directions in Optima-type decision science tools.

Avoiding Inefficiency

Evidence exists of significant inefficiencies in health worldwide (Medeiros and Schwierz 2015). The concept of efficiency in health involves implementing the right services, in the right places, and in the right ways (World Bank 2017). Health systems operating efficiently yield the best possible health and financial protection outcomes for individuals and their populations with the resources available.

Inefficiencies are very common in most health systems and include the following (see also box 1.1):

- Providing the wrong services through overuse (providing services that may do more harm than good, or are high-cost but low-impact and waste resources or deflect investments for health systems) and underuse (failing to use effective, high-impact, and affordable interventions when they are needed) (Brownlee et al. 2017; Glasziou et al. 2017)
- Providing the right services in the wrong settings or for the wrong populations by, for example, relying on secondary or tertiary settings rather than primary health care, or expecting vulnerable and marginalized populations to use sites for the mainstream general population, which are not sensitized to their needs
- Doing the right service poorly through, for example, leakages and waste through the supply chain, commodities left to expire in poor conditions, or delivering services at much greater expenditure than necessary.

The magnitude of commonly occurring inefficiencies is astoundingly high, with most countries wasting an estimated 20–40 percent of their

---

BOX 1.1

Ten Sources of Inefficiency in Health Care

1. *Medicines*: Underuse of generics and higher than necessary prices for medicines
2. *Medicines*: Use of substandard and counterfeit medicines
3. *Medicines*: Inappropriate and ineffective use
4. *Health care products and services*: Overuse or supply of equipment, investigations, and procedures
5. *Health workers*: Inappropriate or costly staff mix; unmotivated workers
6. *Health care services*: Inappropriate hospital admissions and length of stay
7. *Health care services*: Inappropriate hospital size (low use of infrastructure)
8. *Health care services*: Medical errors and suboptimal quality of care
9. *Health system leakages*: Waste, corruption, and fraud
10. *Health interventions*: Inefficient mix/inappropriate level of strategies

Source: Chisholm and Evans 2010.

health resources, thereby missing opportunities to use resources more efficiently to achieve much more (World Bank 2017). As an example, the World Health Organization estimates that less than one-quarter of funds for health in Africa is spent on the highest-impact health services (*Lancet Global Health* 2016). An estimated cost saving of 10–60 percent is possible from a range of improvements in drug procurement, distribution, and prescribing practices—which would free up funds to provide additional health services across populations. Inefficiencies in health spending are not limited to lower-income settings; they are also commonly reported in high-income countries that are members of the Organisation for Economic Co-operation and Development (OECD) (Hollingsworth 2003).

There are generally three types of efficiency in econometrics: (1) allocative efficiency refers to a resource allocation approach that maximizes health or well-being outcomes for populations (or other set of outputs that people value the most) by using the most cost-effective mix of interventions; (2) technical efficiency is achieved when a set of inputs achieves the maximum possible output(s); and (3) production efficiency occurs when the inputs used to produce this output have the least cost (Hollingsworth 2008). This introduction and book cover allocative efficiency.

There is evidence that allocative efficiency analytics lead to improved health. A notable early example is the Oregon experiment that used cost-effectiveness data to allocate US federal Medicaid health funds in prioritizing medical services to cover the state's population (Ndeffo Mbah and Gilligan 2011). Many high-income countries, such as Australia, Canada, Sweden, and the United Kingdom, systematically use cost-effectiveness criteria for defining health care packages, at least for pharmaceuticals and some well-defined medical consultations, diagnostics, procedures, and other benefits. A prominent example is the National Institute for Health and Care Excellence (NICE), which provides recommendations for the English and Welsh National Health Systems; it formed NICE International, which has now broken away as the international Decision Support Initiative (iDSI), supporting lower-income countries in building capacity and setting priorities for health benefits packages.

Improved allocative efficiency has been seen in lower-income settings. For example, Tanzania defined its essential health benefits package in 1997 on the basis of district-level cost-effectiveness data and population sizes. Consequently, child mortality decreased by 40 percent in the following five years (Stinnett and Paltiel 1996). Chile based its 2003 health reform plan, known as AUGE, on the diseases accounting for 75 percent of the nation's disease burden and the most effective interventions. Public spending on health increased considerably to high-impact programs and led to improved health outcomes (Flessa 2000). Decisions based on a systematic evaluation of Thailand's health benefit system reallocated funds to save many lives, without a change to the total budget (Chalabi et al. 2008; Flessa 2003). Examination of the content and cost of interventions within Mexico's health benefits package identified additional resource requirements to improve equity and financial protection, and also led to resource mobilization (Blumstein 1997). These examples of improvements in resourcing and allocative efficiency have been informed or driven by traditional analytics of cost-effectiveness calculations. The next section discusses this approach. The following section discusses the introduction of Optima, which arose because of urgent needs to improve responses to HIV epidemics and other communicable diseases.

Shortcomings of Traditional Cost-Effectiveness Analyses

CEA is a widely accepted analytical method used in choosing health interventions that offer good value for money by providing greater health benefit at lower costs than other interventions. The value of a health outcome is expressed by calculating an estimated incremental cost per additional outcome obtained or averted (that is, an individual obtains extra healthy life years or avoids dying or living with illness). Metrics involving cases averted are most suitable for resource allocation within a single disease (vertical analyses) because it is easier to compare direct health benefits gained from different interventions on a single disease than it is to measure health benefits gained for multiple interventions across different diseases. When resource allocation decisions are to be made across multiple disease areas or the entire health system, however, then QALYs or DALYs should be used because they encompass mortality and morbidity aspects (Drummond et al. 2005). Interventions are ranked in a league table in increasing value of their incremental cost-effectiveness ratios. Health outcomes are assumed to be maximized if the selection begins with the most cost-effective intervention at full coverage and then moves down the list to successively less cost-effective interventions until the budget is exhausted.

Although CEAs do provide a mechanism for allocating resources, they have considerable and important limitations including their inability to account for interactions between interventions and other objectives like equity in health, well-being, and financial risk protection. Failure to include these elements in health-resourcing decisions can lead to decisions that have catastrophic outcomes for the poor and marginalized subpopulations within a society. An emerging approach that attempts to address this is extended cost-effectiveness analysis (ECEA) (see, for example, Levin et al. 2015; Verguet et al. 2015; Verguet et al. 2016; Watkins et al. 2016). The goal of ECEA is to find a balance between the interventions that cost-effectively avert illness and death and interventions that afford financial risk protection or decrease the health gap between the poorest and the richest strata of society. CEAs, and ECEAs, can provide useful guidance with respect to their primary purpose of maximizing population health for simple, noninteracting health technology assessment (HTA). They have considerable shortcomings, however, in their ranking and estimation of benefits; these shortcomings become increasingly apparent as the system of assessment becomes more complex and dynamic and as there are interactions between interventions. CEA and its extensions do not usually take the following aspects into account:

- The interrelationship between causes of burden of disease and associated health interventions. CEAs consider interventions as independent, thereby neglecting their interactions.
- The fact that priority setting may change at different funding levels once priority populations may be covered to address certain objectives, or due to decreasing cost-effectiveness because of the nonlinearities of service scale, for example because of exponentially higher marginal costs of reaching the final hard-to-reach 20 percent, or dynamics of burden of disease
- The dynamic nature of burden of disease due to wider primary prevention, epidemiological, or population-wide impacts of the health services being implemented (for example, the impact of vaccination or treatment on transmission of infection)
- The nonlinear relationship between cost and coverage of interventions, by not calculating the marginal costs of scaling up or scaling down a service
- The changing nature of financing for interventions, such as starting costs and diminishing returns, or the fact that health services cannot instantly be either scaled up or scaled down
- The pragmatic reality that health services or systems may have many different types of constraints. For example, the logistical capacity of infrastructure, the feasible operational platforms, human resourcing, or supply chain mechanisms may lead to upper or lower constraints on service scale; services could be funded by different sources with different funding restrictions and requirements; and ethical or political constraints may place requirements on system services.
- The decision-maker may have multiple simultaneous objectives and a need to assess all dynamic, interactive, complex factors in a holistic system toward attaining these objectives.

For these reasons, traditional CEA is inadequate for guiding most resource allocation decisions.

The Optima Model for Choosing Interventions

The Optima approach was designed to address the limitations of traditional CEA approaches. Two principles set the Optima approach apart from historical approaches: (1) it considers all quantifiable factors in a decision system together as a whole along with the actual resources that are available; and (2) it includes an optimization algorithm to calculate the analytical best resource allocation decision to address any number of weighted objectives simultaneously while factoring logistic, political, ethical, and economic constraints in the system. Whereas traditional CEAs commonly deem most interventions cost-effective by typical willingness-to-pay thresholds, Optima analyses determine what intervention mix is most cost-effective and affordable in the context of the level of resourcing available and other factors in the system—most notably, the specific objectives of importance to the decision-maker and real-world constraints.

Traditional CEAs can be extended by incorporating an epidemiological framework that accounts for interacting and dynamic effects as well as programmatic cost functions. This extension can be achieved by using mathematical models calibrated to the burden of disease in all subpopulations and links to relationships between marginal costs and programmatic coverage attained in target subpopulations. CEAs can also be extended by defining and using relationships between programmatic coverage in targeted subpopulations and the relevant outcomes related to reducing the disease burden. These additional components advance analyses to create closer links with programmatic realities. Once established, these analytical frameworks, including epidemiological models and programmatic relationships, are well-suited to comparing the projected effects of alternative budget allocation to specific programs, populations, and areas, and to assessing an intervention's impact on a population. Such models can better capture changes in burden of disease, or different cost-effectiveness ratios at different programmatic coverage levels or in the context of different mixes of other interventions in operation. To reflect the deliverability of services as they are applied, cost functions of any shape can be defined in the model as appropriate and as data will allow. These frameworks can be used to estimate the "best" (or "good") health financing allocations across interventions. They can also be used to decide what goes into a specific disease response intervention package or a health benefits package.

Even without consideration of multiple objectives and decision system constraints, just assessing interacting interventions and using an optimization algorithm make a major difference to analytical outcomes. If a disease is being addressed to some extent by one intervention, then a second intervention that attempts to address the same disease may not have the same incremental impact compared to if the second intervention was operating in isolation without the first. These interactions are particularly acute for communicable diseases that affect different key population subgroups disproportionately and for which there are many types of prevention, diagnostic, and treatment interventions available. In conventional CEA (using league tables), each intervention is assessed in isolation or compared to the status quo without dynamic interactions of other interventions being scaled up or down.

In a recent study, Chiu et al. (2017) questioned the validity of this assumption when investigating the response to the HIV epidemic in South Africa at close to full coverage of the most cost-effective interventions. They showed that, when the most cost-effective interventions of condom distribution, medical male circumcision, and ART were sequentially scaled up to high but feasible coverage levels, the incremental cost-effectiveness ratios (ICERs) of the remaining interventions increased up to 400-fold and their order in the league table changed (see figure 1.1) (Chiu et al. 2017).

This finding demonstrates that interactions between interventions are important, especially when other interventions exist that achieve similar outcomes, leading to strongly diminishing returns. For example, for protecting against sexually transmitted HIV, if nearly all sexual acts are protected by condoms, then medical male circumcision, pre-exposure prophylaxis (PrEP), and treatment as prevention will all be less effective incrementally than if any of them was the only protective intervention. Mathematical optimization, by contrast, gives much more realistic cost-effectiveness ratios that account for the interacting effects of programs and dynamic influences on burden of disease for different programmatic coverage levels (figure 1.1). This example demonstrates the importance of a framework to include interacting interventions coupled with an optimization. Using the Optima approach, it is possible to take this example further still by including multiple policy objectives and constraints.

The Optima approach to improving allocative efficiency involves the following key analytical steps (figure 1.2):

1. Assess the burden of disease over time, for each population group, and for each disease state. This assessment is done through data syntheses combined with epidemiological modeling.
2. Identify the interventions, including different service delivery modes and implementation options that have the potential to reduce incidence, morbidity, and mortality. For these interventions, specify the efficacy and effectiveness as well as the costs required to deliver services to different coverage levels.
3. Define strategic objectives and national priority targets—as well as the budgetary, logistic, ethical, and political constraints related to achieving these objectives—across the entire population and by disease area.

Figure 1.1   Rank and Comparison of ICERs between a Conventional League Table Approach and Use of an Optimization Routine That Includes Interactions between Services and Dynamic Effects

a. Rank of ICERs

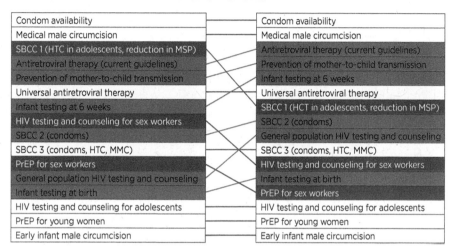

b. Comparison of ICERs

Cost per DALY averted

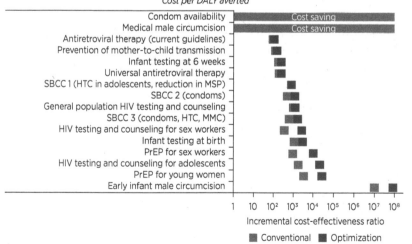

Source: Based on Chiu et al. 2017. Available under the Creative Commons Attribution 4.0 IGO license (CC BY 4.0 IGO) http://creativecommons.org/licenses/by/4.0/.

Note: DALY = disability-adjusted life year; HTC = HIV testing and counseling; HIV = human immunodeficiency virus; ICER = incremental cost-effectiveness ratio; MMC = medical male circumcision; MSP = multiple sexual partners; PrEP = pre-exposure prophylaxis; SBCC = social and behavior change communication.

Figure 1.2 Four Key Steps to the Optima Approach for Decision Science Analytics

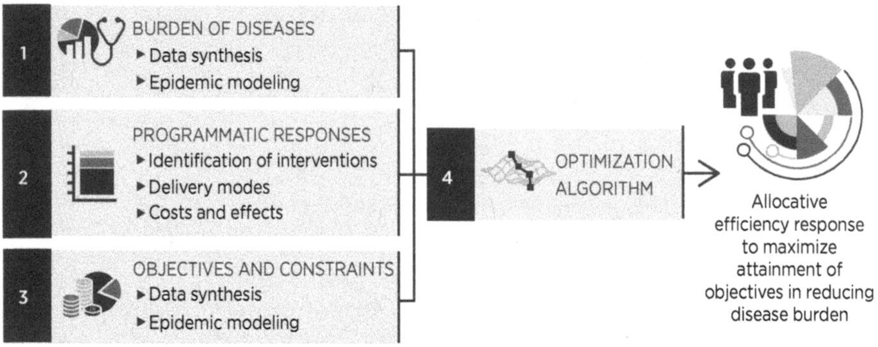

Source: World Bank.

4. Use a formal mathematical optimization algorithm around the constructs from the previous steps to assess the optimal allocation of a given level of resources to best achieve the objectives to reduce disease burden, subject to the defined constraints.

Further methodological details of the Optima approach have previously been published (Kerr et al. 2015), and full technical information on methods is described in a separate chapter of this book. The following subsections provide a summary of dominant concepts for assessment of services in the Optima approach.

Understanding the Burden of Disease(s)

Packages of services are provided in response to the disease burden among the population. All analyses must be grounded in all available knowledge on where the burden of disease occurs—which subpopulation groups are affected and the extent of morbidity and mortality. Public health surveillance data must drive understanding of the morbidity and mortality of diseases among subpopulations. These data, however, do not capture all indicators of importance; therefore, the data can be supplemented by quantitative epidemiological models that extend the implications of available data to infer levels and trends in indicators when all surveillance data are combined into a single framework. Interventions are assessed on the basis of the epidemiological model projections of burden of diseases in subpopulations, according to continuation of the status quo or simulation of any conceivable combination of interventions.

Establishing Cost Functions

A dominant driver of resource optimization is the set of relationships between (1) the cost of service delivery, (2) the resulting coverage levels of these services among targeted populations, and (3) how these coverage levels of services influence behavioral, clinical, and epidemiological outcomes. Such relationships are required to understand how incremental changes in spending directly or indirectly affect the burden of disease. In their first year of operation, most programs typically have initial setup costs, followed by a more effective scale-up with increased funding. Attaining very high coverage levels, however, requires reaching the most difficult-to-reach groups, which requires increased incremental investment for demand generation and related activities (that is, there is a saturation effect with increased funding). In subsequent years, programs may operate at scale without initial setup costs.

The Optima approach typically uses a logistic function fitted to available historical expenditure data or mapped to operational budgets of unit costs, coupled with information about logistical or feasibility constraints for saturation levels, to represent cost-coverage and coverage-outcome curves. An example is shown in figure 1.3 with decreasing and then increasing marginal costs.

Figure 1.3 Example of a Cost Function with Changing Marginal Cost with Scale of Program Implementation

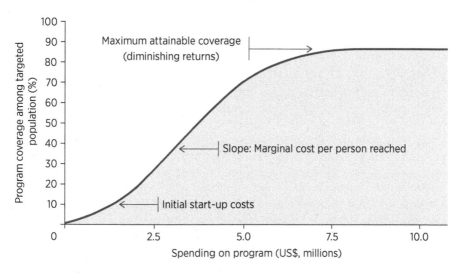

Source: Optima Consortium for Decision Science.
Note: US$ = US dollar.

Defining an Objective Function

National and global strategic health targets, along with other goals of decision-makers, can be formulated into an "objective function"—a quantitative representation of the objectives (goals) of a health response. Objective functions can be a combination of gains in health, financial protection, and equity, and other chosen social values represented by a suitable measure. Some social values like quality of life are already included in the optimization when using DALYs or QALYs as a measure of health outcomes. Other types of social/ethical values can be formally introduced as constraints. For example, "rule of rescue" can involve never defunding emergency care for life-threatening health conditions, even when there is only a small chance of saving a life. Other political, ethical, logistic, and budgetary constraints can be specified within the optimization algorithm to enable all relevant criteria to be included in an objective assessment. Equity and financial risk protection indexes can be defined, along with health metrics, and then the decision-maker can assess the trade-offs associated with different intervention packages. An objective function may also incorporate weights to determine the relative importance of the various goals to the decision-maker. Establishing appropriate time horizons and discounting rates are important to setting appropriate objective functions to reflect the priorities of decision-makers and the societies they represent. Building a formal objective function with weights assigned to different types of outcomes is usually an interactive process that relies upon stakeholder engagement. Health priority targets (national health strategic plans) or global SDG targets can help establish the combination of factors and weights in an objective function.

Using an Optimization Algorithm

Optimization algorithms explore the space of possible interventions at different coverage levels of each intervention, within the budget and other constraints, and find the combination of interventions and their coverage levels that produces the greatest gains in the objective function. Without an optimization algorithm, it is computationally inefficient and practically impossible to find the best analytical solution through scenario simulation of every possible parameter combination in the intervention-coverage space. Many optimization algorithms could be used around the epidemiological model calibrated and informed by setting-specific data, and the cost functions with effectiveness data, to calculate the resource allocation that will be the best solution of the objective function (figure 1.4). In this method, the most cost-effective mix of interventions and their optimal combination of coverage levels to achieve a predefined set of health-related

Figure 1.4   Schematic of an Optimization Algorithm in Two Dimensions of Health Services

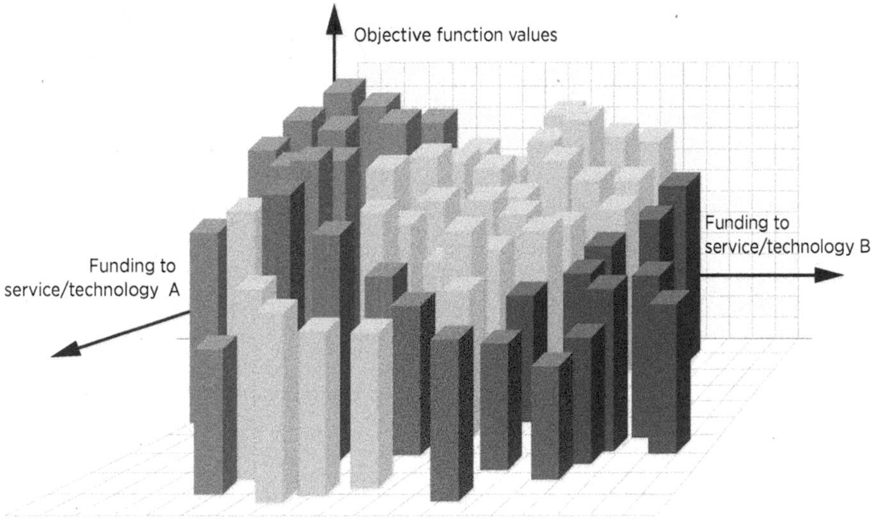

Source: Optima Consortium for Decision Science.

Note: Rather than sample all possible scenarios, optimization algorithms efficiently find a path toward the mathematical best solution against the objective function.

goals are determined. In comparison with scenario analysis, mathematical optimization chooses and rechooses funding allocations according to a set of decision rules, calculates the impact using the epidemiological and costing modules, determines if the selected allocation is a global best solution against the objective, and, if not, repeats the process until the mathematical best solution is found. In this situation, the solution would be the health benefits package theoretically best for this setting given its epidemiological context, infrastructure, costs, objectives, and constraints.

The Optima team has explored various commonly used algorithms but has developed its own adaptive stochastic descent (ASD) algorithm (Brownlee et al. 2017). ASD uses simple principles to form probabilistic assumptions about (1) which parameters have the greatest effect on the objective function, and (2) optimal step sizes for each parameter. The Optima team has shown that, for a certain class of optimization problems (namely, those with a moderate to large number of scalar parameter dimensions—especially if some dimensions are more important than others, as is common with Optima applications), ASD is capable of reaching the optimal solution of the objective function with fewer computational resources than classic optimization methods, such as the Nelder–Mead nonlinear simplex (Glasziou et al. 2017), Levenberg–Marquardt gradient descent (*Lancet Global Health* 2016), simulated annealing (Hollingsworth 2003), and genetic algorithms (Hollingsworth 2008).

Questions Answered through an Optima Analysis

Numerous health policy, program, and research questions can be addressed with the Optima approach. A primary question addressed by Optima analyses is, how can available funding be optimally allocated across the combination of possible interventions, targeted to the right people in the right places at the right time in the right ways, given real-world constraints, to yield the greatest outcomes for a defined objective mix of maximizing health, equity, and financial risk protection? Although previous Optima analyses have not used data to address financial risk protection properly, work is progressing on that important priority.

The following questions are also commonly addressed:

- How close will the country get to its National Health Strategic Plan's targets
  o With the current volume of funding, allocated per current expenditure?
  o With the current volume of funding, reallocated optimally?
- Over the National Health Strategic Plan period (or over a longer period), per current program implementation practices and costs,
  o How much total funding is required to meet the targets?
  o What is the minimum funding required, if allocated optimally between programs, to meet the targets?
- What benefits can be achieved via implementation efficiency gains?
- How would disease burdens look if past investment had not taken place, and what is the estimated cost-effectiveness of the past response?
- What is the expected future impact of policy or program implementation scenarios (with and without investment in specific programs)?

Evolution of Optima Tools

The response to the global HIV epidemic has been unprecedented. It has also changed the ways much of the world approaches global health financing. Since the early 2000s, high-income countries have transferred large sums of money to lower-income countries to provide emergency HIV prevention and treatment programs. Through programs such as the Global

Fund to Fight AIDS, Tuberculosis and Malaria (the Global Fund) and PEPFAR (the US President's Emergency Plan for AIDS Relief), over US$8 billion is made available each year to more than 100 countries (Bitran 2013). The volume and rapid scale-up of this investment has undoubtedly resulted in tremendous health and economic savings (Afridi and Ventelou 2013; Amico et al. 2012; Nunnenkamp and Öhler 2011; Piva and Dodd 2009). This extraordinary emergency response commenced at a time when triple-combination highly active antiretroviral therapy (HAART, now known as ART) had recently become widely available in high-income countries yet the number of individuals in need of therapy far exceeded the supply of antiretroviral drugs in lower-income countries. The 3-by-5 initiative (attaining 3 million people on HAART by 2005) of the World Health Organization (WHO) provided impetus for the world to commit to the goal of expanding access to therapy (WHO and UNAIDS 2003).

Even under the most optimistic scale-up, the need for ART in many countries has far exceeded the supply. Thus, difficult decisions had to be made as to how to allocate a scarce supply of ART. The Optima group started to emerge at that time to provide guidance around these questions of allocation of scarce resources. Epidemiological models were coupled with optimization algorithms to design ART allocation strategies that are as equitable as possible across geographical hot/cold spots (Wilson and Blower 2005a, 2005b, 2006) or, in contrast, were designed to have greatest epidemiological impact through targeting, particularly to geographical centers with the greatest disease burden, by demographic characteristics, or both (Wilson, Coplan, et al. 2008; Wilson, Kahn, and Blower 2006). These approaches were also extended to provide guidance around choices of health care facilities for stockpiling antiretrovirals and distributing them among different sized catchment regions (Wilson and Blower 2007). The Wilson-Blower method for antiretroviral optimization was applied to, and adopted in, different parts of Sub-Saharan Africa (see, for example, Malangu 2005), and these approaches informed WHO committees addressing ART rollout. These methods provided insights into potential epidemiological impact and inequity in access but did not include costing components or allocation of funding for programs. The methods were used for research activities and not deployed for use as public goods for general use or for country ownership to address their policy questions.

The team then expanded this foundational Optima approach to develop the following missing components.

Country-specific models as public goods: Learning from the important country engagement and ownership processes conducted by others—such as through the Asian Epidemic Model, now AIDS Epidemic Model (AEM) (Brown and Peerapatanapokin 2004), and the process of the Joint United Nations Programme on HIV/AIDS (UNAIDS) with countries through the use of Spectrum (Stover, Brown, and Marston 2012; Stover et al. 2008)—the Optima team invested in the creation of country-specific public goods. With funding and other support from development partners including Australia's Department of Foreign Affairs and Trade (DFAT), the World Bank, and the National Health and Medical Research Council, HIV epidemic models with accompanying software user interfaces were developed specifically for Australia (see, for example, Wilson, Hoare, et al. 2008), Cambodia (the Cambodian HIV Epidemic Model [CHEM]) (Heymer 2011), Indonesia (the HIV in Indonesia Model [HIM]) (Wilson et al. 2011), Papua New Guinea (Gray et al. 2011; Gray et. al. 2012; Gray et al. 2014), and the Philippines (Farr and Wilson 2010). Stakeholder involvement in these countries was of crucial importance. Despite some enthusiasm and initial use in the respective countries, these models were not maintained as tools used routinely in these countries for the longer term. This situation is likely due to only moderate capacity in these countries to use the models and a shortage of personnel located in the countries' national AIDS commissions or ministries of health dedicated to use modeling analyses in an integrated way into planning and decision-making processes.

Incorporating economic assessments: People who inject drugs (PWID) are among the most vulnerable and marginalized groups of people affected by HIV epidemics. Despite the evidence of their effectiveness for reducing HIV among PWID (Bastos and Strathdee 2000; Gibson, Flynn, and Perales 2001; Jenkins et al. 2001; Palmateer et al. 2010; Wodak 2006; Wodak and Cooney 2005), harm reduction programs can regularly be under threat—largely for political reasons. Economic arguments have been essential to demonstrate not only that the programs provide large health benefits and are cost-effective but also that they are cost-saving with considerable return on investment. No scientific case exists for defunding harm reduction. The Optima team conducted a comprehensive study with every state/territory jurisdiction of Australia to calculate the return on investment of harm reduction programs (Kwon et al. 2009; Kwon et al. 2012; Wilson et al. 2009); this study supported their continuation or in some locations led to their considerable scale-up and to widespread operational targets set as guided by modeling. It also led to further economic assessments of harm reduction, supporting countries and regions, and the building of United Nations scientific consensus statements.

Importance of the region of Eastern Europe and Central Asia: This study, and other international research studies by the same research group, received attention from the World Bank and UNAIDS, which facilitated greater international uptake of this approach. Eastern Europe and Central Asia (EECA) is one of only two regions of the world with increasing HIV epidemics after 2010. In this region, PWID have been most affected, and it is among PWID that the increasing epidemics have initially occurred. It was decided, therefore, that it could be highly useful to conduct similar studies on the cost-effectiveness of harm reduction for countries in EECA. Building on the public goods generated for other countries and the economic analyses for PWID in Australia, a generic global public good model and software interface were developed and launched for calculating the cost-effectiveness of harm reduction. Led by UNAIDS, a large collaborative multiyear study was conducted across nine countries in the EECA region—Armenia, Belarus, Estonia, Georgia, Kazakhstan, Moldova, the Russian Federation, Tajikistan, and Ukraine (Wilson et al. 2018). Anecdotal evidence has suggested that this initiative kept these crucial programs operational in some countries and facilitated some additional investments for them, albeit still at levels lower than ideal.

Large significance of the small country of Armenia: The harm reduction evaluation study led to a request from the government of Armenia and UNAIDS country office in Armenia for the leader behind Optima to draft what became the National Programme on the Response to HIV Epidemic in the Republic of Armenia for 2013–16, working with the Armenian National Center for AIDS Prevention. This national plan accelerated the broader use of ART in Armenia, with demonstrated impact of ART's effectiveness in the country (Mallitt et al. 2014). Furthermore, in the process of setting aspirational but attainable targets for the national strategic plan and in creating the accompanying operational plan about how these goals can be achieved, epidemic modeling and resource optimization were used (Armenia 2013). Armenia became the exemplar country for how a national strategic and operational plan can best be developed by involving country-specific data, stakeholders, modeling, and resource optimization. Although forms of resource optimization (of ART drugs) had been conducted 5–10 years earlier, and bodies of work were building to this point, this study with, and for, Armenia in 2011 could be considered the first application of a full study that addressed the primary question for which the Optima approach has now become known. Subsequent HIV investment cases using the Optima approach have been conducted for Armenia in 2013–14 (Kerr and Wilson 2014) and in 2015–16 (Kelly et al. 2016), including a major study summarized as a chapter of this book.

The Optima group knew that this process and analytical support could be extremely helpful to countries and that a major gap needed to be filled. Building on the foundation of the previously developed country-specific models (specifically building on HIM) and the experience from Armenia, the Optima team set out to develop an HIV model that included resource optimization and could be applied generically to any country through upload of the country's data and calibration of the model to those data.

What emerged was Prevtool, an HIV modeling tool that could conduct analyses of HIV program cost-effectiveness and uniquely HIV resource optimization (Eaton et al. 2014; Naning et al. 2014). Prevtool was later renamed Optima HIV to reflect better the purpose and use of the tool.

The Launch of Optima HIV

In 2013, Optima HIV was launched as an open-access, web-based application for accessing the Optima team's HIV model. This new product was accompanied by an expanded vision that included the following:

- Substantial technical advancements to the model, based on learned experiences from country case studies, with complete flexibility of innovative features to address any problem expected to arise in the conduct of HIV investment cases
- Application in generalized epidemic settings, addressing unique issues of time horizons with time-varying optimization needs, and geospatial targeting
- Pushing the boundaries to blur the lines between allocative efficiency and technical efficiency in the same study
- Development of a state-of-the-art, web-based, graphical user interface for the model
- Building capacity around the world to use the new model and interface product as a true global public good
- Facilitating its widespread use in each region of the world.

The Dissemination of Optima HIV

The Optima HIV software has since been used in approximately 40 countries in applications with ministries of health for guiding target setting, investment cases for operations of national strategic plans, and Global Fund Concept Notes. It has also been applied to over 50 countries in research studies as well as to inform the Association of Southeast Asian Nations (ASEAN) Health Ministers Summit, Hanoi 2015, and the United Nations General Assembly 2014 (Prasada Rao 2015; UNAIDS 2014). Optima analyses have moved beyond choosing the right programmatic areas to also guiding the right implementation choices (see, for example, Zhang et al. 2015), which is an area of increasing focus. Optima analyses have directly influenced health resource allocation, shifting funding to the most cost-effective mix of programs for countries to be on track to reduce new infections and deaths by 10–30 percent compared to previous programmatic responses. Country and regional workshops have built up capacity for using the Optima approach and the Optima HIV model in most regions.

With the expansion of capacity in the use of the Optima approach brought about by the new Optima HIV software, the need arose to expand the base of the Optima group. The core home of the Optima group has been the Burnet Institute in Australia. (The group was formerly at the University of New South Wales where precursor models for implementing the Optima approach were developed.) Other academic institutions have joined in partnership to form the Optima Consortium for Decision Science: University College London, the University of Bern, the University of Geneva, the University of Sydney, and the University of Copenhagen have groups that are also currently part of the consortium's Optima activities.

Rather than a country-by-country approach, a regional effort to using the Optima approach and Optima tools has created greater networking and learning experiences between countries in the same region, improved uptake, and efficient and coordinated activities between funders, development partners, countries, and technical supporters. The EECA region was the first group of countries to adopt this approach, to examine the allocative efficiency of their HIV responses collectively as a region. It is therefore appropriate that this book highlights that the EECA region has been at the forefront of investment case analytics. Other regions have since followed.

Conclusions and Future Directions

The World Bank's Health, Nutrition, and Population Global Practice has a Global Solutions Group focusing on decision and delivery science. This group seeks to develop global decision and delivery science tools and to apply them to the World Bank's global health and nutrition portfolio, which includes health, nutrition, and health-sensitive, multisectoral investments in approximately 150 countries worldwide. As part of its efforts to improve the efficiency and effectiveness of its health responses, the World Bank has used several tools, including the different Optima tools, as part of a package of technical support to countries. Typically, the modeling process has been part of the broader policy and program dialogue on HIV, TB, and nutrition allocative and implementation efficiency.

The EECA region has been a pioneer in the extensive use of these tools to improve the allocative efficiency of its HIV and TB programs. This book shows the potential of what can be done with a model like Optima and how it can support real-life improvements in policy and more efficacious budget allocations.

Other organizations that have supported and used Optima include the US Centers for Disease Control and Prevention (CDC), PEPFAR, the Global Fund, UNAIDS, and WHO.

Future directions for optimization modeling include the following:

Mathematical optimization for expansion to other disease burdens beyond HIV: In a context of flatlining global and domestic health and development investments, improvements in allocative and implementation efficiency are tantamount to budget increases that do not require additional resources from finance ministries or development assistance. Although most countries acknowledge the need to invest in allocative efficiency, changing allocations is challenging in the absence of evidence and political will. Moreover, political interests and epidemiological complexities make it challenging to invest in the right mix of programs. Mathematical optimization tools such as Optima and others seem to have shown that it could be useful in filling some of this gap for country decision-makers. Beyond HIV, Optima has, for example, been developed for and used in TB, nutrition, hepatitis C, and malaria programs. Other optimization approaches are also now being developed by other modeling groups, further building the global knowledge base on what it will take to maximize the health impact for the money.

Mathematical optimization to develop health benefits packages: As part of the SDGs, universal health coverage (UHC) by 2030 is an important goal. Because of limited resources, however, not all services can be provided, and decision-makers must decide which ones to include in publicly funded health benefits packages (HBPs). More than 60 low- and middle-income countries have some form of HBP (Chalkidou et al. 2016), with many more moving to develop HBPs. Established HBPs vary greatly in terms of benefits included, coverage levels, and HBP budgets as a proportion of overall public expenditure (Giedion, Alfonso, and Díaz 2013). Substantial global evidence has been building on program and cost-effectiveness of priority health interventions (for example, through the Disease Control Priorities initiative) with the goal of influencing program design and resource allocation at global and country levels. Other evidence—including local data on disease burden, costs, intervention coverage and quality, and outcomes and local priorities—is available to support country-level decision-making. Within ministries of health, increasing capacity also exists for health technology assessment (HTA) for defining HBPs. The methods for forming these packages, however, are not standardized and are often not informed by good data and real-world constraints or formally organized against strict criteria. Mathematical modeling methods can help HTA units view generic globally recommended HBPs as a baseline reference and then customize their own package based on local factors and policy objectives. Moreover, allocative efficiency only goes so far. There is need to design health packages that not only allocate efficiently to maximize health but also factor weightings toward equity and financial risk protection.

Mathematical optimization for choosing service delivery modalities and implementation cascades: The complexity of health decision-making can be simplified by using the lens of the care cascade, which sequentially asks four questions about a patient's journey through the continuum of care:

1. Is a patient diagnosed if he or she has a health condition?
2. Is the patient linked to appropriate health care?
3. Is the patient adherent to the required care regimen?
4. Does the patient achieve disease control?

Failure at each stage precludes success at the next, which means the cascade of care may tumble rapidly, with failures compounded from tier to tier. The concept of the cascade of care holds great promise for tackling entrenched chronic primary health care challenges. Simple visualization of cascade break points can pinpoint choke points and bottlenecks, as well as identify key remedial steps. More complex analytic tools permit comparison of the cost-effectiveness of different corrective cascade interventions. The fact that the cascade captures the temporal progression of care means that improvement in the first tiers—diagnosis and linkage—can be achieved rapidly, making the cascade an important tool for rapid performance improvement and measurement.

Mathematical optimization for human development: Faced with existing and emerging disease threats, an ever-expanding armory of health technologies, and associated delivery challenges, the health sector has devoted more attention to allocative and implementation efficiency than other sectors have. Challenges, lessons, tools, and implications from health applications can be tailored for other sectors. Mathematical optimization approaches could be considered for use in human development writ large, such as for improvements in the Human Capital Index.

Participation in efforts to address the ongoing challenges of costs and cost-coverage curves: One of the foundational challenges of mathematical optimization efforts is the need for rich and expansive data about the costs and coverage of programs and how those change in terms of the program level of maturity, the marginal costs of service delivery, and other exogenous factors that may influence service delivery temporally. The cost-coverage curves are the "vulnerable underbelly" of such models. Ongoing effort is needed to ensure that these data are collected, curated, and updated to improve the ability of modelers to estimate solutions of use to policy makers. No tool or technique can replace the value of good quality data with which to parameterize the model.

Beyond mathematical optimization, movement toward incorporation of big data analytics: Beyond the stochastic modeling and evolutionary algorithms approaches described in this book, the field of big data analytics and artificial intelligence has exploded with promise in the field of health. The next generation of mathematical and quantitative approaches to support decision-makers in addressing their pernicious health challenges will draw on these methods. Underscoring such approaches will remain the need for an intimate understanding of the problem and the systems and context within which they are to be used and a willingness to explore new options for solving old challenges.

Note

* The authors wish to thank the many team members from the Optima Consortium for Decision Science and its partner academic institutions who have contributed to the refinement of implementation in the Optima approach, its technical development, and extensions of its many modules and algorithms, as well as the application of Optima models. Special thanks are expressed to the additional cocreators of Optima (Cliff Kerr and Robyn Stuart) who also reviewed this chapter.

References

Afridi, M., and B. Ventelou. 2013. "Impact of Health Aid in Developing Countries: The Public vs. the Private Channels." *Economic Modelling* 31 (March): 759–65.

Amico, P., B. Gobet, C. Avila-Figueroa, C. Aran, and P. De Lay. 2012. "Pattern and Levels of Spending Allocated to HIV Prevention Programs in Low- and Middle-Income Countries." *BMC Public Health* 12: 221.

Armenia. 2013. "National Programme on the Response to HIV Epidemic in the Republic of Armenia for 2013–2016." Unpublished report, Government of Armenia, Yerevan.

Bastos, F. I., and S. A. Strathdee. 2000. "Evaluating Effectiveness of Syringe Exchange Programmes: Current Issues and Future Prospects." *Social Science & Medicine* 51 (12): 1771–82.

Bitran, R. 2013. "Explicit Health Guarantees for Chileans: The AUGE Benefits Package." UNICO Studies Series 21, World Bank, Washington, DC.

Blumstein, J. F. 1997. "The Oregon Experiment: The Role of Cost-Benefit Analysis in the Allocation of Medicaid Funds." *Social Science & Medicine* 45 (4): 545–54.

Brown, T., and W. Peerapatanapokin. 2004. "The Asian Epidemic Model: A Process Model for Exploring HIV Policy and Programme Alternatives in Asia." *Sexually Transmitted Infections* 80 (Suppl. 1): i19–i24.

Brownlee, S., K. Chalkidou, J. Doust, A. G. Elshaug, P. Glasziou, I. Heath, S. Nagpal, V. Saini, D. Srivastava, K. Chalmers, and D. Kornestein. 2017. "Evidence for Overuse of Medical Services Around the World. *Lancet* 390 (10090): 156–68.

Burki, T. 2014. "Elimination on the Agenda for Hepatitis C." *Lancet Infectious Diseases* 14 (6): 452–53.

Chalabi, Z., D. Epstein, C. McKenna, and K. Claxton. 2008. "Uncertainty and Value of Information when Allocating Resources within and between Healthcare Programmes." *European Journal of Operational Research* 191 (2): 530–39.

Chalkidou, K., A. Glassman, R. Marten, J. Vega, Y. Teerawattananon, N. Tritasavit, M. Gyansa-Lutterodt, A. Seiter, M. P. Kieny, K. Hofman K, and A. J. Cuyler. 2016. "Priority-Setting for Achieving Universal Health Coverage." *Bulletin of the World Health Organization* 94 (6): 462–67.

Chisholm, D., and D. Evans. 2010. "Improving Health System Efficiency as a Means of Moving towards Universal Coverage." Background Paper 28 for the 2010 World Health Report, World Health Organization, Geneva.

Chiu, C., L. F. Johnson, L. Jamieson, B. A. Larson, and G. Meyer-Rath. 2017. "Designing an Optimal HIV Programme for South Africa: Does the Optimal Package Change When Diminishing Returns Are Considered?" *BMC Public Health* 17 (1): 143.

Cohen, M. S., Y. Q. Chen, M. McCauley, T. Gamble, M. C. Hosseinipour, N. Kumarasamy, J. G. Hakim, J. Kumwenda, B. Grinsztejn, J. H. Pilotto, S. V. Godbole, S. Mehendale, S. Chariyalertsak, B. R. Santos, K. H. Mayer, I. F. Hoffman, S. H. Eshleman, E. Piwowar-Manning, L. Wang, J. Makhema, L. A. Mills, G. deBruyn, I. Sanne, J. Eron, J. Gallant, D. Haylir, S. Swindells, H. Ribaudo, V. Elharrar, D. Burns, T. E. Taha, K. Nielsen-Saines, D. Celentano, M. Essex, T. R. Fleming, and HPTN 052 Study Team. 2011. "Prevention of HIV-1 Infection with Early Antiretroviral Therapy." *New England Journal of Medicine* 365 (6): 493–505.

Drummond, M. F., M. J. Sculpher, G. W. Torrance, B. J. O'Brien, and G. L. Stoddart. 2005. *Methods for the Economic Evaluation of Health Care Programmes*, 3rd ed. Oxford: Oxford University Press.

Eaton, J. W., N. A. Menzies, J. Stover, V. Cambiano, L. Chindelevitch, A. Cori, J. A. Hontelez, S. Humair, C. C. Kerr, and D. J. Klein. 2014. "Health Benefits, Costs, and Cost-Effectiveness of Earlier Eligibility for Adult Antiretroviral Therapy and Expanded Treatment Coverage: A Combined Analysis of 12 Mathematical Models." *Lancet Global Health* 2 (1): e23–e34.

Farr, A. C., and D. P. Wilson. 2010. "An HIV Epidemic Is Ready to Emerge in the Philippines." *Journal of the International AIDS Society* 13:16.

Flessa, S. 2000. "Where Efficiency Saves Lives: A Linear Programme for the Optimal Allocation of Health Care Resources in Developing Countries." *Health Care Management Science* 3 (3): 249–67.

Flessa, S. 2003. "Priorities and Allocation of Health Care Resources in Developing Countries: A Case-Study from the Mtwara Region, Tanzania." *European Journal of Operational Research* 150: 67–80.

Fonner, V. A., S. L. Dalglish, C. E. Kennedy, R. Baggaley, K. R. O'Reilly, F. M. Koechlin, M. Rodolph, I. Hodges-Mameletzis, R. M. Grant. 2016. "Effectiveness and Safety of Oral HIV Preexposure Prophylaxis for All Populations." *AIDS* 30 (12): 1973–83.

GBD 2015 DALYs and HALE Collaborators. 2016. "Global, Regional, and National Disability-Adjusted Life-Years (DALYs) for 315 Diseases and Injuries and Healthy Life Expectancy (HALE), 1990–2015: A Systematic Analysis for the Global Burden of Disease Study 2015." *Lancet* 388 (10053): 1603–58.

GBD Disease 2015 Disease and Injury Incidence and Prevalence Collaborators. 2016. "Global, Regional, and National Incidence, Prevalence, and Years Lived with Disability for 310 Diseases and Injuries, 1990–2015: A Systematic Analysis for the Global Burden of Disease Study 2015." *Lancet* 388 (10053): 1545–1602.

GBD 2015 SDG Collaborators. 2016. "Measuring the Health-Related Sustainable Development Goals in 188 Countries: A Baseline Analysis from the Global Burden of Disease Study." *Lancet* 388 (10053):1813–50.

Gibson, D. R., N. M. Flynn, and D. Perales. 2001. "Effectiveness of Syringe Exchange Programs in Reducing HIV Risk Behavior and HIV Seroconversion Among Injecting Drug Users." *AIDS* 15 (11): 1329–41.

Giedion, U., E. A. Alfonso, and Y. Díaz. 2013. "The Impact of Universal Coverage Schemes in the Developing World: A Review of the Existing Evidence." UNICO Studies Series 25, World Bank, Washington, DC.

Glasziou, P., S. Straus, S. Brownlee, L. Trevena, L. Dans, G. Guyatt, A. G. Elshaug, R. Janett, and V. Saini. 2017. "Evidence for Underuse of Effective Medical Services Around the World." *Lancet* 390 (10090): 169–77.

Görgens, M., J. Petravic, D. J. Wilson, and D. P. Wilson. 2017. "See the Bigger Picture: Resource Optimization Tools to Inform HBP Design." In *What's In, What's Out: Designing Benefits for Universal Health Coverage*, edited by A. Glassman, U. Giedion, and P. C. Smith. Washington, DC: Center for Global Development.

Gray, R. T., N. Lote, J. M. Murray, D. P. Wilson, A. Vallely, J. Kaldor, and P. Siba. 2012. "The Papua New Guinea HIV Model: Explaining the Past, Describing the Present, and Forecasting the Future of the HIV Epidemic in PNG." Kirby Institute, University of New South Wales, Sydney.

Gray, R. T., A. Vallely, D. P. Wilson, J. Kaldor, D. MacLaren, A. Kelly-Hanku, P. Siba, and J. M. Murray. 2014. "Impact of Male Circumcision on the HIV Epidemic in Papua New Guinea: A Country with Extensive Foreskin Cutting Practices." *PLoS One* 9 (8): e104531.

Gray, R. T., L. Zhang, T. Lupiwa, and D. P. Wilson. 2011. "Forecasting the Population-Level Impact of Reductions in HIV Antiretroviral Therapy in Papua New Guinea." *AIDS Research and Treatment* 2011: 891593.

Heymer, K. J. 2011. "Using Mathematical Modelling to Evaluate Drivers and Predict Trajectories of HIV and STI Epidemics in South East Asian and Australian Populations." Submitted for the degree of doctor of philosophy, University of New South Wales. https://eprints.qut.edu.au/74059/1/whole.pdf.

Hollingsworth, B. 2003. "Non-Parametric and Parametric Applications Measuring Efficiency in Health Care." *Health Care Management Science* 6 (4): 203–18.

Hollingsworth, B. 2008. "The Measurement of Efficiency and Productivity of Health Care Delivery." *Health Economics* 17 (10): 1107–28.

Jamison, D. T., L. H. Summers, G. Alleyne, K. J. Arrow, S. Berkley, A. Binagwaho, F. Bustreo, D. Evans, R. G. Feachem, J. Frenk, G. Ghosh, S. J. Goldie, Y. Guo, R. Horton, M. E. Kruk, A. Mahmoud, L. K. Mohohlo, M. Ncube, A. Pablos-Mendes, K. S. Reddy, H. Saxenian, A. Soucat, K. H. Ulltveit-Moe, and G. Yamey. 2013. "Global Health 2035: A World Converging within a Generation." *Lancet* 382 (9908): 1898–1955.

Jenkins, C., H. Rahman, T. Saidel, S. Jana, and A. M. Hussain. 2001. "Measuring the Impact of Needle Exchange Programs among Injecting Drug Users through the National Behavioural Surveillance in Bangladesh." *AIDS Education and Prevention* 13 (5): 452–61.

Kelly, S. L., A. J. Shattock, C. C. Kerr, R. M. Stuart, A. Papoyan, T. Grigoryan, R. Hovhannisyan, S. Grigoryan, C. Benedikt, and D. P. Wilson. 2016. "Optimizing HIV/AIDS Resources in Armenia: Increasing ART Investment and Examining HIV Programmes for Seasonal Migrant Labourers." *Journal of the International AIDS Society* 19 (1): 20772.

Kerr, C. C., R. M. Stuart, R. T. Gray, A. J. Shattock, N. Fraser-Hurt, C. Benedikt, M. Haacker, M. Berdnikov, A. M. Mahmood, S. A. Jaber, M. Görgens, and D. P. Wilson. 2015 "Optima: A Model for HIV Epidemic Analysis, Program Prioritization, and Resource Optimization." *Journal of Acquired Immune Deficiency Syndrome* 69 (3): 365–76.

Kerr, C. C., and D. P. Wilson. 2014. "HIV Investment in Armenia: Analysis & Recommendations." Unpublished technical report for the Government of Armenia.

Kwon, J. A., J. Anderson, C. C. Kerr, H. H. Thein, L. Zhang, J. Iversen, G. J. Dore, J. M. Kaldor, M. G. Law, L. Maher, and D. P Wilson. 2012. "Estimating the Cost-Effectiveness of Needle-Syringe Programs in Australia." *AIDS* 26 (17): 2201–10.

Kwon, J. A., J. Iversen, L. Maher, M. G. Law, and D. P. Wilson. 2009. "The Impact of Needle and Syringe Programs on HIV and HCV Transmissions in Injecting Drug Users in Australia: A Model-Based Analysis." *Journal of Acquired Immune Deficiency Syndrome* 51 (4): 462–69.

Lancet Global Health. 2016. "Financing for Health: Where There's a Will." *Lancet Global Health* 4 (10): e663.

Levin, C. E., M. Sharma, Z. Olson, S. Verguet, J. F. Shi, S. M. Wang, Y. L. Qiao, D. T. Jamison, and J. J. Kim. 2015. "An Extended Cost-Effectiveness Analysis of Publicly Financed HPV Vaccination to Prevent Cervical Cancer in China." *Vaccine* 33 (24): 2830–41.

Malangu, N. 2005. "Estimating the Number of Antiretroviral Treatment Facilities Based on the Wilson-Blower Method." *PLoS Medicine* 2 (8): e270.

Mallitt, K. A., S. R. Grigoryan, A. S. Papoyan, H. C. Wand, and D. P. Wilson. 2014. "Access to Antiretroviral Therapy and Survival in Eastern Europe and Central Asia: A Case Study in Armenia." *Journal of the International AIDS Society* 17: 18795.

Medeiros, J., and C. Schwierz. 2015. *Efficiency Estimates of Health Care Systems.* European Economy Economic Papers 549. Brussels: Directorate General Economic and Financial Affairs, European Commission.

Naning, H., C. Kerr, A. Kamarulzaman, S. Osornprasop, M. Dahlui, C. W. Ng, and D. P. Wilson. 2014. "Return on Investment and Cost-Effectiveness of Harm Reduction Program in Malaysia." World Bank, Washington, DC.

Ndeffo Mbah, M. L., and C. A. Gilligan. 2011. "Resource Allocation for Epidemic Control in Metapopulations." *PloS ONE* 6 (9): e24577.

Nunnenkamp, P., and H. Öhler. 2011. "Throwing Foreign Aid at HIV/AIDS in Developing Countries: Missing the Target?" *World Development* 39 (10): 1704–23.

Palmateer, N., J. Kimber, M. Hickman, S. Hutchinson, T. Rhodes, and D. Goldberg. 2010. "Evidence for the Effectiveness of Sterile Injecting Equipment Provision in Preventing Hepatitis C and Human Immunodeficiency Virus Transmission among Injecting Drug Users: A Review of Reviews." *Addiction* 105 (5): 844–59.

Piva, P., and R. Dodd. 2009. "Where Did All the Aid Go? An In-Depth Analysis of Increased Health Aid Flows Over the Past 10 Years." *Bulletin of the World Health Organization* 87 (12): 930–39.

Prasada Rao, J. V. R. 2015. "Investing for Results: How Asia Pacific Countries Can Invest for Ending AIDS." Presentation to the Asia Pacific Intergovernmental Meeting on HIV and AIDS, Bangkok, January 29.

Stinnett, A. A., and A. D. Paltiel. 1996. "Mathematical Programming for the Efficient Allocation of Health Care Resources." *Journal of Health Economics* 15 (5): 641–53.

Stover, J., T. Brown, and M. Marston. 2012. "Updates to the Spectrum/Estimation and Projection Package (EPP) Model to Estimate HIV Trends for Adults and Children." *Sexually Transmitted Infections* 88 (Suppl. 2): i11–i16.

Stover J., P. Johnson, B. Zaba, M. Zwahlen, F. Dabis, and R. Ekpini. 2008. "The Spectrum Projection Package: Improvements in Estimating Mortality, ART Needs, PMTCT Impact and Uncertainty Bounds." *Sexually Transmitted Infections* 84 (Suppl. 1): i24–i30.

UNAIDS (Joint United Nations Programme on HIV/AIDS). 2014. *Fast-Track: Ending the AIDS Epidemic by 2030*. Geneva: UNAIDS.

United Nations General Assembly. 2015. "Transforming Our World: The 2030 Agenda for Sustainable Development." United Nations document A/Res/70/1, October 21.

Verguet, S., Z. D. Olson, J. B. Babigumira, D. Desalegn, K. A. Johansson, K. E. Kruk, C. E. Levin, R. A. Nugent, C. Pecenka, M. G. Shrime, S. T. Memirie, D. A. Watkinds, and D. T. Jamison. 2015. "Health Gains and Financial Risk Protection Afforded by Public Financing of Selected Interventions in Ethiopia: An Extended Cost-Effectiveness Analysis." *Lancet Global Health* 3 (5): e288–96.

Verguet, S., C. Pecenka, K. A. Johansson, S. T. Memirie, I. K. Friberg, J. R. Driessen, and D. T. Jamison. 2016. "Health Gains and Financial Risk Protection Afforded by Treatment and Prevention of Diarrhea and Pneumonia in Ethiopia: An Extended Cost-Effectiveness Analysis." In *Reproductive, Maternal, Newborn, and Child Health: Disease Control Priorities*, 3rd ed. Vol. 2, edited by R. E. Black, R. Laxminarayan, M. Temmerman, and N. Walker. Washington, DC: World Bank.

Wang, H., M. Naghavi, C. Allen, R. M. Barber, Z. A. Bhutta, A. Carter, D. C. Casey, F. J. Charlson, A. Z. Chen, and M. M. Coates. 2016. "Global, Regional, and National Life Expectancy, All-Cause Mortality, and Cause-Specific Mortality for 249 Causes of Death, 1980–2015: A Systematic Analysis for the Global Burden of Disease Study 2015." *Lancet* 388 (10053): 1459–1544.

Watkins, D. A., Z. D. Olson, S. Verguet, R. A. Nugent, and D. T. Jamison. 2016. "Cardiovascular Disease and Impoverishment Averted Due to a Salt Reduction Policy in South Africa: An Extended Cost-Effectiveness Analysis." *Health Policy and Planning* 31 (1): 75–82.

WHO (World Health Organization). 2015. "The End TB Strategy: Global Strategy and Targets for Tuberculosis Prevention, Care and Control after 2015." Geneva: WHO.

WHO (World Health Organization). 2016a. "Eliminating Malaria." Geneva: WHO.

WHO (World Health Organization). 2016b. "Global Health Sector Strategy on Viral Hepatitis 2016–2021." Geneva: WHO.

WHO (World Health Organization) and UNAIDS (Joint United Nations Programme on HIV/AIDS). 2003. *Treating 3 Million by 2005: Making It Happen, The WHO Strategy*. Geneva: WHO.

Wilson, D. P., and S. M. Blower. 2005a. "Allocating Antiretrovirals in South Africa: Using Modeling to Determine Treatment Equity." *PLoS Med* 2 (6): e155; author reply e186.

Wilson, D. P., and S. M. Blower. 2005b. "Designing Equitable Antiretroviral Allocation Strategies in Resource-Constrained Countries." *PLoS Med* 2 (2): e50.

Wilson, D. P., and S. M. Blower. 2006. "Rational Choices for Allocating Antiretrovirals in Africa: Treatment Equity, Epidemiological Efficiency, and Feasibility." *PLoS Med* 3 (3): e160.

Wilson, D. P., and S. M. Blower. 2007. "How Far Will We Need to Go to Reach HIV-Infected People in Rural South Africa?" *BMC Med* 5: 16.

Wilson, D. P., P. M. Coplan, M. A. Wainberg, and S. M. Blower. 2008. "The Paradoxical Effects of Using Antiretroviral-Based Microbicides to Control HIV Epidemics." *Proceedings of the National Academy of Sciences of the United States of America* 105 (28): 9835–40.

Wilson, D. P., A. Hoare, D. G. Regan, H. Wand, and M. G. Law. 2008. "Mathematical Models to Investigate Recent Trends in HIV Notifications among Men Who Have Sex with Men in Australia." National Centre in HIV Epidemiology and Clinical Research, University of New South Wales, Darlinghurst, Australia.

Wilson, D. P., J. Kahn, and S. M. Blower. 2006. "Predicting the Epidemiological Impact of Antiretroviral Allocation Strategies in KwaZulu-Natal: The Effect of the Urban-Rural Divide." *Proceedings of the National Academy of Sciences of the United States of America* 103 (38): 14228–33.

Wilson D., J. Kwon, J. Anderson, H. H. Thein, M. Law, L. Maher, G. Dore, and J. Kaldor. 2009. "Return on Investment 2: Evaluating the Cost-Effectiveness of Needle and Syringe Programs Among Injecting Drug Users in Australia." National Centre in HIV Epidemiology and Clinical Research, University of New South Wales, Darlinghurst, Australia.

Wilson D. P., P. Riono, C. Kerr, A. Kwon, L. Zhang, J. Kaldor, A. Sutrisna, M. N. Farid, and N. Hadi. 2011. "The HIV in Indonesia Model (HIM)." Software Manual, University of Indonesia, Jakarta. http://optimamodel.com/hiv/applications .html#2011.

Wilson, D. P., Zhang L., C. C. Kerr, A. Uusküla, J. A. Kwon, A. Hoare, K. Sharapka, T. Balabayev, A. Yakusik, E. Gvozdeva, G. Ionascu, D. Otiashvili, T. Grigoryan, A. Soliev, L. Zohrabyan, M. Williams-Sherlock, and C. Avila on behalf of the Technical Working Group to evaluate the cost-effectiveness of needle-syringe programs in Eastern Europe and Central Asia. 2018. "Needle-Syringe Programs Are Cost-Effective in Eastern Europe and Central Asia: Data Synthesis, Modeling, and Economics for Nine Case-Study Countries." Optima Consortium for Decision Science.

Wodak, A. 2006. "Lessons from the First International Review of the Evidence for Needle Syringe Programs: The Band Still Plays On." *Substance Use and Misuse* 41 (6–7): 837–39.

Wodak, A, and A. Cooney. 2005. "Effectiveness of Sterile Needle and Syringe Programmes." *International Journal of Drug Policy* 16 (Suppl. 1): 31–44.

World Bank. 2017. "Second Annual UHC Financing Forum Greater Efficiency for Better Health and Financial Protection." Forum meeting report, Washington, DC, World Bank, April 20–21.

Zhang, L., N. Phanuphak, K. Henderson, S. Nonenoy, S. Srikaew, A. J. Shattock, C. C. Kerr, B. Omune, F. van Griensven, S. Osornprasop, R. Oelrichs, J. Ananworanich, and D. P. Wilson. 2015. "Scaling Up of HIV Treatment for Men Who Have Sex with Men in Bangkok: A Modelling and Costing Study." *Lancet HIV* 2 (5): e200–07.

2

Armenia
Mobilizing an HIV Response When a Key Population Is Mobile

Samvel Grigoryan, Sherrie L. Kelly, Arshak Papoyan, Ruben Hovhannisyan, Trdat Grigoryan, David P. Wilson, Diego Cuadros, and Wendy Heard

Briefly

- Labor migrants make up a considerable portion of people living with human immunodeficiency virus (HIV) in Armenia.
- There is a lack of proven, internationally agreed service delivery models for labor migrants in concentrated epidemic contexts.
- A sensitivity analysis was carried out to determine under what conditions HIV programs for labor migrants can be cost-effective.
- Innovative strategies to reach labor migrants are needed.

Introduction

Armenia is a country with an astonishing history; whoever has walked through the city of Yerevan or visited its museums and restaurants can feel that in Armenia history is present. Today's Armenia is situated in the highlands around the biblical mountain of Ararat, which is where, according to the Bible, Noah landed with his ark. As if the arrival of this early migrant on a boat was to be symbolic, migration would continue to play a key role in Armenian history. The borders of the country itself have shifted and once extended to the Mediterranean Sea. Today, the Armenian diaspora is present in various parts of the world, and Armenian seasonal labor migrants migrate to the Russian Federation, other parts of Eastern Europe, and Central or Western Asia for work.

Identifying and Addressing the HIV Risk

The fact that HIV must have spread to Armenia in the 1980s with an unknown traveler or returning citizen is not unique. It is how HIV spread to virtually all countries around the world. As in most countries of Eastern Europe and Central Asia, a concentrated HIV epidemic evolved in the 1990s, particularly among people who inject drugs (PWID), with HIV prevalence peaking at about 10 percent. What is special about HIV and migration in Armenia is that, after 2005, new diagnoses related to injecting behavior started to decline in Armenia and a growing proportion of new HIV infections was reported among outbound labor migrants. This situation poses a unique challenge for HIV programs: How does a program address a population whose main risk of HIV infection occurs outside the country? Is it possible to identify an HIV response that does justice to the variety of epidemic contexts that outbound labor migrants may be exposed to while abroad? Should the response primarily focus on migrants or on the communities of key populations in Armenia among whom the epidemic could spread—or both?

These are unique questions faced by an allocative efficiency study conducted a few years ago, and there were no simple solutions because no international best practice exists for responding to this type of epidemic. Instead, the study team—consisting of national experts from Armenia, led by the National Center for AIDS Prevention, and mathematical modelers, led by the World Bank and the Burnet Institute—had to perform pioneering analyses. The first step was to collate data and perform an epidemiological analysis. Given that, in 2014, it was estimated that there were 4,000 people living with HIV (PLHIV) in Armenia, the HIV epidemic there was classified as low-level and concentrated.[1] According to available estimates, the epidemic is stabilizing in most key populations including female sex workers (FSWs), men who have sex with men (MSM), and PWID.

To ensure their consistency and relevance, and unless otherwise indicated, the data provided in this chapter relate to the situation in Armenia at the time the analysis was conducted.

New Population Groups Affected by HIV

Seasonal outbound labor migrants are considered one of the key populations most vulnerable to HIV in Armenia. Outbound labor migrants are influenced by certain factors that increase their vulnerability to HIV. Migration can place people in situations of increased vulnerability to HIV and other serious infections by limiting their access to health care and also sometimes to legal services and protection. It can also increase their vulnerability by separating migrants from their families, spouses, and local support networks and by inducing additional social, political, and economic stressors. Social exclusion leaves migrants highly vulnerable to HIV: being far away from their families and regular sexual partners, many outbound migrants may feel released from the social norms they follow when living among friends and family in Armenia. These factors may drive the migrants to engage in high-risk behaviors surrounding HIV. As a rule, legislation in host countries restricts migrants' access to health care services outside of Armenia, so Armenia's outbound labor migrants lack access to basic information about HIV/AIDS (acquired immune deficiency syndrome) or to HIV testing and prevention. The misconception that HIV is passed only from sex workers contributes to the transmission of HIV. Examination of HIV cases registered among outbound labor migrants shows that they report being infected from their noncommercial sexual partners, whom they regarded as trustworthy and with whom they had short- or long-term relations.

Emigration is very prevalent among Armenian citizens. It is estimated that between 80,000 and 100,000 labor migrants, predominantly male, return to Armenia each year, with most (58.3 percent) settling in urban centers. Generally, labor migrants travel to find work in countries with HIV prevalence rates higher than in Armenia. Most migrants (over 90 percent) travel to Russia, where HIV prevalence in the general population (aged 15–49 years) is at least 1 percent. As such, labor migrants returning to Armenia may have been exposed to HIV while working and living in their receiving countries.

Analysis of self-reported HIV diagnoses registered in Armenia from 2004 to 2014 reveals that the main mode of HIV transmission has shifted. The proportion of transmissions via injecting drug use dropped fivefold—from approximately 67 percent to 13 percent. In contrast, the proportion of

Figure 2.1 Self-Reported Modes of HIV Transmission in Armenia, 2004–14

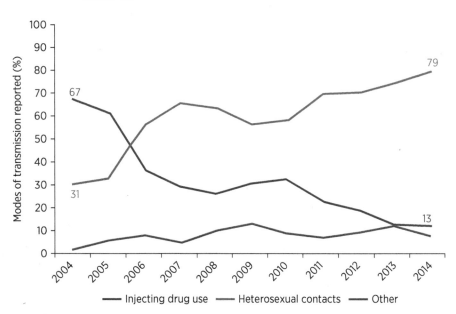

Source: World Bank based on data from the Armenian National Center for AIDS Prevention.
Note: HIV = human immunodeficiency virus.

people infected through heterosexual contact more than doubled from approximately 31 percent to 79 percent (figure 2.1). According to self-reporting, in 2006 heterosexual contact overtook injecting drug use as the primary mode of HIV transmission. During the same 10-year period, most new diagnoses (81 percent) were recorded among seasonal outbound labor migrants and their partners, partners of the previously mentioned risk populations, and those practicing unsafe sexual behaviors (figure 2.2). Potential data limitations include desirability bias in the type of self-reported transmission, leading to underreporting of risk behaviors, particularly among MSM and PWID.

Seasonal outbound labor migrants have emerged as a population group that contributes substantially to the HIV epidemic in Armenia. For example, data on new HIV diagnoses show that over 50 percent of PLHIV registered between 2011 and 2014 were suspected to have been infected outside Armenia. Fifty-nine percent of the new HIV diagnoses registered during 2012–14 were infected abroad, with heterosexual transmission reported as the most common cause. Fourteen percent of registered cases

Figure 2.2 Distribution of Registered HIV Cases, by Population Group Category, Armenia, 2004–14

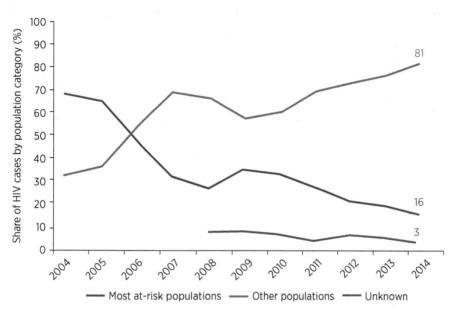

Source: World Bank based on data from the Armenian National Center for AIDS Prevention.

Note: Most at-risk populations include people who inject drugs, sex workers, and men who have sex with men. Other populations include seasonal outbound labor migrants and their partners, partners of those most at-risk, and those practicing unsafe sexual behaviors. HIV = human immunodeficiency virus.

were sexual partners of seasonal migrant laborers. Thus, nearly 75 percent of cases newly registered during 2012–14 were associated with seasonal labor migration.

Soundness of the Data

Self-reported data in the HIV response in many settings around the world have proved to be unreliable. In this case, however, the trend is notable because it is very pronounced in terms of reducing self-reported transmission through drug injecting practices and is supported by declines in the estimated HIV prevalence among PWID. This reduction supports the conclusion that the main mode of HIV transmission has shifted. Table 2.1 provides a summary of HIV/AIDS in Armenia for the years leading up to the allocative efficiency study conducted using the Optima model.

Table 2.1 Summary of HIV/AIDS Prevalence in Armenia, 2000–13

	2000	2005	2010	2011	2012	2013	Source
HIV diagnoses							
Cumulative registered number of people diagnosed with HIV	140	363	971	1,153	1,381	1,619	National Center for AIDS Prevention
Cumulative registered number of people diagnosed with HIV and confirmed to be alive	125	286	740	888	1,076	1,262	
New HIV diagnoses							
Number of people newly diagnosed with HIV, all ages	29	75	148	182	228	238	National Center for AIDS Prevention
Number of people newly diagnosed with HIV, aged 15+ years	29	73	144	180	224	233	
Number of people newly diagnosed with HIV, aged 0–14 years	0	2	4	2	4	5	
Number of people newly diagnosed with HIV, females of all ages	6	15	51	67	70	77	
Number of people newly diagnosed with HIV, males of all ages	23	60	97	115	158	161	
Registered AIDS-related deaths							
Annual registered number of AIDS-related deaths	3	10	23	25	37	42	National Center for AIDS Prevention
Cumulative registered number of AIDS-related deaths	11	46	175	200	237	279	

continued next page

Table 2.1 *(continued)*

	2000	2005	2010	2011	2012	2013	Source
HIV prevalence among key populations (2014)							
HIV prevalence among sex workers (%)	—	0.4	1.2	—	1.3	0.4	IBBS 2014 (National Center for AIDS Prevention 2015)
HIV prevalence among MSM (%)	—	—	2.3	—	2.7	2.1	
HIV prevalence among PWID (%)	14.0	9.3	10.7	—	6.3	4.0	
HIV prevalence among prisoners (%)	—	—	1.5	1.1	1.3	1.1	
HIV prevalence among labor migrants (%)	—	—	—	—	—	—	
Service coverage and use							
Number of people receiving ART	0	28	253	330	452	579	National Center for AIDS Prevention
Number of syringes estimated to have been distributed per PWID	0	0	0	0	0	0	
Number of PWID receiving OST	0	0	0	148	215	301	
Self-reported modes of HIV transmission (% of people newly diagnosed with HIV)							
Heterosexual HIV transmission	31.0	33.0	58.1	69.2	70.6	73.9	National Center for AIDS Prevention
HIV transmission through injecting drug use	62.1	61.0	32.4	23.1	19.3	13.4	
HIV transmission through unsafe blood or blood products	3.4	0.0	0.7	0.0	0.4	0.0	
HIV transmission from mother to child	0	3.0	2.0	1.1	1.3	2.1	

Sources: Based on 2015 data from the Armenian National Center for AIDS Prevention database; Armenia 2015.

Note: ART = antiretroviral therapy; HIV/AIDS = human immunodeficiency virus/ acquired immune deficiency syndrome; IBBS = integrated biobehavioral surveillance; MSM = men who have sex with men; OST = opioid substitution therapy; PWID = people who inject drugs; — = not available.

The Allocative Efficiency Analysis

Trends Predicted by the Analysis

Assuming that HIV-related behaviors and HIV program coverage levels from 2013 remain stable until 2020, the Optima modeling analysis for Armenia had six main findings:

1. Armenia is experiencing a low-level concentrated HIV epidemic. The number of PLHIV was projected to remain relatively stable until 2020 if the 2013 government spending level and allocation are maintained.
2. An estimated 300 people will become infected with HIV, predominantly through sexual transmission and injecting drug use, and 150 AIDS-related deaths will occur by 2020.
3. The epidemic in most population groups is stabilizing. For instance, the model suggests that HIV prevalence in FSWs will stabilize at slightly above 1 percent.
4. HIV prevalence among PWID and prisoners was projected to decline.
5. In contrast, a slight increase in HIV prevalence in coming years was projected among seasonal labor migrants.
6. A slight increase in HIV prevalence also was projected among MSM.

To accompany the findings from the analysis, which were included in a modeling report published in 2015,[2] it was also important to note what data and information were not available. In this case, some questions remain unanswered. For example, to what type of HIV-related risks were outbound migrants exposed? To what extent were outbound migrants becoming infected with HIV? Are self-reported modes of transmission correctly reflecting the reality whereby the primary mode of HIV transmission is now via heterosexual transmission? If so, were the majority of newly infected labor migrants infected as clients of sex workers or was there underreporting of new infections among MSM?

Cost-Effectiveness of HIV Programs Targeting Migrants

The initial modeling analysis provided a useful depiction of the overall HIV epidemic. The key question then remained: How can we determine the optimal use of HIV resources to best respond to this epidemic? Is it better to focus funding on key populations where we know HIV prevalence and incidence are highest, despite relatively small population sizes for these groups and their declining contribution to the overall number of new HIV infections? Or should we instead focus HIV response efforts on seasonal labor migrants, keeping in mind that we know much less about what drives new HIV infections for this group but do know that the number of new infections among this group is now relatively larger than for other subpopulations? Alternatively, how could these strategies be combined?

The team faced another challenge in answering this tricky question. Substantial international evidence can be used to inform assumptions surrounding the cost-effectiveness of standard HIV programs such as antiretroviral therapy (ART), HIV testing, needle syringe programs, and condom promotion for key populations. Such evidence on the effectiveness of HIV programs targeting seasonal labor migrants and the costing data for these programs were not readily available. Therefore, the team inverted the approach, instead asking the following question: Given a certain amount of funding, what level of coverage must be achieved for HIV programs targeting seasonal labor migrants to be considered cost-effective? Findings from this sensitivity analysis are shown in figure 2.3.

Figure 2.3 Cost-Outcome Sensitivity Analysis for Armenia's Seasonal Labor Migrant HIV Testing Programs, Based on the 2013 HIV Budget

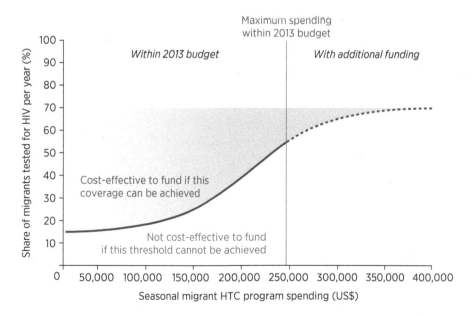

Source: World Bank 2015.

Note: Based on the Armenian government's 2013 budget. HTC = HIV testing and counseling; HIV = human immunodeficiency virus; US$ = US dollar.

This sensitivity analysis surrounding the seasonal labor migrant program suggests a cost-effectiveness threshold. The program would be cost-effective to fund only if high coverage levels could be reached at relatively low costs compared to other HIV programs. For example, with spending of US$200,000, more than 40 percent of migrants would need to be tested annually for this program to be considered cost-effective. Furthermore, because this program was only implemented beginning in 2010, its full epidemiological impact must still be determined. As a result of this limitation, to completely evaluate the impact and understand the effectiveness of this program, several important assumptions had to be made. Additional data must be collected to strengthen the cost-effective evaluation of HIV programs targeting seasonal labor migrants.

Optimally Investing HIV Resources

Following a comprehensive epidemic and cost-effectiveness analysis, an optimization modeling analysis was carried out. The optimization analysis was the cornerstone of the study and resulting report.

Using the same US$3.9 million in annual programmatic HIV government spending reported for 2013, Armenia could avert an additional 290 new HIV infections and 288 AIDS-related deaths between 2015 and 2020 if it allocates resources optimally to minimize both incidence and deaths (figure 2.4). These health outcomes could be achieved by shifting the allocation to ART from 17 percent to 24 percent of the Armenian government's total HIV budget from 2013.

Achieving National Targets

Using the Optima HIV model, the team calculated that the minimal spending required to achieve Armenia's moderate national HIV strategic objectives would be two times the 2013 government spending (figure 2.5). To best achieve these moderate objectives, ART scale-up should be prioritized (figure 2.5).

Optimal allocation of HIV resources to meet national targets was projected to achieve five key results:

1. Optimal investment of approximately US$6 million annually in HIV programs could result in national targets of 50 percent reduction of both HIV incidence and AIDS-related deaths by 2020.
2. Incidence could be reduced to fewer than 200 new HIV infections per year by 2020 (figure 2.6).
3. AIDS-related deaths could be reduced to fewer than 100 annually by 2020 (figure 2.7).

Figure 2.4 Optimal Allocation of 2013 Funding Levels to Minimize Both HIV Incidence and AIDS-Related Deaths in Armenia by 2020

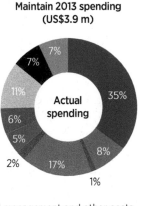

Maintain 2013 spending (US$3.9 m)

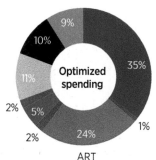

Optimized for both HIV incidence and AIDS-related deaths

■ Fixed management and other costs
■ Prisoner testing and prevention program
■ Prevention of mother-to-child transmission
■ Men who have sex with men testing and prevention program
■ Opioid substitution therapy

■ HIV testing and counseling (general population)
■ Antiretroviral therapy
■ Seasonal migrant testing and prevention program
■ People who inject drugs testing, prevention, and needle-syringe program
■ Female sex worker and client testing and prevention program

Source: World Bank 2015.

Note: Armenian government spending on HIV programs totaled US$3.9 million in 2013. AIDS = acquired immune deficiency syndrome; ART = antiretroviral therapy; HIV = human immunodeficiency virus; m = million; US$ = US dollar.

4. It was projected that a total annual investment in HIV programs of US$6 million from 2015 to 2020 would be necessary to achieve national targets by 2020. It was estimated that increased investment could result in averting an additional 600 new HIV infections and 400 AIDS-related deaths over the 2015–20 period.

5. Assuming that the additional HIV funding estimated to be required to achieve national targets is invested following the optimal resource allocation, the costs per infection and per AIDS-related death averted for Armenia were estimated to be US$18,900 and US$34,700, respectively.

The study found that, when Armenian national targets are achieved, sexual transmission of HIV will be reduced by almost 50 percent and transmission by contaminated syringes used for drug injection will be reduced by almost 65 percent.

Figure 2.5 Minimum Annual Resource Allocation Required to Achieve 2020 National Strategy Targets for Armenia, Compared with Maintaining the 2013 Government Spending Level

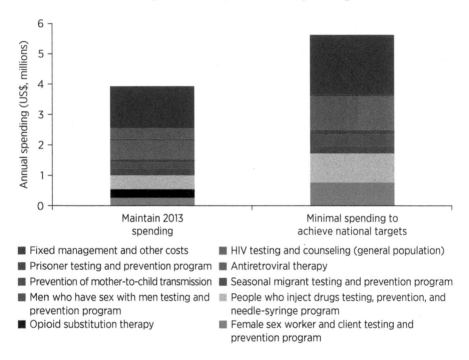

■ Fixed management and other costs
■ Prisoner testing and prevention program
■ Prevention of mother-to-child transmission
■ Men who have sex with men testing and prevention program
■ Opioid substitution therapy
■ HIV testing and counseling (general population)
■ Antiretroviral therapy
■ Seasonal migrant testing and prevention program
■ People who inject drugs testing, prevention, and needle-syringe program
■ Female sex worker and client testing and prevention program

Source: World Bank 2015.
Note: HIV = human immunodeficiency virus; US$ = US dollar.

Figures 2.6 through 2.8 show trends in new HIV infections, AIDS-related deaths, and the number of PLHIV under four different spending scenarios explored as part of the study:

1. Zero spending simulates a scenario with no investment in HIV programs, equivalent to discontinuing all programs.
2. Maintaining 2013 spending implies maintaining the government spending level and HIV program allocations as last reported in 2013.
3. Minimal spending to achieve national targets is the level required to achieve at least a 50 percent reduction in new HIV infections and AIDS-related deaths by 2020.
4. Minimal spending to achieve ambitious targets refers to the ambitious target of "Getting to Zero," defined as an 85 percent reduction in HIV incidence and AIDS-related deaths by 2020.

Figure 2.6 Impact of Different Investment Scenarios on New HIV Infections in Armenia, 2010–20

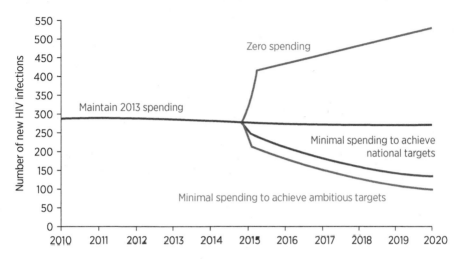

Source: World Bank 2015.

Note: Maintain 2013 spending refers to Armenian government spending. HIV = human immunodeficiency virus.

Figure 2.7 Impact of Different Investment Scenarios on AIDS-Related Deaths in Armenia, 2010–20

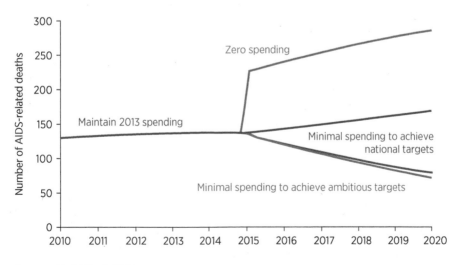

Source: World Bank 2015.

Note: Maintain 2013 spending refers to Armenian government spending. AIDS = acquired immune deficiency syndrome.

Figure 2.8 Total Number of People Living with HIV in Armenia under Different Spending Scenarios, 2010–20

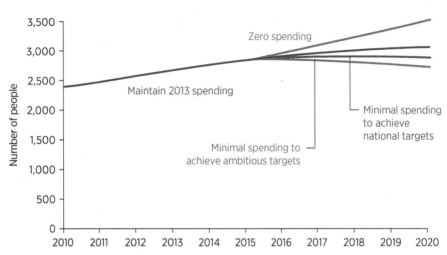

Source: World Bank 2015.
Note: Maintain 2013 spending refers to Armenian government spending. HIV = human immunodeficiency virus.

Table 2.2 provides the annual HIV resource allocations for 2015–20 for two optimization results presented previously: optimized allocations of 2013 government spending (figure 2.4) and minimal spending to achieve national targets (figure 2.5). The 2013 spending allocations are included as a reference for comparison because they served as the baseline scenario (maintaining 2013 spending).

To reach the impact goals of Armenia's National Strategic Plan would require doubling annual government spending on direct programs from US$2.5 million to US$5.1 million (or US$6.4 million including indirect costs). This amount would imply increasing the 2013 total budget by approximately 60 percent. Alternatively, it would require reducing the cost per person reached by nearly 40 percent for all programs. Increasing budgets by 60 percent or cutting costs may both be unrealistic individually, but combining resource mobilization and technical efficiency gains could achieve national targets.

An extra US$2.5 million on top of the Armenian government's 2013 budget of US$3.9 million (or corresponding cost reductions) would avert 1,800 new infections compared to zero spending; it would also avert 700 new infections by 2020 compared to the 2013 government spending without optimization. Optimized allocation of US$3.9 million would still avert an estimated 1,500 new infections compared to zero spending—or 300 new

Table 2.2 Average Annual Resource Allocations for Three Spending Scenarios, Armenia, 2015–20

US dollars

Indicator	2013 spending allocation maintained	2013 spending allocation optimized to minimize new HIV infections and AIDS-related deaths	Minimal spending to achieve national targets
Annual HIV program spending (targeted HIV programs only)	2.5 million	2.5 million	5.1 million
Cumulative spending (all targeted and nontargeted HIV programs), 2015–20	17.2 million	18.4 million	34.2 million

Source: World Bank 2015.

Note: Annual resource allocations are through the end of 2019—that is, they are to be completed by 2020. The 2013 spending allocation refers to Armenian government spending. Spending amounts are rounded to the nearest 1,000. HIV = human immunodeficiency virus.

infections compared to maintaining the 2013 government budget without optimization. As discussed, optimization analysis recommends prioritizing the scale-up of the ART program. The reallocated funding along with an addition of approximately US$100,000 would be sufficient to achieve the ART coverage targets proposed in the National Strategic Plan.

Table 2.3 then compares the cost-effectiveness of the different investment options. The cost per HIV infection or per AIDS-related death averted with optimal HIV resource allocation is US$12,700 or US$21,000, respectively.

Conclusions and Recommendations

The following five conclusions and recommendations can be drawn from the analyses undertaken in Armenia.

1. The Optima analysis projects a stable HIV epidemic in most population groups over the 2015–20 study period. The results suggest that past and ongoing HIV programmatic efforts have had a substantial impact on the course of the epidemic compared to a scenario with no spending on HIV programs. Model projections show that maintaining the 2013 government budget allocations from 2015 to 2020 would avert over 40 percent cumulative new HIV infections and 59 percent of AIDS-related deaths compared with a scenario with no HIV program spending.

Table 2.3 Impact and Cost-Effectiveness of HIV Programs in Armenia for Various Spending Scenarios, 2015–20

Cumulative 2015–20	Zero spending	2013 spending allocation maintained	Optimized to minimize new HIV infections and AIDS-related deaths	Minimal spending to achieve national targets
New HIV infections	2,800	1,700	1,400	1,000
AIDS-related deaths	1,600	1,000	700	600
Number of people living with HIV by 2020	3,700	3,100	3,100	2,900
New infections averted	Baseline	1,200	1,500	1,800
AIDS-related deaths averted	Baseline	600	900	1,000
Cost-effectiveness (US$)				
Cost per new infection averted	Baseline	14,700	12,700	18,900
Cost per AIDS-related death averted	Baseline	29,100	21,000	34,700

Source: World Bank 2015.
Note: Annual resource allocations are through the end of 2019—that is, they are to be completed by 2020. The 2013 spending allocation refers to Armenian government spending. Numbers rounded to the nearest 100. AIDS = acquired immune deficiency syndrome; HIV = human immunodeficiency virus; US$ = US dollar.

2. Despite efforts by the government of Armenia to control the epidemic and the considerable impact that the 2013 government budget allocations have shown and will continue to have, optimal resource allocation could further improve the impact on health with no additional resources (using 2013 annual government spending levels).
3. The analysis suggests that the ART program should be prioritized and that the ART budget should increase by another 40 percent over the 2013 funding of US$650,000 allocated for ART, increasing investment in ART to over US$900,000 per year on average.
4. Funding toward the HIV programs with the highest impact should be prioritized over lower-impact programs, such as those targeting the general population.
5. HIV programs targeting outbound seasonal labor migrants returning to Armenia, including testing and other prevention services, were introduced in response to a relative increase in new infections in this group. Because these targeted programs were only fairly recently implemented,

their efficacy has yet to be fully determined. Accordingly, a pilot program should be implemented and its outcomes rigorously evaluated, including uptake of testing and other HIV services among migrants.

In 2012 the Armenian government spent 7.9 percent of its total national budget on health, which was below the global average of 11.7 percent. It was projected that, in order to achieve national HIV targets by 2020, funding for HIV programs needed to increase by over 50 percent. Increasing overall government spending on health could also effectively boost domestic HIV financing by helping to cover existing resource gaps in the HIV response.

These recommendations focus on optimal allocation of HIV resources; however, outstanding questions about HIV programs targeting outbound seasonal labor migrants require additional creative thinking and new solutions. Online communication technology has not yet been fully leveraged in reaching seasonal labor migrants. This group could be recruited online for receiving health communications and service reminder notifications via email and smartphone apps for better treatment adherence. Challenges and treatment adherence needs are currently being better defined.

Actions Taken and Next Steps

To address growing concerns about HIV/STI (sexually transmitted infection) vulnerabilities facing outbound Armenian seasonal labor migrants, the Caucasus Research Resource Center–Armenia—with financial support from the Global Fund to Fight AIDS, Tuberculosis and Malaria—implemented, between November 2012 and March 2013, an evaluation to assess access to prevention services by migrants and also a strategy to design more effective interventions. This analysis revealed that the most effective approach to providing HIV testing to migrants is to combine it with other medical services, because that approach is expected to increase the likelihood that individuals will access HIV testing and agree to be tested.

On the basis of this recommendation, HIV prevention programs targeted at outbound Armenian seasonal labor migrants were designed to include an outreach component to more effectively reach and deliver HIV services to this group at the community level. Local health care workers from rural outpatient clinics undertaking outreach-related responsibilities perform preliminary work: identifying households where migrants reside, meeting with these residents and their partners, counseling them on prevention of HIV and STIs, providing relevant information, and encouraging them to undergo HIV testing. This component is important because outreach workers are the crucial link connecting this targeted population to available HIV services. These workers also play a central role in efforts to ensure that service delivery mechanisms are operating at capacity. It is important to note that HIV service packages targeting migrants are provided free of charge; they are also provided anonymously and confidentially via mobile or rural outpatient clinics. The services include testing for HIV, hepatitis B, hepatitis C, and syphilis; screening for tuberculosis; ultrasound examination; medical counseling; and referral. This approach significantly increases access to services by migrants and coverage of this population for HIV testing, diagnosis, ART, and care.

Notes

1. The lower and upper bounds of the range of HIV estimates were 2,700 and 5,900 PLHIV (UNAIDS 2015).
2. Note that much of this chapter reviews the process and findings of the modeling exercise documented in the report produced for that analysis; as such, the material herein draws significantly on that report. For more detail see World Bank 2015 in the reference list for this chapter.

References

Armenia, National Center for AIDS Prevention. HIV program database. Yerevan.

Armenia, National Center for AIDS Prevention. 2015. "Health Results from the HIV Biological and Bio-behavioral Surveillance in the Republic of Armenia 2014." National Center for AIDS Prevention, Yerevan.

UNAIDS (Joint United Nations Programme on HIV/AIDS). 2015. "HIV Estimates with Uncertainty Bounds 1990–2014." UNAIDS, Geneva.

World Bank. 2015. "Optimizing HIV Investments in Armenia." World Bank, Washington, DC.

3

Belarus
Changing HIV Budgets Based on Allocative Efficiency Analysis

Alena Fisenka, Richard T. Gray, Pavel Yurouski,
Vera Ilyenkova, David P. Wilson, Marelize Görgens,
and Clemens Benedikt

Briefly

- Belarus has experienced a growing epidemic, which is projected to remain concentrated in key populations.
- Belarus conducted an HIV (human immunodeficiency virus) allocative efficiency analysis in 2014–15, which contributed to improved allocations of resources in the National HIV/AIDS (acquired immune deficiency syndrome) Prevention Program (NAP) 2016–20.
- Additional efficiency gains and increased investment in the HIV response are required.

Introduction

An Increased Need for HIV Services amid Constrained Resources

Belarus has faced a significant, two-pronged challenge in its HIV response. The nation needed to simultaneously continue scaling up prevention efforts while also finding ways to provide treatment to a rapidly growing number of people living with HIV (PLHIV). The Joint United Nations Programme on HIV/AIDS (UNAIDS) estimated that the number of PLHIV in Belarus increased from 750 in the year 2000 to 24,000 in 2017. During the same period, new HIV infections increased from fewer than 500 per year in 2000 to 1,800 in 2010 and then continued to grow to reach 2,400 in 2017.[1]

Between 2011 and 2013, the total amount of funding for HIV programming in Belarus increased gradually—even as funding from international sources declined. During this time period international funding decreased by 37 percent, whereas domestic funding rose, primarily due to a 62 percent increase in government funding in 2013 (figure 3.1).

Between 2010 and 2012, Belarus increased the proportion of government spending on health to over 13 percent—thereby allocating more to health than the 2012 global average of 11.7 percent. Despite increases in funding for the HIV response, in a regional comparison Belarus's overall levels of HIV funding remained low relative to the size of its epidemic. Looking at allocations within the HIV budget, in 2013 Belarus devoted 24 percent of its total government HIV budget to fund treatment and care programs for PLHIV. Although the government covered 61 percent of antiretroviral (ARV) treatment costs, no government funds were used for ARV drug costs in that year. Belarus spent approximately US$800 per person living with HIV; the comparable spending rates in six other countries in the region ranged from US$490 to US$2,201.[2]

Figure 3.1 Total Annual Expenditure on HIV Programs, by Source in Belarus

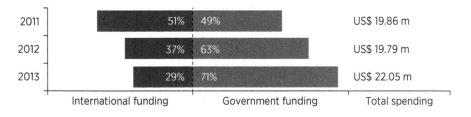

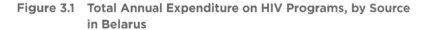

Source: World Bank based on AIDS spending data from UNAIDS.
Note: HIV = human immunodeficiency virus; m = millions; US$ = US dollar.

Two Phases of Analysis

This chapter summarizes the process and several key findings from two related analytical efforts that employed mathematical modeling techniques to better understand the scope of the need and ways to improve program impact and efficiency (figure 3.2). First, in 2014, an allocative efficiency study was conducted to inform the development of the national strategic plan on HIV and the Concept Note developed by Belarus in 2015 for the Global Fund to Fight AIDS, Tuberculosis and Malaria (the Global Fund) (World Bank 2015). Then, in 2016, a second scenario analysis was carried out to estimate the effect of the actual changes in budgets after the allocative efficiency analysis and the national strategic planning process.

The 2014 study was conceptualized by a regional steering group convened by the World Bank and involving the Global Fund, UNAIDS, and the United Nations Development Programme (UNDP). A national technical group convened by UNAIDS was formed in collaboration with the government. Epidemiological, program, and cost data were collected by in-country experts with technical support from UNAIDS, UNDP, and the World Bank using an adapted Microsoft Excel–based Optima data entry spreadsheet.

The 2016 follow-up analysis of reallocations was carried out for 2016–18 as a scenario analysis in Optima. Two scenarios were analyzed in terms of their effect on new HIV infections, deaths, and disability-adjusted life years (DALYs). The first scenario assumed that over the 2016–18 period the same allocations of resources as in 2013 would be applied—in other words, that "business as usual" would continue. The second scenario was built around actual reallocation of resources in Belarus as per the National HIV/AIDS Prevention Program (NAP) 2016–20. The average total annual NAP budget for the years 2016–18 was used as a basis for the reallocation analysis.

Figure 3.2 Timeline of the Two Studies on Belarus's HIV Efforts

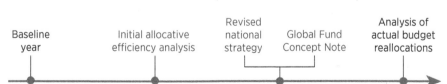

Source: World Bank.

Note: HIV = human immunodeficiency virus.

A Note on Inflation and Data

A specific methodological challenge was how to reflect inflation, which ranged between 16 percent and 21 percent during the 2013–15 period.[3] Inflation might potentially influence the cost of specific future interventions and the comparison of a future distribution of funding to past expenditure. Some activities such as procurement of drugs involve inputs purchased outside the country, whereas other activities depend on local inputs and human resource costs, which may be affected differently by inflation. Four different summaries of 2016–18 budgets were prepared to assess the potential effect of inflation on the distribution of resources between different programs: (1) allocations in Belarussian rubles (hereafter, rubles or Rbl) in absolute terms (2013–18); (2) allocations in 2013 rubles; (3) allocations in 2013 rubles with varied adjustments; and (4) allocations in US dollars. In consultation with national program experts, it was decided that option 3 was closest to the actual development of program costs. In addition, because the relative difference between the four allocations was smaller than the absolute difference, the scenario analysis compared the effect of past and revised allocations at the same level of funding while using the percentages of funding allocated to different programs to distinguish the scenarios (see figure 3.5 later in the chapter). In line with this option, the analysis was carried out in 2013 rubles with inflation adjustments in line with official inflation rate estimates for commodities and an assumed 3 percent annual cost increase in rubles for human resources, training, and other local costs.

To ensure their consistency and relevance, and unless otherwise indicated, the data provided in this chapter relate to the situation in Belarus at the time the analysis was conducted.

Initial Study Results and Their Interpretation

A Concentrated HIV Epidemic

The 2014 epidemiological analysis component within the allocative efficiency study established that Belarus has been experiencing a growing epidemic, which is projected to remain concentrated in key populations. People who inject drugs (PWID) continue to account for approximately half of all new infections. Moreover, although transmission is shifting toward sexual transmission, even in 2030 (assuming constant program coverage and behaviors) over 33 percent of infections are projected to remain among PWID.

Figure 3.3 describes the breakdown of PLHIV, new infections, and deaths in Belarus among different subpopulations. PWID account for approximately

Figure 3.3 Distribution of Estimated HIV, Estimated New Infections, and Estimated AIDS-Related Deaths, by Population Group in Belarus, 2014

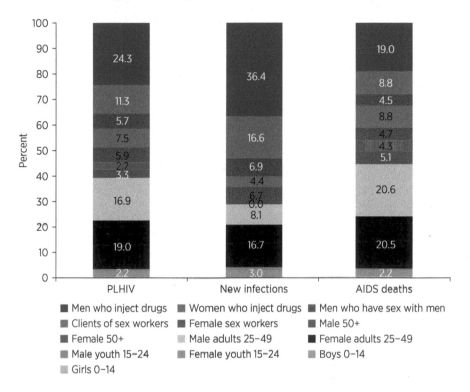

Source: World Bank 2015.

Note: AIDS = acquired immune deficiency syndrome; HIV = human immunodeficiency virus; PLHIV = people living with HIV.

50 percent of all new infections. As of 2014, however, only just over 33 percent of PLHIV were PWID, and fewer than 33 percent of AIDS-related deaths were among PWID, which is partially explained by the higher background mortality among PWID from non-AIDS-related causes.

Actual and anticipated HIV incidence rates per 1,000 person years are shown in figure 3.4. Throughout 2000–30, the model predicts that HIV incidence will remain highest among PWID. This result suggests that, according to projections, drug-injecting behavior is likely to remain a dominant risk factor. HIV incidence rates among female sex workers (FSWs) and their clients will grow moderately. In contrast, according to projections of current trends, HIV incidence rates among men who have sex with men (MSM) are expected to grow rapidly in Belarus.

Figure 3.4 Estimated HIV Incidence Rates in Specific Populations, Belarus, 2000–30

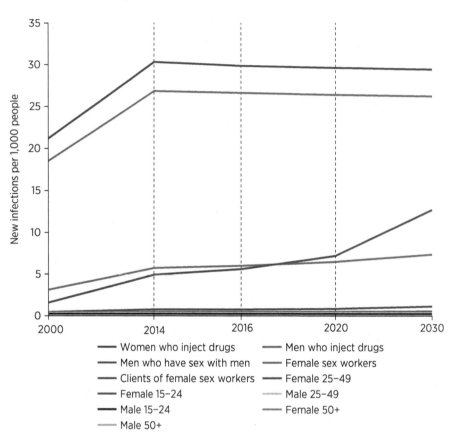

Source: World Bank based on Optima model.
Note: HIV = human immunodeficiency virus.

In Belarus in the early 2000s, the HIV epidemic among MSM was relatively small. According to Optima estimates and recent trends, however, MSM have become a rapidly growing segment of the epidemic and, by 2030, are projected to account for 1 out of every 7 new infections. Experience from other countries in the Europe and Central Asia region has shown that more rapid increases in HIV epidemics among MSM may occur. The epidemic among FSWs and their clients has recently accounted for approximately 1 in 10 new infections, and this share is projected to remain stable.

Large proportions of HIV acquisition in the general population in Belarus likely are due indirectly to transmission in three key populations: female sexual partners of men who inject drugs, female partners of MSM, and clients of sex workers. Therefore, new HIV infections among key populations and their sexual partners will also continue to increase—unless sustained reductions in new HIV infections among key populations are achieved.

HIV Funding before Allocative Efficiency Analysis

In 2013, HIV spending in Belarus was allocated to a relatively broad range of diverse priorities. No single program area received more than 20 percent of HIV spending (figure 3.5). Fifteen percent of total HIV spending was

Figure 3.5 Total National HIV Program Spending, by Expenditure Area, Belarus, 2013

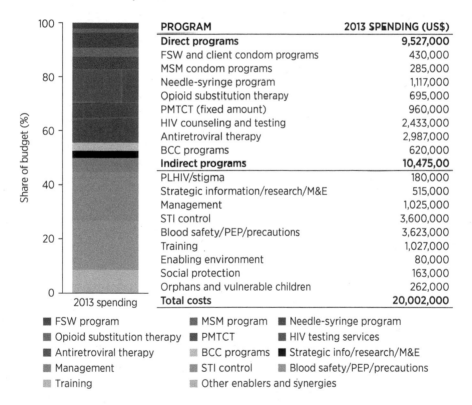

PROGRAM	2013 SPENDING (US$)
Direct programs	**9,527,000**
FSW and client condom programs	430,000
MSM condom programs	285,000
Needle-syringe program	1,117,000
Opioid substitution therapy	695,000
PMTCT (fixed amount)	960,000
HIV counseling and testing	2,433,000
Antiretroviral therapy	2,987,000
BCC programs	620,000
Indirect programs	**10,475,00**
PLHIV/stigma	180,000
Strategic information/research/M&E	515,000
Management	1,025,000
STI control	3,600,000
Blood safety/PEP/precautions	3,623,000
Training	1,027,000
Enabling environment	80,000
Social protection	163,000
Orphans and vulnerable children	262,000
Total costs	**20,002,000**

- FSW program
- MSM program
- Needle-syringe program
- Opioid substitution therapy
- PMTCT
- HIV testing services
- Antiretroviral therapy
- BCC programs
- Strategic info/research/M&E
- Management
- STI control
- Blood safety/PEP/precautions
- Training
- Other enablers and synergies

Source: World Bank based on Belarus government AIDS spending assessment data.

Note: BCC = behavior change communication; FSW = female sex worker; HIV = human immunodeficiency virus; MSM = men who have sex with men; M&E = monitoring and evaluation; PEP = post-exposure prophylaxis; PLHIV = people living with HIV; PMTCT = prevention of mother-to-child transmission; STI = sexually transmitted infection; US$ = US dollar.

allocated to antiretroviral therapy (ART), which supported 5,200 PLHIV. This supported population accounted for approximately one-fifth of all PLHIV and thereby left a substantial coverage gap. Twelve percent of HIV spending was allocated to HIV testing for different populations, and another 12 percent was allocated to dedicated programs for key populations. Five percent of funding was allocated to prevention of mother-to-child transmission (PMTCT) and 3 percent to general population behavior change communication (BCC).

More than 50 percent of HIV spending was allocated to cross-cutting expenses, which are referred to as indirect programs in figure 3.5 because their direct effect on impact level goals of reducing HIV incidence and mortality is unknown. These programs were not included in the mathematical optimization.

Recommendations of the Allocative Efficiency Study

The optimization and scenario analyses carried out in the original allocative efficiency study in 2014–15 produced the following policy-relevant findings:

Scaling up ART. The first consistent finding of these analyses was the critical role of scaling up ART, which would substantially affect both incidence and deaths. The analyses using the Optima model indicated that ART could be scaled up through increased initiation of ARV support for people already known to be living with HIV and through increased HIV testing and counseling (HTC) for key populations. HIV testing for the general population was not found to be among the most cost-effective strategies for initiating treatment.

Focusing on PWID. A second consistent finding was the continued need for scaling up services for PWID. From an HIV prevention perspective, the Optima analyses found that needle and syringe exchange programs (NSPs) would be the most cost-effective investment to further reduce rates of needle-sharing and thereby to reduce the risk of infection with HIV. These programs would also prevent infection with hepatitis viruses and other blood-borne pathogens. Opioid substitution therapy (OST) also offers critical benefits for HIV prevention, treatment adherence, and health in general, and should be scaled up as well according to model estimates.

Targeting high-impact programs. A third consistent finding was that Belarus could increase the impact of its HIV program by reallocating funds from general population, management, and other cross-cutting expenses to increase the share of investment going into the previously mentioned high-impact programs. The analyses suggested also that Belarus could enhance impact by increasing the total funding available to the HIV response so that high-impact programs could be scaled up further. With optimized allocations of the same amount of funding available over the period 2015–20 as in 2013 (US$19.7 million), new HIV infections could be reduced by 7 percent and deaths by 25 percent. The analyses also established the optimized mix and cost of programs to achieve national targets (figure 3.6), which for the purpose of this exercise were defined

Figure 3.6 Comparison of 2013 Spending with Optimized Allocation of Resources, Belarus

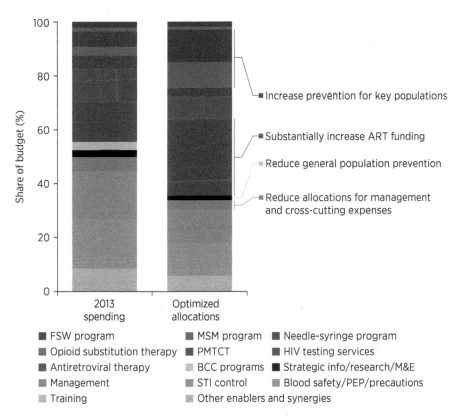

Source: World Bank based on Belarus government AIDS spending assessment data and the Optima model.

Note: ART = antiretroviral therapy; BCC = behavior change communication; FSW = female sex worker; HIV = human immunodeficiency virus; MSM = men who have sex with men; M&E = monitoring and evaluation; PEP = post-exposure prophylaxis; PMTCT = prevention of mother-to-child transmission; STI = sexually transmitted infection.

as impact targets for HIV incidence and deaths: reducing incidence by 45 percent, reducing deaths by 65 percent, and reducing mother-to-child transmission to below 1 percent. The analyses suggested that, to fully achieve these targets, approximately US$58 million would be required, which is nearly three times the 2013 investment level. The large funding requirement for fully achieving national targets was driven primarily by the very large necessity for HIV testing services (HTS) to achieve the specified ART coverage. Considering available funding and given unit costs, fully achieving current targets was considered ambitious.

Reducing new infections and deaths. Doubling the investment in high-impact programs while keeping management and other cross-cutting costs stable would require 148 percent of the total 2013 spending (US$29.5 million). Compared to 2013 allocations, over the 2015–20 period, the 148 percent level would reduce new infections by 43 percent and deaths by 51 percent. This allocation of resources was deemed both feasible and beneficial. Therefore, it was considered one of the core findings of the allocative efficiency study.

The optimized allocation implied substantial increases in ART, NSP, and OST allocations in both amount and percentage. BCC programs for the general population would be defunded. HTS, PMTCT, and management costs would remain stable. The analysis estimated that, through this optimized allocation, by 2020, 10,000 new infections and 5,100 deaths could be averted as compared to business as usual (that is, maintaining 2013 levels of allocations).

Alternative funding, higher efficiency. The analyses also recommended mobilizing additional resources through options including seeking other funding sources for programs such as sexually transmitted infection (STI) control and blood safety, which have major benefits beyond HIV. In practice, the most promising option for achieving these additional impacts was considered to be a combination of measures: more focused allocations, increased investment, reduced unit costs in some programs, and identification of alternative and cofinancing from non-HIV budget lines for programs such as STI control, blood safety, and OST.

Box 3.1 summarizes the 10 main implications of the epidemic and optimization analyses carried out as part of the 2014–15 Belarus HIV allocative efficiency study.

BOX 3.1

Ten Priority Recommendations of the 2014–15 Allocative Efficiency Study for Belarus

1. The epidemics among the key populations—people who inject drugs (PWID), men who have sex with men (MSM), and female sex workers and their clients—account for approximately two-thirds of all new HIV infections in Belarus and need to remain the core focus of HIV programs.
2. It is critical for Belarus to continue to prioritize the ongoing anti-retroviral therapy (ART) scale-up and substantially increase the funding allocation to ART.
3. Addressing the HIV-related and wider health needs of PWID remains a critical priority for Belarus.
4. To address the growing HIV epidemic among MSM, programs for this population need to increase in coverage.
5. Focused programs for sex workers should be sustained and reach the sex workers at the highest risk of HIV.
6. Programs for the general population are much less cost-effective compared to programs for key populations and should receive reduced allocations.
7. If alternative funding for blood safety and sexually transmitted infection programs could be identified, without any loss of the full HIV budget of US$19.7 million, the alternative funding would free up US$7.2 million.
8. It is worth conducting additional implementation efficiency analysis focused on the programs that absorb the largest pro-portion of funding (ART, opioid substitution therapy, and PWID/needle and syringe exchange programs; management; and other costs).
9. A number of complementary health priorities require contin-ued attention and should be allocated additional funding out-side HIV budgets; these priorities include harm-reduction programs for PWID, and particularly opioid substitution therapy.
10. Domestic and international resource mobilization for HIV pro-grams should remain a priority. It may be necessary to increase funding by 10–50 percent compared to 2013 levels, given the growing epidemic and the need to reduce HIV incidence and deaths by 40–50 percent.

Reallocating Funds Based on Findings

Informing Core National Planning Processes

The findings of the HIV allocative efficiency analysis in Belarus were applied in two interrelated planning and budgeting processes: the development of the new National HIV/AIDS Prevention Program (NAP) 2016–2020 and the development of a three-year Global Fund Concept Note covering the 2016–18 period.

The main principles of the government policy on HIV/AIDS had been set out in the first NAP for 2000–2005 in line with international declarations and commitments at the time. Because the NAP remains the cornerstone and the main guidance document for the renewed vision of the HIV response, the scope of the allocative efficiency analysis was to inform the fourth NAP for 2016–20, which was developed through a wide-ranging dialogue involving key national players, international agencies, PLHIV, and representatives of key affected populations. The resulting overall goals of the NAP 2016–20 have been defined in line with the UNAIDS Fast Track targets:

- To decrease the number of new HIV infections
- To decrease the number of AIDS deaths
- To create a supportive and enabling environment to address stigma and discrimination and legal barriers to achieve universal access to HIV prevention, treatment, and care services

The Concept Note submitted to the Global Fund was based on the NAP for 2016–20, which informed the suggested activities, service packages, coverage indicators, and unit costs included in the note.

Budget Allocations Prioritizing High-Impact Programs

The allocative efficiency study was used and directly referred to in both planning processes. As can be expected, the budget allocations in the national strategy do not exactly match the recommendations of the allocative efficiency study, but the distribution of resources is very similar to the allocations recommended in the study (figure 3.7). In particular, the three main principles of the allocative efficiency study were applied: (1) move more funds into core high-impact programs with a direct pathway to reducing new infections and deaths; (2) scale up treatment; and (3) focus prevention on key populations at highest risk and reduce funding for general populations.

Considering that any mathematical model is a simplification of reality and cannot be exactly and immediately implemented, it is not surprising that the analysis of reallocations also illustrates some variation in how

Figure 3.7 Comparison of 2013 Spending with 2016–18 Budget Allocations, Belarus

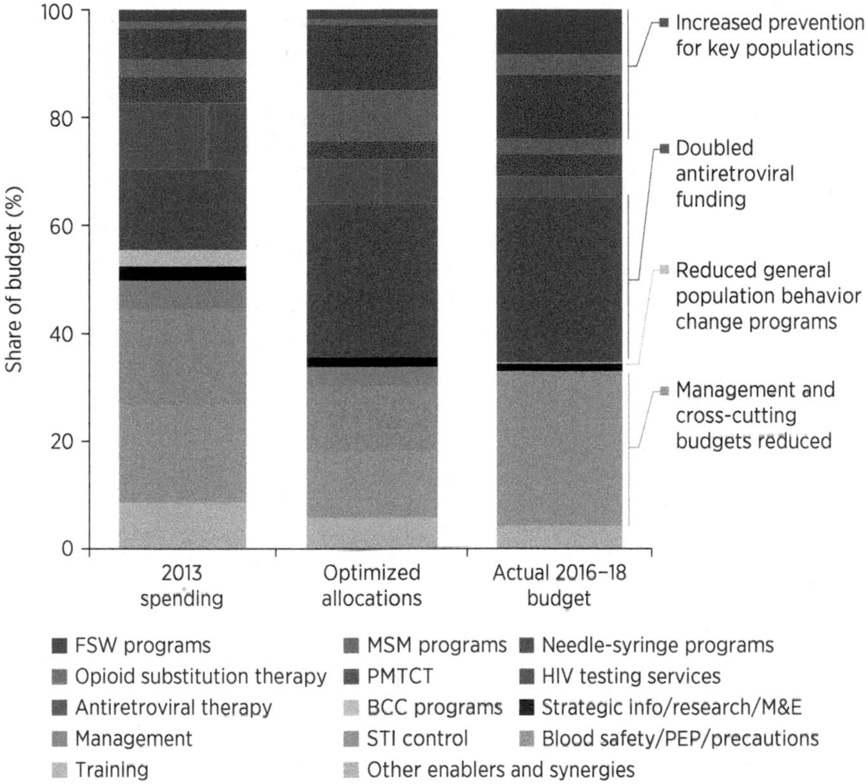

Source: World Bank based on Belarus government AIDS spending assessment data and the Optima model.

Note: The bar for the 2016–18 budget shows the annual average. Spending on prevention for key populations increased from 12 percent to 27 percent. Antiretroviral funding rose from 15 percent to 31 percent. Spending on general population behavior change programs decreased from 3 percent to less than 1 percent. Spending on management and cross-cutting budgets fell from 52 percent to 34 percent. BCC = behavior change communication; FSW = female sex worker; HIV = human immunodeficiency virus; M&E = monitoring and evaluation; MSM = men who have sex with men; PEP = post-exposure prophylaxis; PMTCT = prevention of mother-to-child transmission; STI = sexually transmitted infection.

findings were applied. For prevention among key populations, the optimization analysis had recommended the parallel scaling up of NSPs and OST. The actual allocations in the 2016–18 budget reflect a scaling up of NSPs, whereas OST remained stable at 3 percent of total HIV spending. At the same time, budgets for programs to reach FSWs and MSM were increased. Although this aspect of the actual allocations did not precisely match the allocation recommendations in the model, the results suggest that the reallocation will likely be seen to have had large effects on new HIV infections over the 2016–18 period.

Impact of the New Budget Allocations on HIV Infections and Deaths

Over the 2016–18 period, the actual budget allocations are projected to result in fewer new HIV infections: 9,400 new HIV infections instead of the 12,600 predicted with business as usual. This lower number of infections equals a 26 percent reduction. AIDS-related deaths are expected to be 3,500 instead of 5,300—34 percent less than with business as usual. Figure 3.8 shows the estimated new HIV infections and AIDS deaths in the business-as-usual scenario (2013 distribution of resources continued during 2016–18) and the actual 2016–18 budgets developed by national experts and reflecting allocative efficiency considerations. The effects of improved allocations are sustained after 2018 but insufficient to achieve global end of AIDS targets by 2030.

Figure 3.8 Effect of Changes in Budgets on New HIV Infections and AIDS Deaths, Belarus, 2016–18

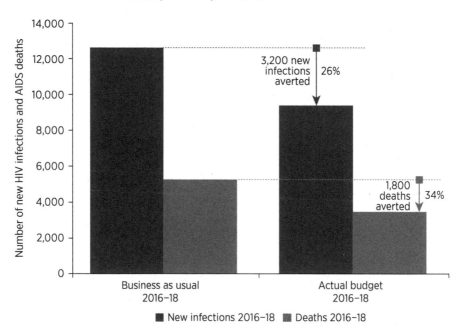

Source: World Bank based on the Optima model.

Note: AIDS = acquired immune deficiency syndrome; HIV = human immunodeficiency virus.

Figure 3.9 Long-Term Effect of Changes in Budgets on New HIV Infections and AIDS Deaths, Belarus

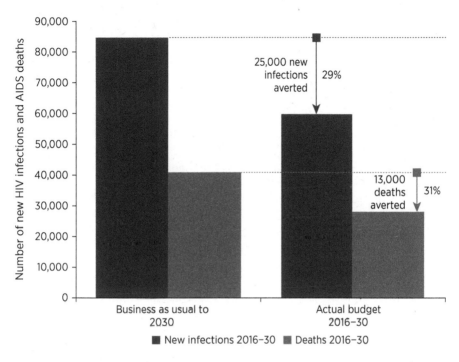

Source: World Bank based on the Optima model.

Note: Optimized allocations are projected to avert 92,000 DALYs (18 percent).
AIDS = acquired immune deficiency syndrome; DALY = disability-adjusted life year;
HIV = human immunodeficiency virus.

Figure 3.9 shows the long-term effects of the revised budget allocations. In this analysis, effects of the 2013 (business-as-usual) allocation are compared to the actual allocations in the 2016–18 budgets and an assumption is made that from 2019 these two different allocations will continue up to 2030. This analysis suggests that effects of the revised allocations will be sustained up to 2030. The number of new HIV infections incurred between 2016 and 2030 is projected to be 59,600 with revised budget allocations, compared to 84,400 with business as usual. Assuming actual 2013 budget allocations continue, an estimated 28,000 AIDS deaths are expected to occur between 2016 and 2030, compared to 41,000 with business as usual. Thus, a continuation of actual 2013 allocations would produce a 31 percent reduction in AIDS deaths compared to continuation of business-as-usual allocations.

This analysis shows that optimized allocation of resources—if sustained—will continue to produce positive results, which illustrates the value of engaging in analysis of budget allocations. The long-term analysis also suggests, however, that revised budget allocations will be insufficient to achieve global end of AIDS targets in Belarus by 2030. With the improved actual allocations, 3,100 new HIV infections would be incurred annually between 2016 and 2018, and an average of 4,200 new infections would be incurred annually between 2019 and 2030. This increase is largely due to the fact that the number of people who require ART will continue to increase and 2016–18 budget levels will be insufficient to sustain high ART coverage. This projection therefore also suggests that, in the context of its increasing HIV epidemic, either Belarus's HIV response budget needs to continue increasing beyond 2018 or further reductions in unit costs of ART need to be identified.

Strengthening Cascades and Integration

Through budget reallocations, Belarus has made a major step forward in increasing the efficiency and sustainability of its HIV response. Because Belarus's concentrated HIV epidemic continues to grow, however, even improved allocations at current levels of investment will not be sufficient to achieve epidemic control. The large treatment gap will require both an increase in resources and the simultaneous exploration and use of implementation efficiency gains. A key instrument that Belarus could apply in improving implementation efficiency is HIV treatment cascade analysis. Available data suggest major breakpoints in the HIV treatment cascade (figure 3.10).

Despite the continued scaling up of ART that has occurred, the pace of the growth of the epidemic since 2005 means that the treatment gap has remained large. For this reason, a critical need exists to reduce HIV transmission among key populations. This reduction could involve a strengthened cascade from knowing key population sizes, to reaching key populations with programs including outreach, and to retaining key populations in focused prevention services. The treatment cascade can also benefit from a focus on testing key populations and their sexual partners. In addition, enhanced referrals for ART and adherence support will be required. This range of requirements along the prevention and treatment cascades calls for revised and integrated outreach approaches to key populations.

The contribution of HIV to years of life lost in Belarus increased from 0.3 percent to 0.8 percent between 2000 and 2015,[4] which makes HIV the fastest-growing infectious disease; but the bulk of disease burden in Belarus remains in noncommunicable diseases. Infectious diseases such as HIV and tuberculosis remain closely interlinked with noncommunicable disease risk

Figure 3.10   Trends in Number of People Living with HIV and Basic Treatment Cascade, Belarus, 2014

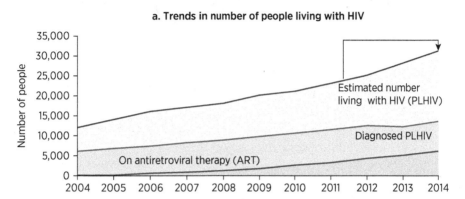

a. Trends in number of people living with HIV

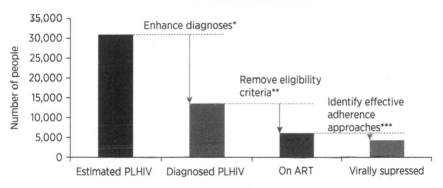

b. Basic treatment cascade

Sources: World Bank based on UNAIDS 2016 estimates, national HIV program database, and estimate produced for this book (viral suppression).

Note: To reduce new infections and slow the rate of increase in the need for treatment, key population cascades should be strengthened: identify, engage, and retain key populations in HIV and health services. In panel b, * = the gap between the estimated number of people living with HIV and the number of people diagnosed with HIV would shrink with enhanced diagnoses focused on key populations and their partners; ** = the gap between the number of people on antiretroviral therapy and the number of people diagnosed with HIV would shrink with enhanced referrals and the removal of eligibility criteria for antiretroviral therapy; *** = the gap between the number of people who are virally supressed and the number of people on antriretrovial therapy would shrink if effective adherence approaches are identified for specific contexts and key populations. ART = antiretroviral therapy; HIV = human immunodeficiency virus; PLHIV = people living with HIV.

factors such as drug and alcohol use. Achieving HIV and tuberculosis targets by 2030 is unlikely to be achieved in isolation; it will need to be part of broader strategies to address risk factors in health and to achieve universal health coverage including preventive elements.

Conclusions

Belarus conducted an HIV allocative efficiency analysis in 2014–15, which contributed to improved allocations of resources in its NAP for 2016–20. The improved allocations were estimated to have immediate and long-term benefits, reducing new HIV infections and AIDS deaths by approximately one-third. With the expiration of the 2016–18 Global Fund grant, however, additional efficiencies and investments are required going forward. These investments could be based on an update of the allocative efficiency analysis in 2019–20. More broadly, the requirements of a sustained HIV response need to be explored, including scale-up of ART for all PLHIV and modalities to sustain community outreach to ensure high access and uptake of HIV prevention, treatment, and other key health services among key affected populations.

Notes

1. Based on UNAIDS 2018 estimates.
2. This figure was arrived at by dividing the total spending included in the country Optima spreadsheet by the total number of PLHIV according to UNAIDS HIV estimates.
3. Based on World Bank National Accounts Data. For more information, see http://data.worldbank.org/indicator/NY.GDP.DEFL.KD.ZG?locations=BY.
4. Based on Institute for Health Metrics and Evaluation's Global Burden of Disease Study 2015 Data Visualizations, retrieved from http://vizhub.healthdata.org /gbd-compare/.

Reference

World Bank. 2015. "Optimizing Investments in Belarus for the National HIV Response." World Bank, Washington, DC.

4

Bulgaria
Transitioning to Domestic Financing of HIV Programs amid High Costs

*Tonka Varleva, Hristo Taskov, Tsveta Raycheva,
Emilia Naseva, Petar Tsintsarski, Nina Yancheva,
Vyara Georgieva, Laura Grobicki, Jolene Skordis-Worrall,
Feng Zhao, and Nejma Cheikh*

Briefly

- Bulgaria is transitioning to domestic financing for its human immunodeficiency virus (HIV) response.
- A relatively high proportion of available HIV funding has been spent on antiretroviral therapy (ART) in Bulgaria compared to other countries, but coverage remained below 30 percent at the time of the study.
- Antiretroviral drug prices have been much higher than in countries in the region that are not members of the European Union.
- Reducing ART costs is critical for scaling up treatment and ensuring sustainability of the HIV response.

Introduction

At the Crossroads of Two Epidemics

Bulgaria is at the crossroads of two epidemics with different dynamics and different underlying driving forces. According to data from the European

Center for Disease Prevention and Control (ECDC), the epidemic in the region of Eastern Europe and Central Asia is the fastest-growing HIV epidemic in the world, and the largest proportion of the new infections belongs to people who inject drugs (PWID) (ECDC and WHO Regional Office for Europe 2016). At the same time, the epidemic in Central and Western Europe continues to grow mainly among men who have sex with men (MSM).

HIV Prevalence among Key Populations

The epidemic in Bulgaria is concentrated among PWID and MSM (Varleva, Raicheva et al. 2015; Varleva, Tsintsarski et al. 2015). Integrated biobehavioral surveillance (IBBS) 2016 results show that HIV prevalence among MSM had increased to 3.9 percent compared to 0 percent in 2012, and most of the HIV-positive cases identified in the survey (13 out of 17 in total) were interviewed in Sofia, the capital city, where HIV prevalence has been recorded at 12.7 percent (Bulgaria 2016). Sofia was chosen as one of the cities in the Sialon II project, which culminated in a report on biobehavioral surveys among MSM in 13 European cities. That report estimated that the prevalence among MSM in Sofia was 3.0 percent, but the confidence interval (CI) was quite wide (95 percent CI 0.9–9.1) (Mirandola et al. 2016). The HIV prevalence among PWID was 10.6 percent (IBBS 2012 data) and has been nearly constant over the years since 2006.

The Roma population is at higher risk of HIV infection than other ethnicities in the country. This higher risk is mainly due to the elevated risk among young Roma men who have sex with men, inject drugs, sell sex, or some combination of the three activities—all of which place them in other key populations and are attributable to their poverty, higher unemployment rate, lower health literacy, and social isolation (Varleva, Kabakchieva et al. 2015).

The epidemic among female sex workers (FSWs) has stabilized around 1 percent (Varleva, Boneva et al. 2015). The general population in Bulgaria has been less affected by HIV, but the epidemic is expected to grow because of the concentration of HIV cases in key populations like MSM and PWID, which implies continued HIV transmission from members of these populations to their female sexual partners.

A total of 2,474 HIV cases were registered between 1986 and 2016, with the number of new cases registered each year increasing gradually throughout that period to 207 new cases registered in 2016. The rise is due to the expansion of HIV testing by actively providing voluntary counseling and HIV testing services among the key populations. During this same time period, the male-to-female ratio of diagnosed individuals changed from 3:1 to 4:1. Mode of transmission data for 2010–16 show MSM accounting for a growing share of all diagnosed cases (up from 20 percent to 49 percent) and PWID accounting for a smaller percentage over the same time period (a drop from 34 percent to 10 percent) (Varleva and Toneva 2017).

Since 2004, the Prevention and Control of HIV/AIDS (acquired immune deficiency syndrome) program has been implemented with a grant from the Global Fund to Fight AIDS, Tuberculosis and Malaria (the Global Fund). This program made it possible to complement the national response to the AIDS epidemic and ensure that the country has an integrated and balanced approach through (1) prevention, (2) treatment, and (3) care and support for the people affected by HIV. The program ensures geographical equity and high coverage levels—not only in meeting the targets agreed with the Global Fund but also in the implementation of national-scale interventions (map 4.1).

Nongovernmental organizations (NGOs) have implemented the prevention activities. In doing so, they have gained significant and unique expertise and skills for HIV prevention and control—working among key populations, developing administrative and managerial skills, and also gaining public and social significance. NGOs offer a wide range and high quality of services, care, and support, based on experience and evidence. The acquired skills and knowledge, as well as preexisting relationships of trust between the NGOs and the target groups, create opportunities for timely assessment of the specific needs of the target groups and the adaptation of the services to meet their needs.

Bulgaria has been a member of the European Union (EU) since 2007, but it has one of the weakest economies in the EU.[1] The government's ability to fund HIV prevention activities is limited. During the 2004–17 period, the Global Fund supported HIV/AIDS prevention activities, whereas the government focused on funding antiretroviral therapy (ART) and most of the opioid substitution therapy (OST) programs.

Intervention Strategy and Funding Impact

The establishment and implementation of good practices for effective interventions among the highest-risk groups have served as a bulwark against the development of a larger epidemic in the country. The expected overall increase in the epidemic appears to be driven by incidence and prevalence among PWID and MSM—key populations that currently receive only a small portion of prevention funding. Although improvements have been made regarding condom use, interventions targeting these key populations need to be strengthened. Prevention programs

Map 4.1 **Mapping the Implementation in Bulgaria of the Prevention and Control of HIV/AIDS Program Financed by the Global Fund to Fight AIDS, Tuberculosis and Malaria**

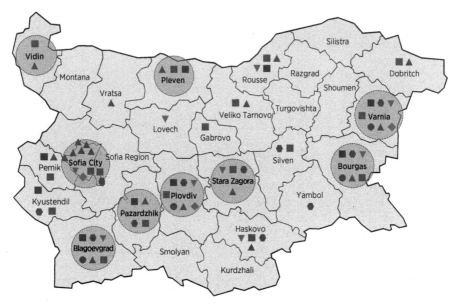

HIV prevention carried out by NGOs among:

- ■ Injecting drug users
- ▼ Sex workers
- ● Men who have sex with men
- ◆ People living with HIV
- ● Roma and Sinti communities
- ■ Young people
- ▲ Voluntary counseling and testing center
- ◯ Local coordination centers

Source: Bulgaria 2014a. © Bulgarian Ministry of Health. Reproduced with permission of the Bulgarian Ministry of Health; further permission required for reuse.

Note: In addition to the projects shown on the map, programs have also been provided in Sofia for injecting drug users and men who have sex with men. HIV/AIDS= human immunodeficiency virus/acquired immune deficiency syndrome; NGO = nongovernmental organization.

targeting these populations are most at risk of defunding as Bulgaria transitions out of Global Fund support, because in the past these programs have been funded with donor funds. An optimized allocation of current funding may reduce long-term financial commitments to the HIV response by containing HIV incidence and prevalence. All of these arguments underscore the importance of ensuring the continuation of prevention activities among all key populations.

With the ending of the Global Fund–supported Prevention and Control Program in 2017, the new National Program for Prevention and Control of HIV/AIDS and STIs (sexually transmitted infections) 2017–2020 (Bulgaria 2017) stood to continue the prevention activities among key affected populations, albeit at a smaller scale. The reduction in the prevention activities began in 2016 as Global Fund support decreased. As of 2016, most of the OST programs were private and paid for by the patients themselves, whereas 9 out of 30 were funded by the Bulgarian government and local municipalities. Domestic public funding is the main source of HIV spending and has grown substantially since 2007 (figure 4.1).

The MSM population accounts for the largest proportion of new infections, but prevention programs targeted specifically to MSM account for only about 1.7 percent of HIV spending. The HIV epidemic among PWID is relatively stable in Bulgaria because of significant and prolonged efforts to reach this population. The key PWID and MSM populations should be reached as far as possible with strong preventive efforts, complemented by a comprehensive HIV testing and treatment program. HIV prevalence among FSW clients may increase if the prevention activities are cut. The Roma population and young people should also be covered with prevention activities.

Figure 4.1 HIV Spending in Bulgaria, by Funding Source, 2007–14

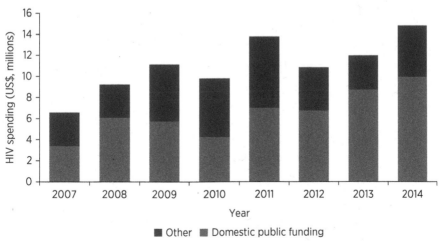

Source: World Bank based on Bulgaria 2014b and other Bulgarian Ministry of Health data.
Note: HIV = human immunodeficiency virus; US$ = US dollar.

Funding Analysis Study

Study Findings

Recognizing the need to effectively manage the transition from Global Fund support, the World Bank was asked to conduct a study exploring whether the existing domestic funding for HIV/AIDS programming could be allocated more efficiently. The study was conducted in 2015 using the Optima allocative efficiency model populated with relevant data for Bulgaria. The findings showed that, without the prevention programs, an additional 1,150 new infections (19 percent) would occur by 2030, leading to additional treatment and health costs of approximately US$60 million.

To ensure their consistency and relevance, and unless otherwise indicated, the data provided in this chapter relate to the situation in Bulgaria at the time the analysis was conducted.

The allocative efficiency analysis also suggested a need to increase investment in programs for MSM and PWID at higher levels than the financing provided by the Global Fund, including needle and syringe exchange programs (NSPs) and OST. It also found that increasing coverage of MSM programs could be particularly beneficial given the high number of new infections in this key affected population.

The study found that the allocative efficiency of Bulgaria's programming supported by the Global Fund could be improved by increasing investment in key populations through ART and prevention programs—aimed not only at MSM and PWID but also at all other key affected populations, including young people. This improvement could reduce new infections, deaths, and future costs.

Better Targeting Prevention for Key Populations

Spending on HIV prevention and treatment may not be benefitting those most in need. Model-based estimates have suggested increasing HIV incidence and prevalence among key high-risk populations, in particular among MSM.

Although the increase in prevalence among male and female PWID is expected to be small, the Optima analyses suggest that there remains a need to invest in programs for PWID, including NSPs and OST (figure 4.2).

If future funding falls below the 2014 level, optimization suggests that ART, OST, PWID, and MSM programs should have first priority. This prioritization is due to several factors. First, ART is essential to minimize AIDS-related deaths and helps reduce HIV incidence. Second, for prevention, increasing condom use among MSM and PWID is epidemiologically

Figure 4.2 Comparison of Actual and Optimized Allocation of 2014 Spending Levels to Minimize Both New Infections and Deaths in Bulgaria for the Period 2015–30

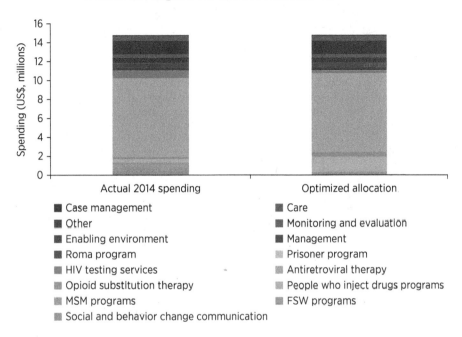

Source: World Bank 2017.
Note: FSW = female sex worker; HIV = human immunodeficiency virus; MSM = men who have sex with men; US$ = US dollar.

important because of the key role of these two populations in HIV transmission. Finally, these results also reflect the fact that the model construct protects funding for ART and OST services.

Other Scenarios Assessed in the Optima Exercise

As discussed previously, the Optima modeling analysis was used to assess HIV outcomes through 2030 in the following scenarios: (1) if 2014 spending levels and allocations were maintained and (2) if the 2014 spending levels were maintained but reallocated to maximize efficiency. It was also used to compare the trajectory of the HIV epidemic by 2030 in Bulgaria under the 2014 HIV response against the likely trajectories in three alternative HIV response scenarios that are not constrained by a budget but are determined solely by targets. The following three scenarios were identified through consultation with local stakeholders and were used for comparison:

1. Test and treat: This scenario assumed that, by 2020, 90 percent of people living with HIV (PLHIV) will be aware of their status and 90 percent of the diagnosed PLHIV will be on ART.
2. Attaining combined targets for prevention and treatment: This scenario assessed the trajectory of the HIV epidemic if the country aims for reaching global goals for all key populations.
3. Defunding all preventive programs: This scenario explored possible impacts of defunding all prevention programs for the key populations (including HIV testing services [HTS] programs).

Because the final National HIV Strategic Plan targets had not been confirmed at the time the modeling was conducted, the analysis was run to establish how much funding would be required to (1) contain the existing incidence and death values, (2) reduce new infections and deaths by 20 percent, and (3) reduce new infections and deaths by 50 percent.

Figure 4.3 shows actual 2014 spending, the optimized allocation of 2014 spending, and the minimum spending required with an optimal allocation to achieve the three targets described previously. The model results suggest that maintaining the 2015 incidence and death values could be achieved with an annual budget of US$26.2 million—nearly twice the 2014 budget. Achieving the second target (reducing new infections and deaths by 20 percent) would require an estimated annual budget of about US$39 million. Reducing new infections and deaths by 50 percent could be achieved with an annual budget of about US$47.5 million.

To achieve these targets, the model analysis recommended increased investments in ART, OST, MSM, PWID, prisoner, and HTS programs. In particular, it called for a substantially increased investment in PWID and MSM programs. For example, the model suggested increasing investment in MSM fourfold to stabilize outcomes, and eightfold to reduce incidence and deaths by 20 percent. Reducing incidence and deaths by 50 percent would entail a tenfold increase in funding.

In the modeling analysis, the number of HIV cases on treatment increases over the years as the total number of registered cases rises. Over the same time, the gap between the number of patients and the number of patients on treatment decreases, in alignment with efforts to comply with the global 90-90-90 targets (Varleva and Toneva 2017).

Drug and Treatment Costs

The average price of ART for a patient with HIV per year in Bulgaria is €8,139. At the same time, the prices are lower in other EU Member States

Figure 4.3 Minimum Annual Programmatic Spending Required to Meet Proposed National Strategy Targets, Bulgaria

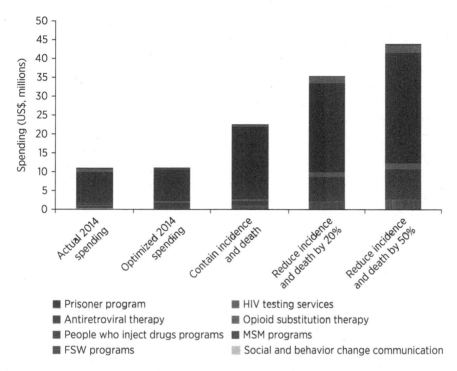

Source: World Bank 2017.

Note: FSW = female sex worker; HIV = human immunodeficiency virus; MSM = men who have sex with men; US$ = US dollar.

(with significantly higher gross domestic product per capita rates) including Italy, the Netherlands, Spain, and the United Kingdom (Dimitrova et al. 2011; Dimitrova et al. 2013; ECDC 2017a).

Antiretroviral treatment for patients in Bulgaria is conducted in accordance with standards approved by the World Health Organization (WHO). The treatment of HIV-positive patients in Bulgaria is also regulated by a normative document, the Methodological Indication for Antiretroviral Treatment of Adults with HIV Infection. This document was updated in 2016 by order of the minister of health (Bulgaria 2016), with methodological guidance based on version 8.0 of guidelines from the European AIDS Clinical Society (EACS 2015). In accordance with those guidelines, all HIV-positive individuals in Bulgaria can receive ART if they wish to do so. In addition, the recommended first-line regimens in Bulgaria are similar to those in the EACS guidelines; only one tier mode—EVG/COBI/TDF/FTC—was missing from these regimes.[2] All of the other tier modes are available and applied with the appropriate indications. The proportion of regimens based on integrase inhibitors is lower, however, which is related to the higher cost of these medications. The TAF, COBI, and, respectively, TAF/FTC, TDF/FTC/RPV, TAF/FTC/RPV, EVG/COBI/TAF/FTC, and DRV/COBI have not yet been registered in Bulgaria as of the time of writing.[3] All other antiretroviral drugs are available and are also used in appropriate alternative treatment regimens.

Reducing the average annual cost of treatment per patient, through lower drug prices or the inclusion of generic medicines, could both generate savings in the state budget and increase inclusion in therapy of newly diagnosed HIV-positive individuals (at an average estimated rate of 200 new individuals provided with ART per year). In addition, starting people on ART in a timely manner would help preserve the individual's health and reduce HIV transmission to sexual and injecting partners. Reducing drug prices would also allow for a part of the savings to be invested in prevention programs for the most vulnerable communities and groups (MSM, injecting drug users, sex workers, and so on) as well as in voluntary counseling and testing programs for HIV and other sexually transmitted infections.

Model Findings

The Optima model findings and conclusions are in line with the following ECDC recommendations considered by the country for implementation:

- Adopt the "Test and Treat" policy (discussed earlier) in all countries in the region, in line with the European AIDS Clinical Society and WHO guidelines.
- Reduce barriers to accessing treatment, including inadequate treatment program coverage, as well as weak referral mechanisms and links to other health and support services; also prevent stigma and discrimination among key populations and by health care professionals.
- Identify opportunities to reduce the costs of antiretroviral drugs to ensure that all countries in the region can finance treatment for all people living with an HIV diagnosis in the medium term and longer term (ECDC 2017a, 2017b).

One way to reduce the price of medications might be to purchase a larger number of packages for treatment on the basis of an agreement with neighboring EU member states. If successful, this practice would free up financial resources to buy medicines to help achieve the Joint United Nations Programme on HIV/AIDS (UNAIDS) target of 90 percent of all individuals diagnosed with HIV receiving sustained ART by 2020 (UNAIDS 2014).

Another possibility would be to cover ART under the National Health Insurance Fund (NHIF). The NHIF controls the drug prices on the basis of the Document for Regulation and Registration of Medicinal Products Prices, Conditions, Rules, and Criteria for Incorporation, Changes, and/or Exclusion of Medicinal Products from the Positive Medicinal List, as well as the terms and rules for operation set forth by the price and reimbursement committee (Bulgaria 2011). Article 8 states that the producer price of medicines procured through the NHIF "may not be higher than the Bulgarian lev (BGN) equivalent of the lowest price for the same medicinal product paid by society health insurance funds of Romania, France, Estonia, Greece, Slovakia, Lithuania, Portugal, and Spain."

A problem here may arise for HIV-positive individuals who are not insured, despite the decision of the TEMC (Regional Expert Medical Committee) to include some of them in the health insurance system. It will also be necessary to respect the confidentiality of all recipients in connection with the issuing mechanism of protocols by specialists for costly treatment and the receipt of medications from the pharmacy.

Allocative Efficiency Analysis Recommendations

The key recommendations from the 2015 Optima analysis include the following:

1. As of the time of the 2015 report, the Bulgarian government had implemented an effective HIV response, managing a concentrated HIV epidemic. The government may be able to better allocate HIV spending to achieve even greater results in minimizing HIV incidence, prevalence, and HIV-related deaths.
2. To assess HIV epidemic trends, the study used Optima's epidemic module, calibrated to HIV prevalence data points available for different subpopulations in Bulgaria, including key populations. The model was also calibrated to data points on the number of people on ART from available data sources and in consultation with Bulgarian experts. Analyses using this model highlighted a strong risk that prevalence and incidence will continue to increase overall in Bulgaria, despite the then-current efforts to contain the epidemic.
3. The expected overall increase in the epidemic appeared to be driven by incidence and prevalence among PWID and MSM, key populations that received only a small portion of prevention funding as of 2014. Although improvements had been made regarding condom use, interventions targeting these key populations needed to be strengthened. Prevention programs targeting these populations were found to be

most at risk while transitioning out of Global Fund support, because these programs had been funded in the past with donor funds.

4. An optimized allocation of 2014 funding could reduce long-term financial commitments to the HIV response by containing HIV incidence and prevalence. Most important, the analysis suggested that optimized allocations of the 2014 spending level—despite increasing treatment coverage—would not increase long-term costs, because of the reductions in new HIV infections achieved through optimized allocations compared to business as usual.

5. Diverting funding away from HIV testing in the general population, toward prevention among MSM and PWID would improve efficiency. This could reduce new infections, deaths, and future costs.

6. The epidemic among the FSW population has been relatively contained because of significant and prolonged efforts to target this group. Wider experience with the epidemic and knowledge of the limitations of mathematical modeling suggest, however, that this finding should be interpreted with caution for the following reasons: (1) the gains from past spending on this population may be eroded over time and (2) investing in programs for this population produces wider public health benefits, for example in relation to other sexually transmitted infections, not captured in an HIV model.

7. Although the Optima analyses advocate for the increased targeting of MSM and PWID, such targeting alone would not be sufficient to contain the epidemic, even at increased funding levels. Key populations should be reached as far as possible with strong preventive efforts, complemented by comprehensive test-and-treat programs.

8. Additional domestic resources will be needed to sustain the HIV response after the withdrawal of Global Fund support. Funding for HIV in Bulgaria increased after 2007. Apart from ART, however, preventive programs and programs focused on key populations have been primarily funded by international donors. The withdrawal of international funding without a concurrent increase in domestic resources will therefore have a significant negative impact on the HIV epidemic in Bulgaria.

9. Transitional funding mechanisms need to be explored with the aim of raising domestic funding to at least the level of the 2014 total budget for the HIV response. International donor funding must be replaced with alternate funding, and all funding should be spent on an optimal mix of programs targeted at key populations and the scale-up of ART delivery.

10. Effective ART scale-up is needed, with a strong focus on HIV diagnosis in key populations. Coverage must be increased if global targets are to be met; in 2017, 43 percent of Bulgaria's estimated 2,800 PLHIV received treatment, compared with a global target of 81 percent by 2020.

11. Comparing the unit costs of care in Bulgaria with data from other countries in the region suggests that greater technical efficiency in spending might be achieved through strategies to reduce the average spend per person reached, which is particularly relevant for ART programs. Care should be taken, however, that these strategies do not compromise the quality of prevention or treatment, and further analyses of technical efficiency are needed before more robust conclusions can be reached.

Conclusions

The Bulgarian government has implemented an effective HIV response, managing a concentrated HIV epidemic. Since Global Fund support for prevention activities ended, the amounts spent on HIV prevention have declined dramatically. With an increasing number of HIV-positive individuals and the high cost of therapy, these expenses are expected to require a steadily increasing share of the state budget. Savings from reducing the cost of treatment could be directed to preventive activities among target populations. These activities would reduce future costs for ART by reducing the rate of HIV transmission and decreasing the spread of the infection to the general population. Better allocation of HIV spending would help minimize HIV incidence, prevalence, and HIV-related deaths.

One key to preserving a low incidence of HIV infection and ensuring the sustainability of the HIV response is to maintain anonymous and free HIV counseling and HIV testing services close to people who need them most, in particular the key and priority populations for the national response. These services should include access to medical professionals and the use of mobile medical units and direct outreach prevention work to vulnerable communities and groups with services such as counseling and the distribution of protective equipment and health education information materials. A successful strategy must include and provide adequate funding for efforts to promote knowledge of HIV status through testing, linking testing to access to care, and providing motivation and support for adherence to treatment. Treatment must also be provided in a timely manner in order to preserve the health of the individual and to prevent HIV transmission to the person's sexual partners. The professional and well-intentioned attitude of health care professionals toward people from key communities and a lack of discrimination and stigma are also important prerequisites for the successful implementation of preventive programs aimed at reducing the risk of HIV prevalence among the general population. Better allocation of HIV spending will ensure minimization of HIV incidence and prevalence as well as of HIV-related deaths.

Notes

1. Gross domestic product per capita, consumption per capita, and price level indexes (2016) from Eurostat (European Statistical Office of the European Commission).
2. EVG/COBI/TDF/FTC = elvitegravir/cobicistat/tenofovir disoproxil fumarate/ emtricitabine.
3. DRV = darunavir; RPV = rilpivirine; TAF = tenofovir alafenamide.

References

Buglaria, NHIF (National Health Insurance Fund). 2011. "НАРЕДБА ЗА РЕГУЛИ-РАНЕ И РЕГИСТРИРАНЕ НА ЦЕНИТЕ НА ЛЕКАРСТВЕНИТЕ ПРОДУКТИ, УСЛОВИЯТА, ПРАВИЛАТА И КРИТЕРИИТЕ ЗА ВКЛЮЧВАНЕ, ПРОМЕНИ И/ ИЛИ ИЗКЛЮЧВАНЕ НА ЛЕКАРСТВЕНИ ПРОДУКТИ ОТ ПОЗИТИВНИЯ ЛЕКАРСТВЕН СПИСЪК И УСЛОВИЯТА И РЕДА ЗА РАБОТА НА КОМИСИ-ЯТА ПО ЦЕНИ И РЕИМБУРСИРАНЕ." (Document for Regulation and Registration of Medicinal Products Prices, Conditions, Rules, and Criteria for Incorporation, Changes, and/or Exclusion of Medicinal Products from the Positive Medicinal List). NHIF, Sofia.

Bulgaria. 2014a. "Country Progress Report on Monitoring the 2013 Political Declaration on HIV/AIDS, the Dublin Declaration and the Universal Access in the Health Sector Response." Report submitted to UNAIDS. Government of Bulgaria, Sofia.

Bulgaria, Ministry of Health. 2014b. "National HIV/AIDS Spending Report 2014." Ministry of Health, Sofia.

Bulgaria, Ministry of Health. 2016. "Methodological Indication for Antiretroviral Treatment of Adults with HIV Infection." Updated order dated June 3, Ministry of Health, Sofia. Available online in Bulgarian at https://www.mh.government. bg/media/filer_public/2016/06/07/zapoved-rd-01-193-03-06-2016-metodichesko -ukazanie-hiv-infekciq.pdf.

Bulgaria. 2017. "НАЦИОНАЛНА ПРОГРАМА ЗА ПРЕВЕНЦИЯ И КОНТРОЛ НА ХИВ И СЕКСУАЛНО ПРЕДАВАНИ ИНФЕКЦИИ В РЕПУБЛИКА БЪЛГАРИЯ 2017 - 2020 г." (National Program for the Prevention and Control of HIV and Sexually Transmitted Infections in the Republic of Bulgaria, 2017–2020). Government of Bulgaria, Sofia.

Dimitrova, M., G. Petrova, T. Cervenjakova, N. Jancheva, M. Stefanova, M. Manova, A. Savova, and A. Stoimenova. 2011. "Budget Impact Model of New Antiretroviral Biotechnology Medicines for Treatment of HIV/AIDS Patients in Bulgaria." *Biotechnology & Biotechnological Equipment* 25 (3): 2547–54.

Dimitrova, M., G. Petrova, M. Manova, A. Savova, N. Jancheva, T. Cervenjakova, K. Mitov, and M. Stefanova. 2013. "Economic Impact of the Highly Active Antiretroviral Pharmacotherapy on Cost and HIV/AIDS Control in Bulgaria." *Biotechnology & Biotechnological Equipment* 27 (1): 3599–3604.

EACS (European AIDS Clinical Society). 2015. "Guidelines: Version 8.0." EACS, Brussels.

ECDC (European Center for Disease Prevention and Control). 2017a. *HIV Treatment and Care—Monitoring Implementation of the Dublin Declaration on Partnership to Fight HIV/AIDS in Europe and Central Asia: 2017 Progress Report*. ECDC Special Report. Stockholm: ECDC.

ECDC (European Center for Disease Prevention and Control). 2017b. *Technical Missions: HIV, STI and Viral Hepatitis in Bulgaria*. Mission Report. Stockholm: ECDC.

ECDC (European Center for Disease Prevention and Control) and WHO (World Health Organization) Regional Office for Europe. 2016. *HIV/AIDS Surveillance in Europe 2015*. Stockholm: ECDC.

Mirandola, M., L. Gios, N. Sherriff, I. Toskin, U. Marcus, S. Schink, B. Suligoi, C. Folch, and M. Rosińska, eds. 2016. "The Sialon II Project: Report on a Bio-behavioural Survey Among MSM in 13 European Cities." Cierre Grafica.

UNAIDS (Joint United Nations Programme on HIV/AIDS). 2014. *90-90-90. An Ambitious Treatment Target to Help End the AIDS Epidemic*. Geneva: UNAIDS.

Varleva, T., S. Boneva, E. Naseva, T. Yakimova, V. Georgieva, M. Zamfirova, H. Taskov, and B. Petrunov. 2015. "Report of Integrated Bio-behavioural Surveillance of HIV among Males and Females Sex Workers, 2004–2012." Programmes Financed by the Global Fund to Fight AIDS, Tuberculosis and Malaria, Bulgarian Ministry of Health, Sofia.

Varleva, T., E. Kabakchieva, E. Naseva, T. Yakimova, V. Georgieva, M. Zamfirova, H. Taskov, and B. Petrunov. 2015. "Report of Integrated Bio-behavioural Surveillance of HIV among 18–25 Year-Old Males in Roma Community, 2005–2012." Programmes Financed by the Global Fund to Fight AIDS, Tuberculosis and Malaria, Bulgarian Ministry of Health, Sofia.

Varleva, T., Ts. Raicheva, E. Naseva, T. Yakimova, V. Georgieva, M. Zamfirova, H. Taskov, and B. Petrunov. 2015. "Report of Integrated Bio-behavioural Surveillance of HIV among People Who Inject Drugs, 2004–2012." Programmes Financed by the Global Fund to Fight AIDS, Tuberculosis and Malaria, Bulgarian Ministry of Health, Sofia.

Varleva, T., P. Tsintsarski, E. Naseva, T. Yakimova, V. Georgieva, M. Zamfirova, H. Taskov, and B. Petrunov. 2015. "Report of Integrated Bio-behavioural Surveillance of HIV among Men Who Have Sex with Men, 2006–2012." Programmes Financed by the Global Fund to Fight AIDS, Tuberculosis and Malaria, Bulgarian Ministry of Health, Sofia.

Varleva, T., and V. Toneva. 2017. "Updated Epidemiological Data about the Spread of HIV-Infection in Bulgaria during the Period 1986–2016." Paper presented at the Fifth National Symposium of Exotic Infectious and Parasitic Diseases, Tsigov Chark, Bulgaria, May 19–21.

World Bank. 2017. "Optimizing Investments in Bulgaria's HIV Response." World Bank, Washington, DC.

5

Georgia
An HIV Epidemic among Men Who Have Sex with Men

*Ketevan Stvilia, Irma Khonelidze,
Hassan Haghparast-Bidgoli, Cliff C. Kerr,
Feng Zhao, and Marelize Görgens*

Briefly

- Georgia is experiencing a rapidly expanding epidemic among men who have sex with men (MSM), with estimated human immunodeficiency virus (HIV) prevalence for this population ranging from 13 percent to 20 percent.
- An allocative efficiency study identified MSM as a priority, along with antiretroviral therapy (ART) and sustaining program coverage for people who inject drugs (PWID); it also found that new modalities for reaching MSM with HIV services need to be explored.
- Although the epidemic among PWID in Georgia is relatively well contained, programming targeting PWID should be maintained because even modest reductions in allocations for needle and syringe exchange programs could increase infections among PWID.

Introduction

Georgia—"the land of Colchis"—is a small ancient country. It sits on the south slopes of the greater Caucasus, stretching between the Black and Caspian Seas, representing a kind of keystone of the borderlands between Europe, the Middle East, and Asia.

Among its many gifts to mankind, Georgia domesticated the first cultivated grapevines, as well as wheat, some 8,000 years ago. Historically, because of its special geographic location, Georgia was part of a trade route connecting East and West. The wealth of the Silk Road has flowed through Georgia, enriching its merchants and cities. Today, the country is restoring its historical mission by regaining its place in intensive trade routes and population migration in the region and, at the same time, becoming increasingly attractive for tourists. The downside of this development is the fact that Georgia is becoming a transit country for illegal drugs and part of international trafficking routes, which increases the risk that the HIV epidemic will spread in this small country of 3.7 million people.[1]

Since the first case of HIV infection was detected in 1989 in a female who became infected from her husband of African origin, Georgia has experienced a concentrated but growing HIV epidemic. After that first case, new HIV diagnoses in the country increased steadily, reaching 10.9 per 100,000 in 2013 (Georgia 2014). Between the onset of the epidemic and the end of 2015, a total of 5,412 cases were registered[2]—an increase of 49 percent compared to the total of 3,641 cases registered by the end of 2012. At that time, at least 33 percent of people living with HIV (PLHIV) in Georgia were not aware of their status, as indicated by the findings of an integrated biobehavioral surveillance survey (IBBSS) (Georgia 2015; Curatio International Foundation and Tanadgoma 2013b).[3]

Low detection rates lead to late presentation for treatment. A 2014 study[4] found that approximately 50 percent of people newly diagnosed with HIV in Georgia already had acquired immune deficiency syndrome (AIDS), and up to 70 percent of newly HIV-diagnosed patients had CD4 cell counts of less than 350 cells/mm³. The late presentation adversely affects treatment outcomes and significantly increases short-term mortality risk. Despite this relatively high rate of people who present late for treatment, mortality among HIV patients in Georgia has decreased substantially since the country made treatment available to all PLHIV who are eligible and diagnosed (Georgia 2015).[5]

HIV Prevalence in Key Populations

The HIV epidemic is concentrated among key populations: people who inject drugs (PWID), female sex workers (FSWs), and men who have sex with men (MSM).

From the early 1990s until 2004, the HIV epidemic in Georgia was driven largely by injecting drug use and migration to neighboring countries, particularly Ukraine and the Russian Federation where the HIV epidemic developed quickly. Migration by Georgian PWID and the common practices among PWID of using homemade drugs as well as sharing drug preparation and injecting equipment were particularly important components of this trend (Gotsadze, Chawla, and Chkatarashvili 2003). During that period, HIV prevention interventions in Georgia mainly focused on PWID and mostly took the form of harm reduction programs—that is, needle and syringe exchange programs (NSPs) and opioid substitution therapy (OST). Budget allocations for these programs constituted a considerable share of the total national HIV program budget; programs for other key populations were relatively small in scale.

Prevalence trends have since shifted. Research-based evidence indicates a sharp increase in HIV prevalence among MSM. For example, IBBSS evidence found that the prevalence rate for MSM in Tbilisi increased from 7 percent in 2010 to 13 percent in 2013 (Curatio International Foundation and Tanadgoma 2016). By contrast, HIV prevalence among PWID and sex workers has been contained under 5 percent.

National Data before the Allocative Efficiency Study

In 2014, estimates of the number of PLHIV in Georgia ranged between 6,315 and 6,800 (World Bank 2015).[6] Regarding antiretroviral therapy (ART), Georgia followed World Health Organization (WHO) 2013 treatment guidelines (commencing treatment when a patient's CD4 count drops below 500 cells/mm^3) and adopted a universal access approach (WHO 2013). Doing so enabled Georgia to achieve a relatively high coverage of ART in regional comparison, consisting of 37 percent of the total number of PLHIV at that time (Georgia 2015a).[7] The estimated prevalence rate among the general population was 0.07 percent in 2013 (Georgia 2014). Table 5.1 shows the HIV epidemic data for Georgia applied for the model in the 2015 allocative efficiency analysis, which was conducted using the Optima model (World Bank 2015).[8]

To ensure their consistency and relevance, and unless otherwise indicated, the data provided in this chapter relate to the situation in Georgia at the time the analysis was conducted.

Table 5.1 Georgia: Summary of Key National HIV Data, 2000–13

	2000	2005	2010	2011	2012	2013	Source
HIV new diagnoses							
Number of people newly diagnosed with HIV, total	79	242	455	424	526	490	National AIDS Center database
Registered HIV-related deaths							
Annual registered number of deaths due to AIDS, total	34	84	129	157	147	110	National AIDS Center database
HIV prevalence among key populations (2014)							
HIV prevalence among sex workers (%)	—	1.3	19	—	1.3	0.6	IBBSS (2014 data included in 2013 column)
HIV prevalence among MSM (%)	—	4.3	7.0	—	13.0	—	
HIV prevalence among PWID (%)	1.1	1.5	2.4	—	3.0	—	
Service coverage and use	—	—	—	—	—	—	
Number of people receiving ART	0	150	830	1,122	1,456	1,847	National AIDS Center database, OST program database
Estimated number of PWID receiving OST	0	0	1,920	1,760	2,080	4,635	
Estimated key population sizes (most recent year, up to 2014)							
FSW	—	—	—	—	—	6,525	IBBSS (2014 data included in 2013 column)
PWID	—	—	—	—	—	45,000	
MSM	—	—	—	—	—	17,215	

Sources: Curatio International Foundation and Public Union Bemoni 2013; Curatio International Foundation and Tanadgoma 2011, 2012, 2013a, 2013b, 2014a, 2014b; National AIDS Center database.

Notes: AIDS = acquired immune deficiency syndrome; ART = antiretroviral therapy; FSW = female sex worker; HIV = human immunodeficiency virus; IBBSS = integrated biobehavioral surveillance survey; MSM = men who have sex with men; OST = opioid substitution therapy; PWID = people who inject drugs; — = not available.

The 2015 Allocative Efficiency Analysis

Increasing Incidence

With the trends at the time of analysis, the 2014 levels of funding, and 2014 allocations to programs maintained, the total number of PLHIV has

Figure 5.1 Calibration of People Living with HIV and Number of New HIV Infections per Year, Georgia

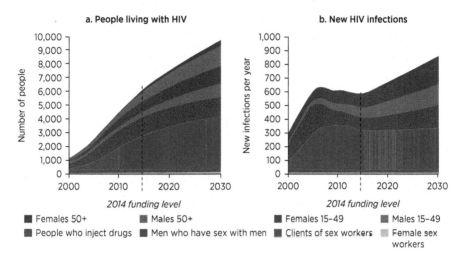

a. People living with HIV

b. New HIV infections

■ Females 50+   ■ Males 50+

■ People who inject drugs   ■ Men who have sex with men

■ Females 15–49   ■ Males 15–49

■ Clients of sex workers   ▨ Female sex workers

Source: World Bank 2015.

Note: HIV = human immunodeficiency virus.

been projected to increase to 7,865 by 2020 and to 9,913 by 2030 (figure 5.1). This projection is based on an expected increase in incidence and a projected decrease in the death rate among PLHIV due to the positive effect of ART.

The model predicts that incidence will increase between 2014 and 2030: from 580 new infections per year in 2014 to 679 new infections per year in 2020 and 860 per year by 2030 (figure 5.1, panel b). Much of the expected increase in incidence is driven by the share of transmission attributed to unprotected sex between MSM, including those who also have sex with women, and their partners. Low condom use between MSM and commercial partners is therefore a particular cause for concern.[9] Among MSM who also have sex with women, the high probability of sex with female partners also raises concerns about their potential role in bridging HIV transmission to the general population.

As a result, overall HIV prevalence has been projected to increase from modeled estimates of 0.18 percent in 2014 to 0.23 percent in 2020 and to 0.28 percent by 2030. Prevalence in the MSM population increased from 7 percent in 2010 to 13 percent in 2012, and the model has predicted an increase to 18.25 percent by 2020 and to 20.3 percent by 2030. HIV prevalence is expected to virtually stabilize in other key populations.

Impact of 2014 Spending Levels

Georgia's gross domestic product (GDP) per capita gradually increased between 2005 and 2015, and, according to the World Bank classification system, the country reached the status of an upper-middle-income country in 2015.[10] As a percentage of GDP, total expenditures for health are comparable to the WHO European regional average and reached 7.42 percent of GDP in 2014 (equaling US$628 per capita), although private sources accounted for 79 percent of those expenditures. Georgia's HIV spending includes the following important characteristics and challenges.

Out-of-pocket private spending as the main source of increased domestic spending. Importantly, from 2006 through 2014, total HIV spending in Georgia increased nearly 140 percent, reaching just under US$14.76 million in 2014 (figure 5.2). During the same period, the share of domestic resources spent on HIV programs in Georgia quintupled, from 10 percent in 2006 to 52.4 percent in 2014 (figure 5.3). As noted, much of this increase in domestic funding has been financed through out-of-pocket (private) expenditure (Georgia 2014).

Transitioning funding, decreasing Global Fund support. The Global Fund to Fight AIDS, Tuberculosis and Malaria (the Global Fund) has been the primary funding partner for key HIV programs in Georgia. As a result of the eligibility and cofinancing requirements of the Global Fund's new funding model, Georgia's external HIV funding is likely to decline. This anticipated decline in funding has led to concern about the sustainability of Georgia's long-term national HIV response. Funding partners are increasingly providing

Figure 5.2 Overall Spending on HIV/AIDS in Georgia, 2006–14

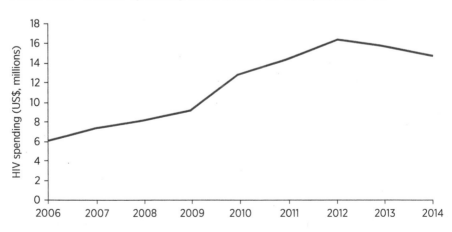

Source: World Bank 2015.

Note: HIV/AIDS = human immunodeficiency virus/acquired immune deficiency syndrome; US$ = US dollar.

Figure 5.3 Funding for HIV in Georgia, by Funding Source, 2006–14

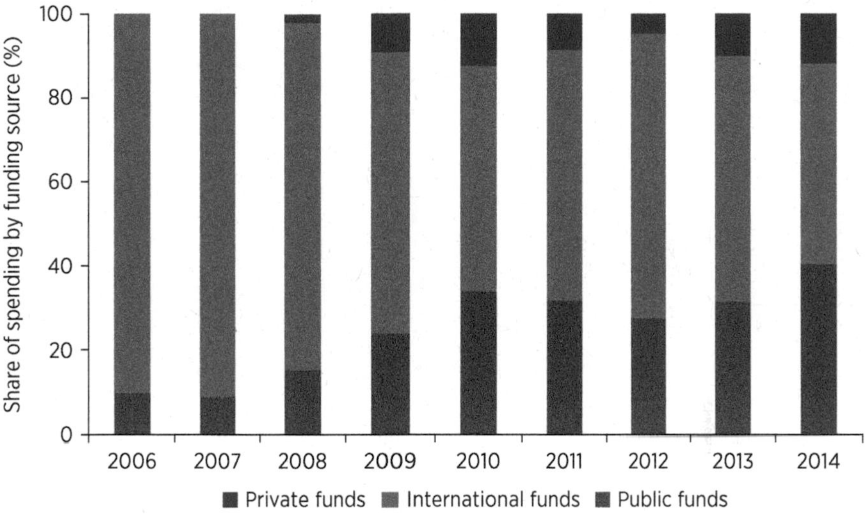

Source: World Bank 2015.

Note: HIV = human immunodeficiency virus.

technical support to help countries establish transitional funding mechanisms that will facilitate the shift from international to domestic financing
of HIV programs.

A focus on prevention, need for programs targeting MSM and FSWs. At the time of
analysis, prevention had been the largest component of HIV spending
(figure 5.4). Within prevention, harm reduction programs for PWID
(including OST and NSPs) represented the largest component, ranging
from 54 percent to 73 percent of prevention expenditure. In 2014,
70 percent of prevention spending was allocated to harm reduction
programs. As noted previously, past investment in programs specifically
targeting MSM and FSWs has been relatively low.[11] These investments
have also varied substantially over time, suggesting a fragile financing climate for individual programs. In 2014, targeted programs for MSM and
FSWs were allocated 5 percent and 3 percent of prevention funding, respectively (figure 5.5) (Georgia 2014, 2015a).[12]

Prevention could be better targeted within and between key populations. HIV prevention and treatment may not cover those in most need (figure 5.5).
Model-based estimates have indicated increasing incidence and prevalence
among males and females between the ages of 15 and 49 (a group that
includes sexual partners of PWID, MSM, and FSWs and their clients) and

Figure 5.4 HIV Expenditure in Georgia, by Type of Spending

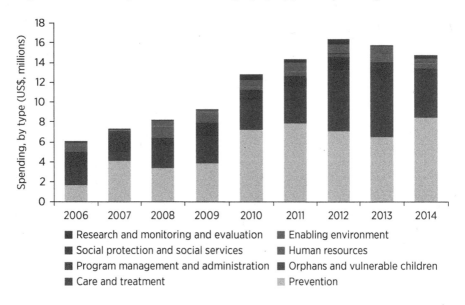

Source: World Bank 2015.

Note: Data taken from the final draft of the National HIV Strategic Plan (March 2015); results should be interpreted accordingly. HIV = human immunodeficiency virus; US$ = US dollar.

some key populations, especially MSM. These estimates suggest that prevention could be better targeted at MSM, including MSM who also have sex with women. The role of this population in bridging HIV transmission to the general population provides a compelling argument for better, and better-targeted, prevention because that would likely produce benefits for both high- and low-risk populations.

Although the increase in prevalence among PWID is expected to be small, the allocative efficiency analyses suggest that investment in programs for PWID is still needed, including NSPs and OST. Given the relatively high cost of OST provision, however, increasing coverage may require further technical efficiency analyses to identify ways to reduce the OST cost averages.

Sources of funding. Reliance on international donors for a substantial portion of HIV financing coupled with an expected reduction in international assistance in the medium to long term constitute key challenges to the sustainability of Georgia's HIV programming. These challenges are expected to be compounded by a rising HIV incidence and require better understanding of the funding needs for 2015 through 2030, using an allocative efficiency analysis.

Figure 5.5 Trends in Spending across Key Priority Prevention and Treatment Programs, Georgia

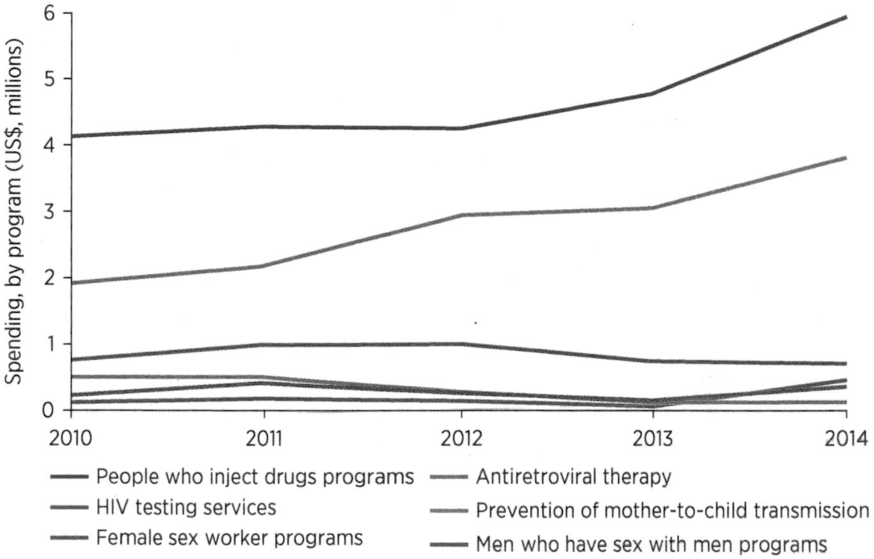

Source: World Bank 2015.

Note: HIV testing services and antiretroviral therapy are programs for the whole population and, as such, include people from key populations. HIV = human immunodeficiency virus; US$ = US dollar.

Key Targets of the Allocative Efficiency Analysis

The 2015 analysis conducted using the allocative efficiency modeling was informed by the country's priorities as highlighted in the National HIV Strategic Plan, which describes the following key impacts and outcomes expected by the end of 2018 (Georgia 2015):

1. Increase domestic funding of the HIV response from 32 percent (2013) to 70 percent (2018).
2. Contain HIV prevalence among PWID, FSWs, and prisoners below 5 percent by 2018.
3. Hold HIV prevalence among MSM below 15 percent by 2018.
4. Reduce the rate of late HIV detection from 70 percent to 35 percent by 2018.
5. Reduce AIDS-related mortality to less than 2 deaths per 100,000 population.

The analysis then used 2014 as its baseline year and focused on four questions:

1. How can Georgia optimize the allocation of its existing HIV funding?
2. What might be gained from increased investment in HIV programming?
3. What is the minimum spending necessary to meet the National HIV Strategic Plan targets?
4. What are the long-term resource needs of the HIV response?

Key Changes to Optimize Spending Allocations

The analysis found that the 2014 distribution of funding is not an optimized allocation that would minimize both new infections and deaths. Optimization of the 2014 budget would avert an estimated 2,969 (15.5 percent) additional HIV infections (mainly among MSM) and 2,238 (36 percent) additional deaths from 2015 to 2030. To achieve these gains, the model suggested the following key changes to optimize allocation of spending at the 2014 budget levels (see figure 5.6):

- ART provision should be increased to 48.7 percent of the budget.
- ART cannot be scaled up unless PLHIV are diagnosed; therefore, it is necessary to continue adequate funding for testing, especially among key populations.
- Spending on low-risk populations (for example, through HIV testing and counseling [HTC] programming) could be more effectively diverted to comprehensive HIV programs that target key populations; however, HTC could continue at lower funding levels (less than 0.1 percent of the total budget), whereas the overall allocation for treatment would increase.
- Investments in MSM programs should be maintained at the level of at least 2.3 percent.
- Investments in and coverage of NSP interventions could be largely maintained, but the proportion of total spending should be reduced from 13.5 percent to 8.5 percent.
- Recommendations for OST spending should be interpreted with caution, because service components such as OST that have significant wider benefits to the PWID population and to national public health may be undervalued by the allocative efficiency model. Efforts should be made to ensure that high unit costs are reduced as far as possible without compromising the quality of care.

Figure 5.6 Comparison of Georgia's Actual 2014 Spending and Optimized Budget Allocation to Minimize Both New Infections and Deaths for the Period 2015–30

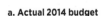

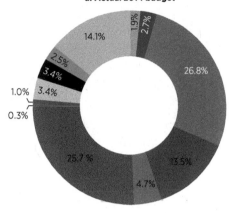

a. Actual 2014 budget

14.1%
1.9%
2.7%
26.8%
2.5%
3.4%
1.0%   3.4%
0.3%
25.7%
13.5%
4.7%

b. Optimized 2014 budget

0.1%
14.1%
2.3%
16.1%
2.5%
3.4%
1.0%   3.4%
0%
8.5%
0%
48.7%

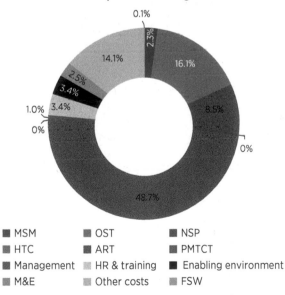

- ■ MSM
- ■ HTC
- ■ Management
- ■ M&E
- ■ OST
- ■ ART
- ■ HR & training
- ■ Other costs
- ■ NSP
- ■ PMTCT
- ■ Enabling environment
- ■ FSW

Source: World Bank 2015.

Note: ART = antiretroviral therapy; FSW = female sex worker; HR = human resources; HTC = HIV testing and counseling; M&E = monitoring and evaluation; MSM = men who have sex with men; NSP = needle and syringe exchange program; OST = opioid substitution therapy; PMTCT = prevention of mother-to-child transmission.

Figure 5.7 shows 2014 spending, the 2018 National HIV Strategic Plan budget, and the minimum spending required to achieve the National HIV Strategic Plan impact targets as determined by the allocative efficiency modeling analysis. The model results suggest that the National HIV Strategic Plan impact could be achieved with approximately 12 percent less funding than the proposed 2018 National HIV Strategic Plan budget. In order to achieve the National HIV Strategic Plan targets, the model findings recommend spending an extra 50 percent on MSM programs, an extra 10 percent on HTC, and an extra 5 percent on ART, while shifting the funding by 25 percent from FSW, 40 percent from OST, and 10 percent from NSP.

Figure 5.7   Minimum Annual Spending Required to Meet Georgia's National HIV Strategic Plan Targets

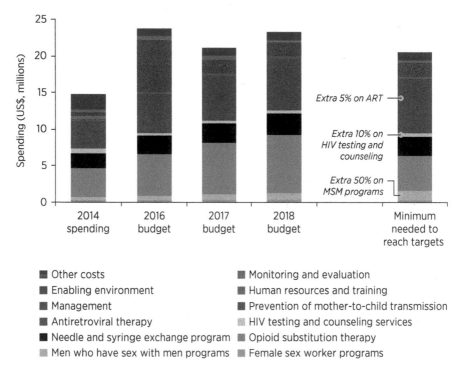

Source: World Bank 2015.

Note: ART = antiretroviral therapy; HIV = human immunodeficiency virus; MSM = men who have sex with men; US$ = US dollar.

The modeling analysis was also used to determine optimal allocations if the total budget is increased to 150 percent of the 2014 spending levels (figure 5.8). This increase would entail spending a total of US$19.1 million on direct programs, whereas the indirect program costs for enablers and management costs are assumed to remain stable.

The larger budget envelope would increase impact by reducing both deaths and new infections (figure 5.9). This increased coverage would require additional resources, technical efficiency gains, or both achieved by reducing the unit costs of programs (without compromising the quality of the outcomes).

Figure 5.8 Comparing the Allocation of Georgia's 2014 Spending against an Optimized Allocation of 150 Percent of 2014 Spending

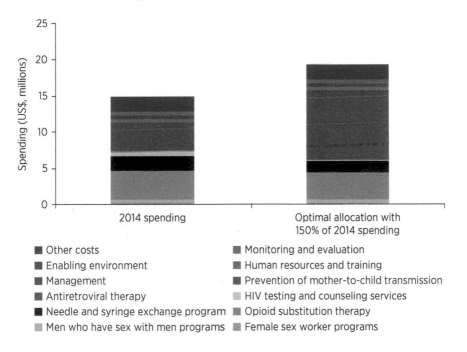

■ Other costs
■ Enabling environment
■ Management
■ Antiretroviral therapy
■ Needle and syringe exchange program
■ Men who have sex with men programs

■ Monitoring and evaluation
■ Human resources and training
■ Prevention of mother-to-child transmission
■ HIV testing and counseling services
■ Opioid substitution therapy
■ Female sex worker programs

Source: World Bank 2015.

Note: HIV = human immunodeficiency virus; US$ = US dollar.

Figure 5.9 Comparing the Impact on Prevalence, Deaths, and New Infections of Actual 2014 Spending against an Optimized Allocation of 150 Percent of the 2014 Budget, Georgia

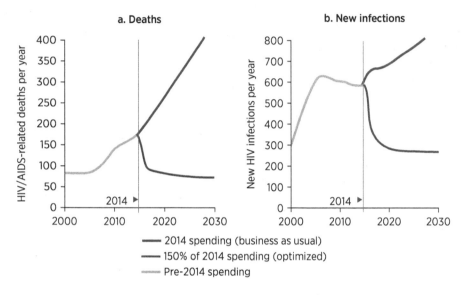

Source: World Bank 2015.
Note: HIV = human immunodeficiency virus.

Allocative Efficiency Analysis Recommendations

There is a strong risk that, despite efforts to contain the HIV epidemic, prevalence and incidence will continue to increase overall in Georgia. The allocative efficiency modeling study produced the following key recommendations (World Bank 2015):

1. The expected overall increase in the epidemic appears to be driven by increasing incidence and prevalence among MSM—a key population that receives only a small portion of the HIV prevention funding. High-risk behaviors in this population, including low condom use, call for significant strengthening of interventions targeting this key population. Increasing the use of condoms with casual and commercial partners is likely to be an effective preventive measure. Additional programs such as pre-exposure prophylaxis (PrEP) also could be considered.

2. The most effective funding allocations for containing the epidemic overall will be those that prioritize the National HIV Strategic Plan targets, improve condom use among MSM, and scale up ART to all

populations in need; additional deterrents, such as high rates of out-of-pocket spending on health care, stigma, and discrimination, can also be minimized by enhancing a rights-based approach to care.

3. Diverting funding away from testing in the general population and to prevention among MSM would improve the efficiency at the 2014 spending levels. The modeling and contextual data suggest that the HIV epidemic among PWID is relatively well contained in Georgia because of significant and prolonged efforts to target this population. Even modest reductions in NSP allocations, however, increase new infections among PWID. As much as possible, therefore, key MSM and PWID populations should be targeted with strong preventive efforts complemented by comprehensive treatment programs.

4. Maintaining annual spending at the 2014 budget levels will not be enough to achieve National HIV Strategic Plan and international targets. For this reason, additional domestic resources will need to be allocated to HIV spending to fill resource gaps in the overall HIV budget envelope. By increasing overall government spending on health, Georgia could increase domestic HIV financing and thereby contribute to covering resource gaps in its HIV response.

5. Comparing the unit costs of care in Georgia with data from other countries in the region also suggests that greater efficiency in spending could be achieved through strategies to reduce the average spending per person reached. This is particularly true for OST programming, which absorbs a substantial portion of HIV prevention spending. Care should be taken, however, to ensure that these strategies do not compromise the existing quality of prevention or treatment. Further technical efficiency analyses should be performed. Another recommendation is to implement provider-initiated testing in an optimal way, considering the high cost of testing and counseling along with low HIV prevalence among the general population.

6. The Global Fund has supported HIV programming in Georgia since 2003, but its support will decrease considerably in the coming years. Despite this decrease, analyses of what is needed to achieve the targets set by the National HIV Strategic Plan have identified a need for continued and even increased investment in an optimized HIV response in Georgia. Gradual takeover by the government of Georgia of Global Fund–supported activities should be well planned to ensure sustainability in access to and quality of services. Guided by allocative efficiency analysis outcomes, additional analysis and detailed planning are needed to better understand the total financial needs of the program and the priority areas for the national HIV response. It is critical that the country defines potential internal and other sources of financing in a timely and well-planned manner.

Actions Taken and Next Steps

To optimize its HIV response, the government of Georgia has already taken the following actions, some of which will need to be followed up with more analysis and further action.

Revised spending allocations, targeting MSM. The recommendations of the allocative efficiency analysis guided the development and implementation of the National HIV Strategic Plan for 2016–18 (Georgia 2015). Both the planned budgets and actual spending reflect the increased allocations for ART and for HIV prevention interventions, the first of all those targeting MSM during this three-year period.

Implementing Treat All, removing ART enrollment criteria. Since December 2015, Georgia has started implementation of the WHO (2016) "Treat All" recommendations, offering ART to all PLHIV regardless of their immune status (CD4 cell count). It was the first among the countries of the Eastern Europe and Central Asia region to do so. Removing ART enrollment criteria has resulted in considerable scale-up of the program. By the end of 2017, 81 percent of all PLHIV with known HIV status were enrolled in ART, and viral suppression was achieved in 87 percent of patients. At the same time, HIV case detection remains the biggest challenge for the HIV National Response. Only 48 percent of the total estimated number of PLHIV were aware of their HIV status. The large number of undiagnosed PLHIV mitigates the gains from the rapid scale-up of ART. Along with accelerating HIV screening among key populations, the country is testing alternative ways to improve HIV case detection, like the rapid scale-up of provider-initiated testing and tandem testing for HIV and the hepatitis C virus (HCV) within the National Hepatitis C Elimination Program, which allows testing of large numbers of individuals at medical facilities. The Hepatitis C Elimination Program was initiated in 2015 with a goal of identifying 95 percent of HCV-positive people and treating 95 percent of them by the end of 2020. The program is supported by US Centers for Disease Control and Prevention and the pharmaceutical company Gilead (which is providing free medicines). This program has become a major driver of different public health programs in Georgia, including HIV programming, thus providing opportunities for development of HCV/HIV integrated cost-effective service delivery models.

Resource centers and piloting PrEP for MSM. To address high HIV prevalence among MSM, the prevention interventions among MSM and transgendered individuals were prioritized in the National Strategic Plan (Georgia 2015, 2018). The LGBT (lesbian, gay, bisexual, and transgender) resource centers established in five large cities in Georgia with support of the Global

Fund HIV Program became the community gathering points where MSM are tested on HIV and receive condoms and lubricants. Georgia was also the first country in the region to start PrEP among MSM. The pilot program was initiated in September 2017 for an initial 100 MSM. If the program gains community support, it will be scaled up and expanded to other key populations as needed.

Increased domestic government spending. Although the government of Georgia strictly followed the funding takeover plan for the activities previously supported through the Global Fund Program during the 2015–17 period and public expenditure on HIV has increased from 55 percent to 67 percent, the country's funding landscape will become more problematic in the future because the Global Fund's country allocation for Georgia is scheduled to decrease by 50 percent during the 2019–22 funding cycle. Along with supporting AIDS treatment, the government of Georgia will need to start investing in HIV prevention interventions for key populations; therefore, additional allocative efficiency analysis would be important to ensure effective allocations of scarce resources.

Notes

1. Data from GeoStat's Country Demographic Data web page (in Georgian), http://www.geostat.ge/?action=page&p_id=151&lang=geo.
2. Data from the National AIDS Center's "HIV/AIDS Epidemiology in Georgia" web page, http://aidscenter.ge/epidsituation_eng.html.
3. Of MSM, 26.2 percent (73 of 278) in 2010 and 33.9 percent (74 of 218) in 2012 reported being tested for HIV in the previous year according to the IBBSS study (Curatio International Foundation and Tanadgoma 2011, 2013b).
4. World Health Organization 2014 National Health Accounts, http://www.who.int/health-accounts/en/.
5. The all-cause mortality rate peaked in 2004, with 10.74 deaths per 100 person years (95 percent CI [confidence interval]: 7.92–14.24); after the widespread availability of ART, this rate significantly decreased to 4.02 per 100 person years (95 percent CI: 3.28–4.87) reported in 2012 (p [probability] < 0.0001). There was more than a threefold decrease in AIDS-related mortality from 6.49 deaths per 100 person years (95 percent CI: 4.34–9.32) in 2004 to 2.05 deaths per 100 person years (95 percent CI: 1.53–2.68) in 2012 (p < 0.0001).
6. Data on prevalence also come from the Joint United Nations Programme on HIV/AIDS (UNAIDS) national HIV estimates files available on Spectrum. For more information, see https://www.unaids.org/en/dataanalysis/datatools/spectrum-epp.
7. UNAIDS national HIV estimates files.
8. Note that much of this chapter reviews the process and findings of the modeling exercise documented in the report produced for that analysis; as such, the

material herein draws significantly on that report. For more detail, see World Bank 2015 in the reference list for this chapter.

9. The proportion of MSM who reported condom use at their last anal insertion with a paid partner was 67 percent (8/12) in 2010 and 50 percent (4/8) in 2012. Given that the denominator for paid partners is very small, this proportion should be interpreted with caution (Curatio International Foundation and Tanadgoma 2013b).

10. Geostat data.

11. Many services for key populations are not allocated in population-specific budgets. As a result, these numbers may not include some spending targeted at the general population that also benefits key populations.

12. Note that these data are from the final draft of the National HIV Strategic Plan (March 2015), and not the final National HIV strategic plan. Results should be interpreted accordingly.

References

Curatio International Foundation and Public Union Bemoni. 2013. "HIV Risk and Prevention Behaviors among People Who Inject Drugs in Six Cities of Georgia: Bio-Behavioral Surveillance Survey in Tbilisi, Batumi, Zugdidi, Telavi, Gori, Kutaisi in 2012." Study Report. Curatio International Foundation, Tbilisi.

Curatio International Foundation and Tanadgoma (Center for Information and Counseling on Reproductive Health). 2011. "Bio-Behavioral Survey among Men Who Have Sex with Men in Tbilisi, Georgia (2010)." Study Report. Curatio International Foundation, Tbilisi.

Curatio International Foundation and Tanadgoma (Center for Information and Counseling on Reproductive Health). 2012. "Bio-Behavioral Surveillance Survey with Biomarker Component among HIV/AIDS Risk Groups, Identifying the Number of Injective Drug Users (IDU), Operations Survey, 2012." Study Report. Curatio International Foundation, Tbilisi.

Curatio International Foundation and Tanadgoma (Center for Information and Counseling on Reproductive Health). 2013a. "HIV Risk and Prevention Behavior among Female Sex Workers in Two Cities of Georgia: Bio-Behavioral Surveillance Survey in Tbilisi and Batumi in 2012." Study Report. Curatio International Foundation, Tbilisi.

Curatio International Foundation and Tanadgoma (Center for Information and Counseling on Reproductive Health). 2013b. "HIV Risk and Prevention Behavior among Men Who Have Sex with Men in Tbilisi, Georgia: Bio-Behavioral Surveillance Survey in 2012." Study Report. Curatio International Foundation, Tbilisi.

Curatio International Foundation and Tanadgoma (Center for Information and Counseling on Reproductive Health). 2014a. "Population Size Estimation of Female Sex Workers in Tblisi and Batumi, Georgia, 2014." Study Report. Curatio International Foundation, Tbilisi.

Curatio International Foundation and Tanadgoma (Center for Information and Counseling on Reproductive Health). 2014b. "Population Size Estimation of Men Who Have Sex with Men in Georgia, 2014." Study Report. Curatio International Foundation, Tbilisi.

Curatio International Foundation and Tanadgoma (Center for Information and Counseling on Reproductive Health). 2016. "HIV Risk and Prevention Behavior among Men Who Have Sex with Men in Tbilisi and Batumi, Georgia: Bio-Behavioral Surveillance Survey in 2015." Study Report. Curatio International Foundation, Tbilisi.

Georgia, NCDC (National Center for Disease Control and Public Health). 2014. "Georgia: Country Progress Report." Global AIDS Response Progress Report, reporting period January 2012–December 2013. NCDC, Tbilisi.

Georgia. 2015a. "Georgia Final Draft National Strategic Plan, 2016–2020." Government of Georgia, Tbilisi.

Georgia, CCM (Country Coordinating Mechanism). 2015b. "Georgian National HIV/AIDS Strategic Plan for 2016–2018." CCM, Tbilisi. http://www.georgia-ccm.ge/wp-content/uploads/HIV-NSP-2016-20181.pdf.

Georgia, CCM (Country Coordinating Mechanism). 2018. "Georgian National HIV/AIDS Strategic Plan for 2019–2022." CCM, Tbilisi.

Gotsadze, T., M. Chawla, and K. Chkatarashvili. 2003. "HIV/AIDS in Georgia: Addressing the Crisis." Working Paper 23, World Bank, Washington, DC.

WHO (World Health Organization). 2013. *Consolidated Guidelines on the Use of Antiretroviral Drugs for Treating and Preventing HIV Infection: Recommendations for a Public Health Approach*. Geneva: WHO.

WHO (World Health Organization). 2016. *Consolidated Guidelines on the Use of Antiretroviral Drugs for Treating and Preventing HIV Infection: Recommendations for a Public Health Approach*, 2nd ed. Geneva: WHO.

World Bank. 2015. "Optimizing Investments in Georgia's HIV Response." World Bank, Washington, DC.

6

Kazakhstan
Achieving Ambitious HIV Targets through Efficient Spending

Andrew J. Shattock, Aliya Bokazhanova,
Manoela Manova, Baurzhan S. Baiserkin, Irina Petrenko,
David P. Wilson, Clemens Benedikt, and Nejma Cheikh

Briefly

- The costs of antiretroviral therapy (ART) vary widely across the region of Eastern Europe and Central Asia. ART drug prices for Kazakhstan have been approximately double the median price in the region.
- Combining allocative and implementation efficiency can increase the impact of existing funding levels.
- By reducing ART costs by 67 percent and management costs by 20 percent, Kazakhstan could achieve ambitious targets of reducing new infections and deaths by 50 percent by 2020.

Introduction

HIV in the Region

Kazakhstan is the world's largest landlocked country. After the fall of the Soviet Union, Kazakhstan achieved independence in 1991. Its main spoken languages are Kazakh and Russian. As of 2016, the population of Kazakhstan was 17,855,384.

Kazakhstan, like other Central Asian countries such as the Kyrgyz Republic, Tajikistan, Turkmenistan, and Uzbekistan, lies along a major drug trafficking route from Afghanistan to the Russian Federation. In Kazakhstan, the availability of inexpensive heroin and a high prevalence of drug use have resulted in a concentrated human immunodeficiency virus (HIV) epidemic among certain at-risk key populations, mostly people who inject drugs (PWID), sex workers, men who have sex with men (MSM), and prisoners.

To ensure their consistency and relevance, and unless otherwise indicated, the data provided in this chapter relate to the situation in Kazakhstan at the time the analysis was conducted.[1]

Impacts of the Spread of HIV in Kazakhstan

In general, the number of new HIV infections in Central Asia rose rapidly in the 1990s and saw another more recent increase. Thus, the number of newly registered HIV cases across the region increased by 6 percent—from 4,404 in 2015 to 4,707 in 2016 (PEPFAR 2016). In Kazakhstan, the number of newly registered HIV cases increased from 2,327 in 2015 to 2,774 in 2016. Injecting drug use and sexual transmission are currently the main routes of HIV transmission in Kazakhstan. The potential for continued rapid spread of HIV, particularly among the injecting drug population, is great because the country is estimated to have as many as 127,800 PWID. About 54 percent of reported HIV cases are due to unsafe injecting drug use; sexual transmission accounts for 41 percent.

Kazakhstan is among the countries in Central Asia that have committed to the Sustainable Development Goals—including Sustainable Development Goal 3 on health, which sets a goal of ending the HIV/AIDS (acquired immune deficiency syndrome) epidemic by 2030. Currently, all Central Asian countries, including Kazakhstan, are also committed to achieving the 90-90-90 targets of the Joint United Nations Programme on HIV/AIDS (UNAIDS): ensuring that by 2020, 90 percent of people living with HIV (PLHIV) will know their status, 90 percent of diagnosed PLHIV will be receiving antiretroviral therapy (ART), and 90 percent of people on ART will have viral suppression (PEPFAR 2016). Kazakhstan faces several challenges in achieving these goals and responding to the spread of HIV in the country.

Many countries are experiencing downward trends in their HIV epidemics after 10–15 years of large global investment (Beyrer and Abdool 2013; Bor et al. 2013; Tanser et al. 2013; UNAIDS 2013a). Some countries, however, now face international donor withdrawal despite epidemics that are not decreasing (Ensirink 2014). Kazakhstan has experienced a decrease in

HIV funding from international donors after achieving upper-middle-income country status in 2006 (UNAIDS 2013b). In future, international aid for HIV is likely to be completely withdrawn from Kazakhstan. Although the government has increased domestic funding for the national response (UNAIDS 2013b), 20 percent of spending in 2012 still came from international donors.[2]

Kazakhstan's gross domestic product (GDP) per capita has exceeded US$12,000. This figure surpasses the GDP per capita of many countries in Eastern Europe and Central Asia, suggesting that Kazakhstan is in a stronger position to fund its HIV response (map 6.1). This economic advantage is diminished, however, by higher costs of procuring ART drugs—with these

Map 6.1   Gross Domestic Product per Capita, Antiretroviral Therapy Unit Costs, and Key HIV/AIDS Program Spending Data, Selected Countries, Eastern Europe and Central Asia

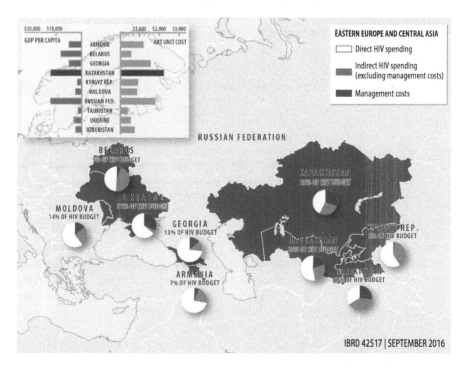

Source: Shattock et al. 2017.

Note: The map depicts only countries for which data were available. The pie charts represent total HIV spending in 2013, and the bar graphs represent national GDP per capita and ART unit costs. The red text represents the proportion of the respective national budget consumed by management costs. ART = antiretroviral therapy; GDP = gross domestic product; HIV/AIDS = human immunodeficiency virus/acquired immune deficiency syndrome.

costs exceeding the regional average for Eastern Europe and Central Asia (of countries for which recent data are available) by 110 percent (map 6.1). This high cost of HIV treatment is primarily driven by the fact that Kazakhstan's upper-middle-income country status excludes its government from voluntary license agreements that pharmaceutical companies negotiate with generic drug manufacturers (MSF 2014). Central Asia—along with Eastern Europe—experiences not only the highest cost of donor-funded ART when procured from originator companies but also the lowest cost when procured from generic manufacturers (Sagaon-Teyssier et al. 2016). This disparity highlights the importance for countries in these regions to have access to the generic ART market. Such high treatment costs in the future would likely hinder the attainment of Kazakhstan's HIV targets—especially after donor withdrawal. It is believed, however, that costs of ART can be substantially reduced through the more efficient pooled procurement processes of the United Nations and the Global Fund to Fight AIDS, Tuberculosis and Malaria (the Global Fund) (Global Fund 2007; UNICEF 2007).

Like other former republics of the Soviet Union, during the 1990s Kazakhstan had an exploding HIV epidemic among PWID (Bobkov et al. 2004; DeHovitz, Uuskula, and El-Bassel 2014; Thorne et al. 2010). This epidemic was driven by the injection of drugs by a high proportion of adults living in towns along major drug trafficking routes (up to 10 percent of the population) (Aceijas et al. 2006). From 2000, the epidemic accelerated, with new HIV infections increasingly reported among heterosexual partners of PWID, female sex workers (FSWs) and their clients, MSM, prison inmates, and migrants (El-Bassel et al. 2014; Thorne et al. 2010). By 2011, heterosexual infection had surpassed injecting drug use as the primary mode of HIV transmission (El-Bassel et al. 2013; ICAP 2011). There were an estimated 23,000 PLHIV in Kazakhstan in 2015 (Kazakhstan 2016). As of 2016, the estimated HIV prevalence was 8.2 percent among PWID, 1.3 percent among FSWs, 3.2 percent among MSM, and 3.9 percent among prisoners (PEPFAR 2016). The priorities of the national strategic plan are to stabilize the epidemic by increasing public awareness of HIV prevention, targeting key populations at higher risk of transmission, continuing to provide access to treatment, and virtually eliminating mother-to-child transmission (Eaton et al. 2014; Sandgren et al. 2008).

Within an HIV response, funding is required for critical enablers to support treatment and prevention programs. These "indirect" costs include management, coordination, enabling environment, training, and capacity-building expenditures. In Kazakhstan, such indirect costs consumed 56 percent of the 2013 HIV budget, with 29 percent of the overall budget allocated to management costs. This proportional allocation to management programs in Kazakhstan is much higher than in many countries in the region of Eastern Europe and Central Asia (map 6.1). Similar findings have previously been reported (Forsythe, Stover, and Bollinger 2009). Although this disparity could be explained partially by potential differences in accounting definitions—with staff and infrastructure costs categorized within indirect or program costs—Kazakhstan likely has opportunities to reduce management costs through implementation efficiencies. Obtaining efficiency gains in essential management programs would provide extra funds for prevention and treatment, allowing Kazakhstan to achieve more with its current resources.

Efficiency Analysis Performed

In an allocative efficiency analysis conducted in 2015 using 2013 budgeting levels and allocations as a baseline, Shattock et al. (2017) used mathematical modeling to explore the potential impact of three types of efficiency gains with respect to Kazakhstan's national targets. The analysis considered simultaneously the impacts of funding the most cost-effective programs to an optimal level (known as allocative efficiency), of decreasing the unit cost of treatment programs (technical efficiency), and of increasing the productivity of indirect programs and overhead costs (implementation efficiency) (Palmer and Torgerson 1999). It further investigated whether ambitious targets could be achieved with such efficiencies.

As described in Kazakhstan's national strategic plan, the priorities of the national HIV/AIDS response are containing the epidemic within key populations, restricting the overall population prevalence to between 0.2 percent and 0.6 percent, and prevention of mother-to-child transmission (PMTCT). The Kazakhstan allocative efficiency study group translated these goals into quantified targets within the Optima allocative efficiency model. The group then interpreted the epidemic targets to mean no further increases in annual newly acquired sexual and injecting HIV infections and no further increases in annual AIDS-related deaths by 2020 compared to 2014 levels. PMTCT was assumed to mean the virtual elimination of mother-to-child transmission as defined by UNAIDS (Mahy et al. 2010; WHO 2010). Ambitious targets were further defined as 50 percent reductions in annual new sexual- and injecting-related transmissions, a 50 percent reduction in annual AIDS-related deaths, and virtual elimination of mother-to-child transmission—all by 2020.

A series of scenarios were then simulated to determine whether Kazakhstan could achieve its national targets—or further, the ambitious targets described above—by 2020 under assumptions of future efficiency gains and total HIV budget. For each scenario three types of efficiency gains were considered: (1) gains in allocative efficiency through optimally redistributing direct funds, (2) gains in implementation efficiency through reducing management costs by reducing administrative and coordination expenses (with surplus funds reallocated to direct programs), and (3) gains in technical efficiency through reducing ART procurement costs in line with unit costs obtained by other countries in the region. The analysis did not consider technical efficiencies of prevention programs. Discussions with country representatives indicated that reductions in future ART costs of up to 60–70 percent were plausible, as were reductions of 20–25 percent in management costs. In order to fully scope the space of potential cost reductions, the study group considered (in percentage point increments) reductions in ART costs from 0 percent to 80 percent, and reductions in management costs from 0 percent to 50 percent. A scenario was simulated for each pairwise combination of ART cost reduction and management cost reduction, with the budget for direct programs in each scenario being optimized through a formal mathematical optimization algorithm (which uses the cost-outcome relationships) representing maximal allocative efficiency (WHO 2015). Two levels of future HIV financing were considered for each simulated scenario. The future annual HIV budget available was restricted to either (1) 2013 levels of funding (where international funds would be replenished from domestic sources) or (2) 2013 levels without international donor funding. In the second case, the 20 percent of the total budget sourced from international donors was assumed to be withdrawn proportionally from direct and indirect programs.[3]

Optimizing Allocations for Specific Targets

Simulating scenarios for each combination of implementation efficiency gain and ART cost reduction assumption allowed for the identification—for both assumptions of future total HIV budget—of the scenarios for which the national and ambitious targets were attained when direct funds were optimally allocated. The study group then identified one key scenario that achieved a desirable outcome (that is, achievement of national or ambitious targets) while still being considered realistic in terms of the efficiency gains required. By comparison with the status quo, this key scenario was analyzed in terms of newly acquired HIV infections averted and AIDS-related deaths averted.

Modeling Analysis Findings

In the absence of optimal allocative, implementation, and technical efficiencies, achieving Kazakhstan's national targets would require a 32 percent (27–42 percent) increase in the HIV budget if the 2013 allocation to direct programs is scaled up proportionally. Although meeting these targets would avert an estimated 4,090 newly acquired HIV infections and 2,950 AIDS-related deaths by 2020 compared to status quo spending, it would require an additional US$75.1 million (US$63.7 million–US$96.4 million), assuming indirect costs remain fixed at US$21.8 million per year.

With no additional annual spending, Kazakhstan can achieve its national targets if either a 44 percent (36–58 percent) reduction in management costs or a 35 percent (30–39 percent) decrease in ART unit costs can be secured, and by also optimally allocating available resources. Alternatively, it could achieve the same targets by combining smaller implementation efficiency gains and ART cost reductions while allocating funds optimally (figure 6.1, panel a). For example, optimal allocative efficiency with a 20 percent decrease in the future cost of ART combined with a 21 percent (15–29 percent) reduction in management costs is estimated to be sufficient to achieve the national targets. The pale yellow area of figure 6.1, panel a, illustrates the combination of efficiency gains that is estimated to lead to achievement of Kazakhstan's national targets if 2013 spending levels remain available. With no additional annual resources, Kazakhstan could fully achieve the ambitious targets by (1) securing at least a 51 percent (49–56 percent) reduction in ART costs, (2) increasing the proportion of the total budget allocated to direct programs by reducing management costs, and (3) optimally allocating available resources across treatment and prevention programs. The orange area of figure 6.1, panel a, illustrates the corresponding combination of efficiency gains estimated to achieve the ambitious targets.

Should the total annual HIV budget be reduced by 20 percent because of international donor withdrawal without replacement from domestic sources, the analysis results indicate that a 35 percent decrease in ART costs would need to be combined with a 32 percent (26–36 percent) reduction in management costs and optimal allocative efficiency for Kazakhstan to realize its national targets (figure 6.1, panel b). The results suggest further that—if substantial implementation efficiency gains (at least 24 percent [19–31 percent] reductions in management costs), substantial technical efficiency gains (at least 70 percent [64–74 percent] reductions in future ART unit costs), and optimal allocative efficiency are attained—Kazakhstan could achieve the ambitious targets without replenishing funds sourced from international donors at the time of the analysis (figure 6.1, panel b)—that is, with only 80 percent of the 2013 HIV budget applied through to 2020.

Figure 6.1 Contour Plot of Thresholds to Achieve National and Ambitious Targets with Varying Levels of Management and Treatment Cost Reductions, Kazakhstan

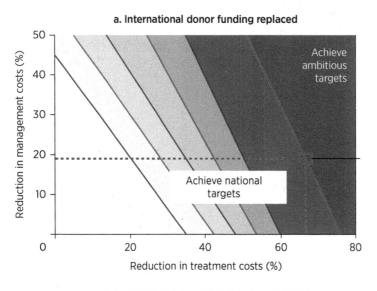

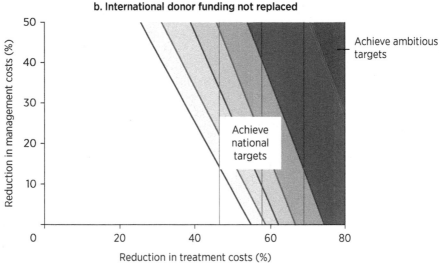

New annual HIV infections and AIDS deaths in 2020 compared to 2014

— No decrease — 10% decrease — 20% decrease
— 30% decrease — 40% decrease — 50% decrease

Source: Shattock et al. 2017.
Note: AIDS = acquired immune deficiency syndrome; HIV = human immunodeficiency virus.

This figure illustrates the estimated reduction in management costs and treatment costs required to achieve (1) national targets (pale yellow/orange region) and (2) ambitious targets (dark orange region) should the annual budget be restricted to either 2013 levels (figure 6.1, panel a) or 2013 levels without international donor funding (figure 6.1, panel b). The colored contours show the thresholds for percentage reductions in both newly acquired HIV infections and AIDS-related deaths by 2020 compared to 2014 levels. The "no increase" contour is the threshold for satisfying the national targets (and is hence the border for the lighter yellow/orange region), whereas the "50 percent decrease" contour satisfies the ambitious targets (and is hence the border for the dark orange region). In each simulation, the proportion of the budget dedicated to direct programs is optimally distributed across programs to minimize incidence, minimize deaths, and virtually eliminate mother-to-child transmission.

Of the array of results that achieved the ambitious targets, the scenario of attaining a 67 percent reduction in the cost of ART along with a 19 percent (14–27 percent) reduction in management costs (with the existing national budget distributed optimally across programs) was identified as being realistic by country representatives and key stakeholders. Henceforth, we refer to this scenario as the "realistic scenario to achieve ambitious targets," or simply the "realistic scenario." The optimally allocated distribution of funds under this realistic scenario is illustrated in figure 6.2 alongside the allocations of the status quo scenario, which represents the 2013 allocation to HIV programs in Kazakhstan. The figure shows the "best-fit" result, whereas table 6.1 presents uncertainty bounds around the optimal allocation of funds in the realistic scenario to achieve ambitious targets.

Summary of Scenario Allocations and Outcomes

Table 6.1 (which covers the period from 2015 through 2020) summarizes the allocation to—and associated coverage of—each modeled program for the status quo scenario and also the combined allocative and implementation efficiency scenario to achieve ambitious targets. The table also contains several key summary epidemiological outcomes from the modeled scenarios. Note that, although total 2015 spending is constrained by the relevant assumption of available budget, spending in consecutive years may vary slightly because of treatment liabilities, where treatment coverage is held constant as a proportion rather than the number of people receiving treatment.

Table 6.1 summarizes a number of key results. In the realistic scenario that achieves the ambitious targets, more funds were directed to programs for key populations: coverage for FSW and client prevention programs

Figure 6.2 Allocations to Kazakhstan's Programs under the Status Quo Scenario and the Realistic Scenario to Achieve Ambitious Targets

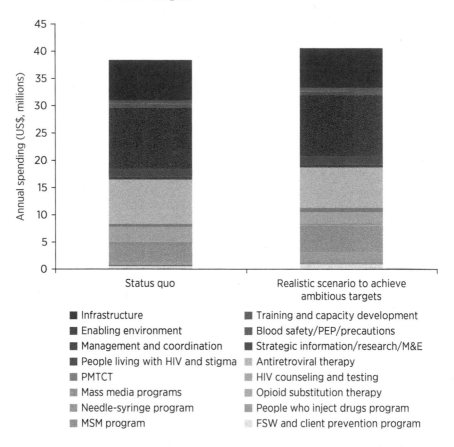

Source: Shattock et al. 2017.

Note: ART = antiretroviral therapy; FSW = female sex worker; HIV = human immunodeficiency virus; M&E = monitoring and evaluation; MSM = men who have sex with men; PEP = post-exposure prophylaxis; PMTCT = prevention of mother-to-child transmission; US$ = US dollar.

increased from 78 percent to 90 percent (85–94 percent); coverage for prevention programs for MSM rose from 8 percent to 19 percent (17–19 percent); coverage in programs for PWID increased from 19 percent to 51 percent (41–54 percent); and coverage in needle and syringe exchange programs (NSPs) rose from 51 percent to 57 percent

Table 6.1 Allocations to Kazakhstan's Programs, Associated Coverage Levels, and Key Epidemiological Outcomes

Analysis to end of 2020	Status quo	Realistic scenario to achieve ambitious targets
Allocation to FSW and client prevention program in 2015 (US$)	604,449	848,673 (737,336–1.0 million)
Allocation to MSM prevention program in 2015 (US$)	128,140	555,350 (376,739–622,025)
Allocation to PWID program in 2015 (US$)	456,213	1.7 million (1.1 million–2.0 million)
Allocation to NSP in 2015 (US$)	3.3 million	4.9 million (4.1 million–5.1 million)
Allocation to OST in 2015 (US$)	73,775	157,946 (73,775–495,909)
Allocation to mass media programs in 2015 (US$)	591,654	211,835 (0–545,436)
Allocation to HIV counseling and testing in 2015 (US$)	2.6 million	2.1 million (2.3 million–3.3 million)
Allocation to PMTCT in 2015 (US$)	551,634	753,810 (710,264–862,413)
Allocation to ART in 2015 (US$)	8.1 million	7.5 million (7.2 million–7.9 million)
Total HIV spending 2015 (US$)	38.3 million	38.3 million
Total direct program spending, 2015–20 (US$)	101.1 million (101.0 million–101.3 million)	110.5 million (107.7 million–116.8 million)
Total indirect program spending, 2015–20 (US$)	130.7 million	116.9 million (110.9 milllion–119.9 million)
Total HIV spending, 2015–20 (US$)	231.9 million (231.7 million–232.0 million)	227.4 million (226.1 million–228.7 million)
FSW and client condom program coverage (%)	78	90 (85–94)
MSM condom program coverage (%)	8	19 (17–19)
PWID condom program coverage (%)	19	51 (41–54)
NSP coverage (%)	51	57 (55–58)
OST program coverage (%)	0.2	0.8 (0–1)
Mass media program coverage (%)	14	6 (0–13)
PLHIV who know their status (%)	82 (81–82)	90 (89–92)
PMTCT program coverage (%)	75	86 (84–90)

continued next page

Table 6.1 *(continued)*

Analysis to end of 2020	Status quo	Realistic scenario to achieve ambitious targets
ART coverage (eligibility: diagnosed and CD4 cell count < 500 cells/mm³) (%)	47 (46–49)	99 (97–99)
Those on treatment who are virally suppressed (%)	87 (85–89)	87 (85–89)
Number on first-line treatment	5,129 (5,094–5,169)	14,667 (14,400–15,374)
Number on second-line treatment	551 (550–552)	1,057 (1,037–1,096)
Number eligible for treatment (eligibility: diagnosed and CD4 cell count < 500 cells/mm³)	11,983 (11,594–12,377)	15,942 (15,711–16,687)
Cumulative new infections 2015–20	9,471 (8,896–10,065)	3,971 (3,920–4,295)
Cumulative AIDS-related deaths 2015–20	6,505 (6,185–6,819)	2,287 (2,200–2,324)
Overall prevalence in 2020 (%)	0.14 (0.14–0.15)	0.13 (0.13–0.14)
Number of PLHIV in 2020	19,171 (18,360–19,998)	17,889 (17,530–18,510)
New infections averted by 2020	Baseline	5,500 (5,052–5,832)
AIDS-related deaths averted by 2020	Baseline	4,218 (4,048–4,466)

Source: Shattock et al. 2017.

Note: AIDS = acquired immune deficiency syndrome; ART = antiretroviral therapy; FSW = female sex worker; HIV = human immunodeficiency virus; MSM = men who have sex with men; NSP = needle and syringe exchange program; OST = opioid substitution therapy; PLHIV = people living with HIV; PMTCT = prevention of mother-to-child transmission; PWID = people who inject drugs; US$ = US dollar.

(55–58 percent). Program coverage also increased for opioid substitution therapy (OST) (from 0.2 percent to 0.8 percent [0.2–1.1 percent]) and PMTCT programs (from 75 percent to 86 percent [84–90 percent]), although coverage of mass media programs decreased from 14 percent to 6 percent (0–13 percent). ART coverage (where those diagnosed with a CD4 count of less than 500 cells per mm³ of blood are eligible [WHO 2015]) increased from 47 percent in the status quo scenario to greater than 90 percent under the realistic scenario to achieve ambitious targets. Because of the assumed decrease in the cost of ART procurement in this scenario, the annual cost of such a program is less (US$7.5 million in 2015) than for the status quo scenario (US$8.1 million in 2015). In addition, with a 19 percent (14–27 percent) reduction in management costs obtained through implementation efficiencies, the percentage of the total HIV budget consumed by indirect costs for 2015–20 is reduced from 56 percent to 51 percent (49–53 percent) under the realistic scenario to achieve ambitious targets compared to the status quo scenario.

The results also indicate that annual newly acquired sexual- and injecting-related HIV infections and AIDS-related deaths will increase in 2020 from 2014 levels under the baseline status quo (figure 6.3). In contrast, annual newly acquired sexual- and injecting-related infections are projected to decrease by 50 percent and 63 percent, respectively, under the realistic scenario of achieving ambitious targets. AIDS-related deaths are estimated to decrease by 71 percent under this scenario. These percentages translate to an estimated 5,500 newly acquired HIV infections and 4,220 AIDS-related deaths being averted under the realistic scenario to achieve ambitious targets compared to the status quo scenario between 2014 and 2020. Virtual elimination of mother-to-child-transmission would also be achieved in the ambitious targets scenario, which was not the case when status quo spending was projected. Because of the epidemiological impact of the realistic scenario to achieve ambitious targets, future treatment liabilities decrease and, over time, the cost of the HIV response begins to decrease accordingly—so much so that between 2015 and 2020 the total cumulative cost of the ambitious targets scenario is estimated to be US$4.5 million less (US$227.4 million) than the status quo scenario (US$231.9 million).

Policy Implications

The government of Kazakhstan has moved to increase domestic responsibility for the HIV budget; between 2007 and 2011 the domestic share of ART funding increased from 7 percent to 100 percent (UNAIDS 2013b). Many other countries have already implemented, or are soon likely to require, a similar transition from international to domestic sources to finance their national HIV responses (Development Continuum Working Group 2015). Historically, however, delays have occurred between external funding withdrawal and domestic funding scale-up (Duric, Leso et al. 2015). Among other factors, delays may be due to political sensitivities surrounding key affected populations such as PWID, FSWs, and MSM (Duric, Leso et al. 2015). In this context of domestic responsibility for key affected population programs, a success story has emerged from Croatia. Following large-scale external support

Figure 6.3 Epidemiological Outcomes under the Status Quo Scenario and Realistic Scenario to Achieve Ambitious Targets in 2020, Compared to 2014

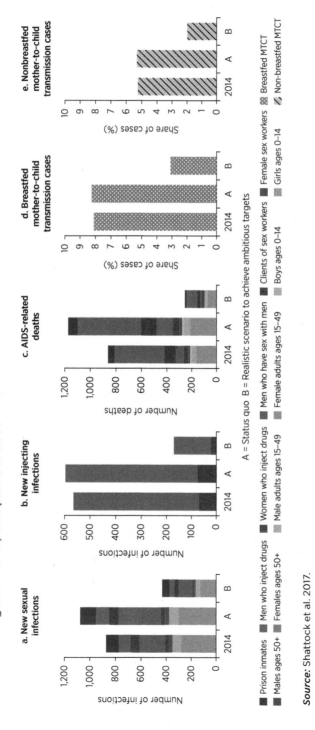

A = Status quo B = Realistic scenario to achieve ambitious targets

Prison inmates ■ Men who inject drugs ■ Women who inject drugs ■ Men who have sex with men ■ Clients of sex workers ■ Female sex workers ■ Breastfed MTCT

Males ages 50+ ■ Females ages 50+ ■ Male adults ages 15–49 ■ Female adults ages 15–49 ■ Boys ages 0–14 ■ Girls ages 0–14 ⊘ Non-breastfed MTCT

Source: Shattock et al. 2017.

Note: Figure illustrates the epidemiological outcomes estimated to arise by implementing the allocation scenarios in figure 6.2 between 2015 and 2020. The first column in each panel represents the value of the indicator in 2014. AIDS = acquired immune deficiency syndrome; MTCT = mother-to-child transmission.

between 2003 and 2006, primarily from the Global Fund, Croatia has since transitioned to a fully domestically financed response and has further scaled up key programs (Duric, Leso et al. 2015). A key factor in Croatia's successful transition to domestic financing was the cooperation between the government and nongovernmental organizations to target resources to otherwise marginalized populations (Duric, Leso et al. 2015). Kazakhstan has also achieved some success in transitioning funding for key affected populations.

The modeling results indicated that, by continuing the 2013 HIV intervention strategy, Kazakhstan would likely have more annual newly acquired infections and AIDS-related deaths in 2020 than 2014. In the absence of allocative, implementation, and technical efficiencies, an estimated 32 percent increase in total HIV budget would be required to achieve national targets. Alternatively, the modeling findings suggested the same targets could be satisfied with no increase in budget by reallocating funding to focus on programs for key affected populations, reducing management costs, reducing ART procurement costs, and consequently increasing treatment coverage. More ambitious epidemiological targets could also be attained without additional overall resourcing. The results suggest that Kazakhstan could potentially reduce new HIV infections and AIDS-related deaths by 50 percent of 2014 levels by 2020 even without replenishment of the 20 percent of the HIV budget expected to be withdrawn. Such an outcome, however, would require substantial implementation efficiency gains and very large reductions in ART costs beyond the levels deemed reasonable by country representatives and key stakeholders.

Allocative efficiency studies have been carried out in many countries to highlight potential inefficiencies in investment approaches (Anderson et al. 2014; Duric, Hamelmann et al. 2015a, 2015b; Fraser et al. 2015; Gouws et al. 2006; Panovska-Griffiths et al. 2014; Wirtz et al. 2013). A 2015 study of the concentrated epidemic in Sudan concluded that reallocating resources from untargeted general population programs to treatment programs, prevention programs for FSWs, and prevention programs for MSM could result in substantial epidemiological gains (Kerr et al. 2015). In light of these findings, the Sudanese government has since shifted funding priorities to closer align with the findings of the study (World Bank 2015). Within Eastern Europe and Central Asia, Armenia has undertaken several studies to assess the allocative efficiency of its HIV response (Kelly et al. 2016; Wilson, Gray, and Hoare 2012), and it has used the evidence to advocate for resources to be targeted toward cost-effective programs for key affected populations such as short-term labor migrants (Agadjanian, Markosyan, and CRRC–Armenia 2013).

Notes on the Modeling

As with all mathematical modeling studies, it is important that these findings be interpreted with an appreciation of the inherent assumptions. The modeling study assumed that it is possible for ART costs to be reduced by up to 80 percent, but whether such reductions in treatment costs are plausible in Kazakhstan is debatable. A 2012 analysis found that implementing partners in Mozambique were able to reduce the mean unit cost of ART by 45 percent between 2009 and 2011 by adjusting inefficient service delivery models (Holmes et al. 2012). Along with more efficient drug procurement via the United Nations and the Global Fund systems, several other factors may synergistically contribute to reduce costs of ART in Kazakhstan. The patent for tenofovir disoproxil fumarate (TDF), a nucleotide reverse transcriptase inhibitor commonly used in fixed-dose combination ART, was set to expire at the end of 2017 (Clayden et al. 2016). Because both originator and generic drug prices typically decrease as associated patents near expiration (Sagaon-Teyssier et al. 2016), it is likely that the cost of purchasing current combinations of ART will decrease. Further, trials have shown that optimizing antiretroviral dosages such that any negative effect on viral suppression is negligible can help to cut the cost of HIV treatment. A number of dose optimization trials comparing the virological efficacy of a reduced dose versus a standard dose of an antiretroviral drug have also been completed (Bunupuradah et al. 2015; Carey 2014), finding that several antiretroviral agents show no difference in virological suppression rates across the different dosages. The implication of reduced antiretroviral dosages on the cost of treatment programs could potentially be substantial.

The analyses in this case considered efficiency gains in both direct and indirect programs. It was assumed that management costs, as indirect costs that absorb a large portion of national funding but cannot be mathematically optimized because of their unquantifiable effect on epidemiological outcomes, can be reduced while still allowing for essential functions to be maintained. A study of the HIV response in Ukraine estimated that costs associated with program staff could be reduced on average by 18 percent while maintaining the same level of outputs (World Bank 2014). In the case of Kazakhstan, the analysis focused on a scenario that incorporates a reduction of approximately 20 percent in management costs—a selection made in line with national expert opinion that it is realistically attainable. It further considered scenarios that assume management costs can be reduced by up to 50 percent of 2013 levels without detrimental effect on the direct treatment and prevention programs that such spending supports. Such results are included to indicate what epidemiological gains may be attainable if such efficiency gains can be achieved. Additional setting-specific work is needed for specific implementation efficiency analyses to understand the plausibility and potential impact of such spending cuts. Further, the results assume that achieving the instant scale-up and scale-down of treatment and prevention programs to optimal levels is plausible. In reality, it may not be plausible if certain logistical, ethical, and political constraints exist that slow or even prevent the scale-up of programs to optimal levels.

The modeling findings suggest that Kazakhstan will not be able to substantially reduce new infections and deaths unless coverages of key prevention and treatment services are scaled up. Achieving the proposed high coverage of effective ART will require extensive demand generation and adherence support. Among PWID, access to OST has been shown to substantially improve adherence to ART (Binford, Kahana, and Altice 2012; Roux et al. 2009) and is thus likely to be an essential condition for a successful treatment program among this key at-risk population. Additional outreach support programs may also be required to increase access and adherence to ART for key populations such as FSWs, MSM, and PWID.

Faced with donor withdrawal and an HIV epidemic that was not decreasing, it was important for Kazakhstan's HIV response to achieve more with limited available resources. This analysis helped guide policy makers in directing available resources to achieve the greatest returns from HIV investments, and ultimately turn the tide of the national epidemic.

Recommendations

The allocative efficiency study produced the following key recommendations for policy makers and planners in Kazakhstan (Shattock et al. 2017):

1. Kazakhstan's investments are already making a great difference in slowing the spread of the HIV epidemic, and the level of investment needs to be sustained. With no programs in place, the HIV epidemic would grow dramatically and a projected 54,000 new infections and 11,100 deaths would occur from 2015 to 2020. Given existing spending and allocations, the epidemic would grow slowly, and 9,500 new infections and 6,500 deaths would occur over 2015–20.
2. By optimizing existing allocations to HIV programs, Kazakhstan could reduce new infections and deaths. Optimized allocation of US$37.8 million (2013 spending) would avert 6 percent of new infections and 22 percent of deaths over 2015–20 compared to the status quo (2013 allocations maintained during the same period). Optimized allocation of 2013 spending would imply increasing coverage of ART from 47 percent to 61 percent (CD4 < 500 cells/mm^3) and of programs for

MSM from 8 percent to 15 percent. Simultaneously, the existing high levels of coverage of NSPs for PWID and existing coverage of OST would be sustained, and savings in the other programs would be made.

3. With additional savings on management costs, Kazakhstan could substantially further increase the impact of the national HIV response. With the same amount of money available as in 2013, saving 20 percent of management costs at existing levels of funding and allocating the resources optimally would avert 18 percent of new infections and 32 percent of deaths, compared to existing allocations.

4. At the 2013 unit costs of programs, achieving the national HIV prevention and treatment targets would require substantial additional investment. To achieve the national targets (no increase in HIV incidence and deaths) would cost US$51.8 million per year—33 percent more than 2013 spending. Achieving the more ambitious targets (reducing new infections and deaths by 50 percent) would cost US$80.1 million, thus requiring substantially increased investment.

5. Reducing the unit cost of ART and scaling up ART to high coverage levels are the key elements required to achieve the national targets at existing spending levels. The unit cost for ART in Kazakhstan has been high compared to other countries in the region, and the effect of a reduction of unit costs by 67 percent (from US$2,280 to US$760 per person reached per year) was explored. Even with such a substantial reduction, ART cost would still be within the range of costs reported by other countries in the region. Combining the ART cost reduction with a 20 percent reduction of management cost and optimized allocation of funds would make it possible to achieve a 50 percent decrease in both HIV incidence and deaths with an annual investment of US$37.7 million—approximately the 2013 funding levels.

6. In Kazakhstan's concentrated HIV epidemic, there is continued need to focus analysis, planning, and implementation on key populations, particularly PWID, MSM, prison inmates, and FSWs and their clients. Under conditions at the time of analysis (constant behaviors and program coverage), new HIV infections are projected to rise by 13 percent and deaths by 32 percent between 2014 and 2020. The epidemics among PWID and MSM are projected to account for two-thirds of new HIV infections and must be core foci of programs.

7. Addressing the HIV epidemic and wider health needs of PWID remains a critical priority for Kazakhstan. NSPs should be sustained with at least 50 percent coverage and further scaled up in the context of comprehensive harm-reduction programs. OST has important effects on HIV prevention and ART adherence and should be provided at substantially larger scale.

8. Addressing the growing MSM epidemic requires an increased coverage of MSM programs. By 2020, MSM are projected to account for approximately 20 percent of new HIV infections. Under 2013 allocations, program coverage would remain low at 8 percent, but it should increase substantially to at least 20 percent. This increased coverage will require pragmatic outreach approaches through informal networks while continuing existing efforts to reduce stigma and discrimination, so that more ambitious targets can be set in future.

9. A reduction in management costs of approximately 20 percent could be explored further in a technical efficiency analysis. Kazakhstan reported management and other costs as 56 percent of total HIV spending. This percentage includes infrastructure costs and can be partially explained by the inclusion of management costs of specific programs.

10. Domestic investment in Kazakhstan's HIV programs is critical to sustain the response, including programs previously covered by the Global Fund, following the country's graduation from Global Fund support.[4] If Kazakhstan can sustain the total level of HIV funding and if the proposed technical efficiency gains can be realized, the country's 2013 level of HIV investment will remain sufficient to achieve the ambitious targets of reducing HIV incidence by 50 percent. If ART costs cannot be reduced, HIV investments must be increased accordingly.

Making Use of the Results

Kazakhstan is among a few countries in the region where ART is fully funded by the government and provided free of charge to patients. The exorbitant cost of ART drugs (on average US$2,280 per patient in 2014) has financially prohibited government scale-up of the HIV treatment program. This high cost of treatment has long been a cause for grave concern for the Kazakhstan Union of People Living with HIV, the Republican Center on Prevention and Control of AIDS (the Republican AIDS Center), and technical partners, notably the US Agency for International Development, the US Centers for Disease Control and Prevention, and UNAIDS.

UNAIDS played a convening role to initiate an extended dialogue between the government, the community of PLHIV, and technical partners to discuss ways to drastically reduce the cost of antiretroviral drugs. There was a growing consensus that the high prices were due to inefficiency in procurement done by a single state-owned procuring agency. As part of this effort, a roundtable in August 2015 focused on ART pricing and the possibility of using alternative methods of procuring antiretroviral drugs, including the UN procurement system, specifically the United Nations Children's

Fund (UNICEF). Participants, including representatives from the Ministry of Health, the Ministry of Finance, the Republican AIDS Center, international donors, and civil society discussed the UNAIDS strategy for reaching the 90-90-90 treatment targets. Issues of ART pricing in the country attracted great interest, including criticism voiced by representatives of Kazakhstan's nongovernmental sector and the Kazakhstan Union of People Living with HIV. After the roundtable, the UNAIDS country office coordinated ongoing discussions with the government that ART prices in the country can be significantly reduced by using the UN procurement mechanism.

Additionally, the UNAIDS office and the Republican AIDS Center effectively used different platforms to introduce the results of the allocative efficiency analysis, in particular the ART price reduction issue. The main outcomes of the study were presented in a session entitled "Improving Efficiency of HIV Investments in EECA (Eastern Europe and Central Asia) Region to End AIDS by 2030" at the Fifth Eastern Europe and Central Asia AIDS Conference, held in Moscow on March 23–25, 2016.

In 2016, a subregional meeting on presenting the results of allocative efficiency and optimized investments for Kazakhstan, the Kyrgyz Republic, and Tajikistan introduced the results of the allocative efficiency studies for each country and discussed optimizing allocation by reducing the currently high unit cost of ART. The UNAIDS executive director also met with the Prime Minister of Kazakhstan, the Chairman of the Kazakhstan Senate, the Minister of Health, the Deputy Minister of Foreign Affairs, and others and addressed the price for ART.

Kazakhstan's achievement on ART price reduction reflected the synergistic efforts of diverse stakeholders: the leadership and commitment of national government, the solidarity of the international community, and the engagement of civil society, most notably PLHIV. Building upon the advocacy campaign with use of allocative efficiency and optimized investments results, the Ministry of Health decided to procure best-value (lower price, ensured quality) ART drugs through the UN system, and in particular through the UNICEF mechanism. The Republican AIDS Center submitted to the UNICEF Supply Division the request for antiretroviral (ARV) procurement services at competitive prices to be provided to the country.

In September 2016, UNICEF and SK-Pharmacy (the main national company for procurement of medicines and medical equipment) signed a memorandum of understanding. In the framework of the memorandum, in 2017, for the first time, 11 ARV medicines were purchased through UNICEF, which allowed for an increase in ART coverage for HIV patients from fewer than 6,000 people before the analysis to approximately 14,500 in 2018; and the savings amounted to about 4 billion tenge (about US$11.7 million).

Notes

1. This chapter relies in part on an article the authors published with other colleagues in 2017 in *PLoS ONE* (Shattock et al. 2017) and on the World Bank (2016) report detailing the findings from the allocative efficiency analysis discussed herein. Portions of this chapter are taken from those sources and are reprinted here with all necessary permissions.
2. Data from the Organisation for Economic Co-operation and Development's Creditor Reporting System database, https://stats.oecd.org/Index.aspx?Data SetCode=CRS1.
3. Data from the Organisation for Economic Co-operation and Development's Creditor Reporting System database, https://stats.oecd.org/Index.aspx?Data Set Code=CRS1.
4. The Global Fund is phasing out support for upper-middle-income countries such as Kazakhstan.

References

Aceijas C. C., S. R. Friedman, H. L. F. Cooper, L. Wiessing, G. V. Stimson, and M. Hickman. 2006. "Estimates of Injecting Drug Users at the National and Local Level in Developing and Transitional Countries, and Gender and Age Distribution." *Sexually Transmitted Infections* 82 (Suppl. 3): iii10–iii17.

Agadjanian, D., K. Markosyan, and CRRC (Caucasus Research Resource Centers)–Armenia. 2013. "Labor Migration and STI/HIV Risks in Armenia: Assessing Prevention Needs and Designing Effective Interventions." Yerevan: CRRC–Armenia.

Anderson S.-J., P. Cherutich, N. Kilonzo, I. Cremin, D. Fecht, D. Kimanga, M. Harper, R. L. Masha, P. B. Ngongo, W. Maina, M. Dybul, and T. B. Hallett. 2014. "Maximising the Effect of Combination HIV Prevention through Prioritisation of the People and Places in Greatest Need: A Modelling Study." *Lancet* 384 (9939): 249–56.

Beyrer, C., and K. Q. Abdool. 2013. "The Changing Epidemiology of HIV in 2013." *Current Opinion in HIV and AIDS* 8 (4): 306–10.

Binford M. C., S. Y. Kahana, and F. L. Altice. 2012. "A Systematic Review of Antiretroviral Adherence Interventions for HIV-infected People Who Use Drugs." *Current HIV/AIDS Reports* 9 (4): 287–312.

Bobkov A. F., E. V. Kazennova, A. L. Sukhanova, M. R. Bobkova, V. V. Pokrovsky, V. V. Zeman, N. G. Kovtunenko, and I. B. Erasilova. 2004. "An HIV Type 1 Subtype A Outbreak among Injecting Drug Users in Kazakhstan." *AIDS Research and Human Retroviruses* 20 (10): 1134–36.

Bor J., A. J. Herbst, M.-L. Newell, and T. Bärnighausen. 2013. "Increases in Adult Life Expectancy in Rural South Africa: Valuing the Scale-up of HIV Treatment." *Science* 339 (6122): 961–65.

Bunupuradah T., S. Kiertiburanakul, A. Avihingsanon, P. Chetchotisakd, M. Techapornroong, N. Leerattanapetch, P. Kantipong, C. Bowonwatanuwong,

S. Banchongkit, V. Klinbuayaem, S. Mekviwattanawan, S. Nimitvilai, J. Sireethorn, P. Supunnee, M. Wisit, B. Warangkana, S. Chaivooth, P. Phanuphak, D. A. Cooper, T. Apornpong, S. J. Kerr, S. Emery, and K. Ruxrungtham, editors. 2015. "Atazanavir/Ritonavir 200/100 mg Is Non-inferior to Atazanavir/Ritonavir 300/100 mg in Virologic Suppressed HIV-Infected Thai Adults: A Multicentre, Randomized, Open-label Trial: LASA." *Journal of the International AIDS Society* 18 (5): 20356.

Carey, D. 2014. "Efavirenz 400 mg Daily Remains Non-inferior to 600 mg: 96 Week Data from the Double-Blind, Placebo-Controlled ENCORE1 Study." *Journal of the International AIDS Society* 17 (4 Suppl. 3): 19523.

Clayden P., S. Collins, M. Frick, M. Harrington, T. Horn, R. Jefferys, E. Lessem, and L. McKenna. 2016. "Drugs, Diagnostics, Vaccines, Preventive Technologies, Research Toward a Cure, and Immune-Based and Gene Therapies in Development." *2016 Pipeline Report: HIV and TB.* http://www.treatmentac tiongroup.org/sites/default/files/2016%20Pipeline%20Report%20Full.pdf.

DeHovitz J., A. Uuskula, and N. El-Bassel. 2014. "The HIV Epidemic in Eastern Europe and Central Asia." *Current HIV/AIDS Reports* 11 (2): 168–76.

Development Continuum Working Group. 2015. "Evolving the Global Fund for Greater Impact in a Changing Global Landscape." Report for the Global Fund Secretariat. Global Fund to Fight AIDS, Tuberculosis and Malaria, Geneva. https://www.theglobalfund.org/media/4151/bm33_developmentcontinuum workinggroup_report_en.pdf?u=636488964340000000.

Duric, P., C. Hamelmann, D. P. Wilson, and C. Kerr. 2015a. "Modelling an Optimised Investment Approach for Tajikistan." UNDP Eastern Europe and Central Asia Series on Sustainable Financing of National HIV Responses, Government of Tajikistan, Dushanbe.

Duric, P., C. Hamelmann, D. P. Wilson, and C. Kerr. 2015b. "Modelling an Optimised Investment Approach for Uzbekistan." UNDP Eastern Europe and Central Asia Series on Sustainable Financing of National HIV Responses, Government of Uzbekistan, Tashkent.

Duric, P., D. Leso, I. Jovovic, and C. Hamelmann. 2015. "Towards Domestic Financing of National HIV Responses: Lessons Learnt from Croatia." UNDP Eastern Europe and Central Asia Series on Sustainable Financing of National HIV Responses, United Nations Development Programme.

Eaton J. W., N. A. Menzies, J. Stover, V. Cambiano, L. Chindelevitch, A. Cori, J. A. Hontelez, S. Humair, C. C. Kerr, D. J. Klein, S. Mishra, K. M. Mitchell, B. E. Nichols, P. Vickerman, R. Bakker, T. Bärnighausen, A. Bershteyn, D. E. Bloom, M. C. Boily, S. T. Chang, T. Cohen, P. J. Dodd, C. Fraser, C. Gopalappa, J. Lundgren, N. K. Martin, E. Mikkelsen, E. Mountain, Q. D. Pham, M. Pickles, A. Phillips, L. Platt, C. Pretorius, H. J. Prudden, J. A. Salomon, D. A. van de Viver, S. J. de Vlas, B. G. Wagner, R. G. White, D. P. Wilson, L. Zhang, J. Blandford, G. Meyer-Rath, M. Remme, P. Revill, N. Sangrujee, F. Terris-Presholt, M. Doherty, N. Shaffer, P. J. Easterbrook, G. Hirnschall, and T. B. Hallett. 2014. "Health Benefits, Costs, and Cost-Effectiveness of Earlier Eligibility for Adult Antiretroviral Therapy and Expanded Treatment Coverage: A Combined Analysis of 12 Mathematical Models." *Lancet Global Health* 2 (1): e23–e34.

El-Bassel N., L. Gilbert, A. Terlikbayeva, E. Wu, C. Beyrer, S. Shaw, T. Hunt, X. Ma, M. Chang, L. Ismayilova, M. Tukeyev, B. Zhussupov, and Y. Rozental. 2013. "HIV among Injection Drug Users and Their Intimate Partners in Almaty, Kazakhstan." *AIDS and Behavior* 17 (7): 2490–500.

El-Bassel N., S. A. Shaw, A. Dasgupta, and S. A. Strathdee. 2014. "Drug Use as a Driver of HIV Risks: Re-emerging and Emerging Issues." *Current Opinion in HIV and AIDS* 9 (2): 150–55.

Enserink M. 2014. "After the Windfall." *Science* 345 (6202): 1258–59.

Forsythe S., J. Stover, and L. Bollinger. 2009. "The Past, Present and Future of HIV, AIDS and Resource Allocation." *BMC Public Health* 9 (Suppl. 1): S1–S4.

Fraser N., C. C. Kerr, Z. Harouna, Z. Alhousseini, N. Cheikh, R. Gray, A. Shattock, D. P. Wilson, M. Haacker, Z. Shubber, E. Masaki, D. Karamoko, and M. Görgens. 2015. "Reorienting the HIV Response in Niger toward Sex Work Interventions: From Better Evidence to Targeted and Expanded Practice." *Journal of Acquired Immune Deficiency Syndromes* 68 (Suppl. 2): S213–S220.

Global Fund (Global Fund to Fight AIDS, Tuberculosis and Malaria). 2007. "Report of the Fifteenth Board Meeting." Global Fund to Fight AIDS, Tuberculosis and Malaria, Geneva.

Gouws E., P. White, J. Stover, and T. Brown. 2006. "Short Term Estimates of Adult HIV Incidence by Mode of Transmission: Kenya and Thailand as Examples." *Sexually Transmitted Infections* 82 (Suppl. 3): iii51–iii55.

Holmes C. B., J. M. Blandford, N. Sangrujee, S. R. Stewart, A. DuBois, T. R. Smith, J. C. Martin, A. Gavaghan, C. A. Ryan, and E. P. Goosby. 2012. "PEPFAR's Past and Future Efforts to Cut Costs, Improve Efficiency, and Increase the Impact of Global HIV Programs." *Health Affairs* 31 (7): 1553–60.

ICAP. 2011. "Epidemiological Profile for HIV/AIDS, Kazakhstan." ICAP, Columbia University, New York.

Kazakhstan, Ministry of Health. 2016. "Country Progress Report on HIV Infection Response–Republic of Kazakhstan." Ministry of Health, Astana. http://www.unaids.org/en/regionscountries/countries/kazakhstan.

Kelly S. L., A. J. Shattock, C. C. Kerr, R. M. Stuart, A. Papoyan, T. Grigoryan, R. Horvannisyan, S. Grigoryan, C. Benedikt, and D. P. Wilson. 2016. "Optimizing HIV/AIDS Resources in Armenia: Increasing ART Investment and Examining HIV Programmes for Seasonal Migrant Labourers." *Journal of the International AIDS Society* 19 (1): 20772.

Kerr C. C., R. M. Stuart, R. T. Gray, A. J. Shattock, N. Fraser-Hurt, C. Benedikt, M. Haacker, M. Berdnikov, A. M. Mahmood, S. A. Jaber, M. Görgens, and D. P. Wilson. 2015. "Optima: A Model for HIV Epidemic Analysis, Program Prioritization, and Resource Optimization." *Journal of Acquired Immune Deficiency Syndromes* 69 (3): 365–76.

Mahy M., J. Stover, K. Kiragu, C. Hayashi, P. Akwara, C. Luo, K. Stanecki, R. Ekpini, and N. Shaffer. 2010. "What Will It Take to Achieve Virtual Elimination of Mother-to-Child Transmission of HIV? An Assessment of Current Progress and Future Needs." *Sexually Transmitted Infections* 86 (Suppl. 2): ii48–ii55.

MSF (Médecins Sans Frontières). 2014. *Untangling the Web of Antiretroviral Price Reductions,* 17th ed. Geneva: MSF.

Palmer, S., and D. J. Torgerson. 1999. "Definitions of Efficiency." *BMJ* 318 (7191): 1136.

Panovska-Griffiths J., A. Vassall, H. J. Prudden, A. Lépine, M.-C. Boily, S. Chandrashekar S, K. M. Mitchell, T. S. Beatie, M. Alary, N. K. Martin, and P. Vickerman. 2014. "Optimal Allocation of Resources in Female Sex Worker Targeted HIV Prevention Interventions: Model Insights from Avahan in South India." *PloS ONE* 9 (10): e107066.

PEPFAR (US President's Emergency Plan for AIDS Relief). 2016. "Central Asia PEPFAR Regional Operational Plan (ROP) 2016: Strategic Direction Summary." https://tj.usembassy.gov/wp-content/uploads/sites/143/2017/05/CAR-ROP16-SDS-May6-2016-final.pdf.

Roux P., M. P. Carrieri, J. Cohen, I. Ravaux, I. Poizot-Martin, P. Dellamonica, and B. Spire. 2009. "Retention in Opioid Substitution Treatment: A Major Predictor of Long-Term Virological Success for HIV-Infected Injection Drug Users Receiving Antiretroviral Treatment." *Clinical Infectious Diseases* 49 (9): 1433–40.

Sandgren E., S. Sandgren, M. Urazalin, and R. Andersson. 2008. "HIV/AIDS Awareness and Risk Behaviour among Pregnant Women in Semey, Kazakhstan, 2007." *BMC Public Health* 8 (1): 295.

Sagaon-Teyssier L., S. Singh, B. Dongmo-Nguimfack, and J.-P. Moatti. 2016. "Affordability of Adult HIV/AIDS Treatment in Developing Countries: Modelling Price Determinants for a Better Insight of the Market Functioning." *JAIDS Journal of the International AIDS Society* 19(1): 20619.

Shattock A. J., C. Benedikt, A. Bokazhanova, P. Duric, I. Petrenko, L. Ganina, S. L. Kelly, R. M. Stuart, C. C. Kerr, T. Vinichenko, S.-F. Zhang, C. Hamelmann, M. Manova, E. Masaki, and D. P. Wilson. 2017. "Kazakhstan Can Achieve Ambitious HIV Targets despite Expected Donor Withdrawal by Combining Improved ART Procurement Mechanisms with Allocative and Implementation Efficiencies." *PLoS One* 12 (2): e0169530. doi:10.1371/journal.pone.0169530.

Tanser F., T. Bärnighausen, E. Grapsa, J. Zaidi, and M.-L. Newell. 2013. "High Coverage of ART Associated with Decline in Risk of HIV Acquisition in Rural KwaZulu-Natal, South Africa." *Science* 339 (6122): 966–71.

Thorne C., N. Ferencic, R. Malyuta, J. Mimica, and T. Niemiec. 2010. "Central Asia: Hotspot in the Worldwide HIV Epidemic." *Lancet Infectious Diseases* 10 (7): 479–88.

UNAIDS (Joint United Nations Programme on HIV/AIDS). 2013a. "AIDS by the Numbers." UNAIDS, Geneva. http://www.unaids.org/sites/default/files/media_asset/JC2571_AIDS_by_the_numbers_en_1.pdf.

UNAIDS (Joint United Nations Programme on HIV/AIDS). 2013b. *Efficient and Sustainable HIV Responses: Case Studies on Country Progress.* Geneva: UNAIDS.

UNICEF (United Nations Children's Fund). 2007. "UNICEF Procurement of HIV/AIDS-Related Supplies." UNICEF. https://www.unicef.org/supply/files/Procurement_of_HA_supplies.pdf.

WHO (World Health Organization). 2010. *Towards the Elimination of Mother-to-Child Transmission of HIV.* Geneva: WHO.

WHO (World Health Organization). 2015. *Consolidated Strategic Information Guidelines for HIV in the Health Sector*. Geneva: WHO.

Wilson D. P., R. T. Gray, and A. Hoare. 2012. "Getting to Zero: HIV Prevention Resource Needs and Optimal Allocations in Armenia." Report prepared for the Global Fund to Fight AIDS, Tuberculosis and Malaria, The Kirby Institute, University of New South Wales, Sydney.

Wirtz A., D. Walker, L. Bollinger, F. Sifakis, S. Baral, B. Johns, R. Oelrichs, and C. Beyrer. 2013. "Modelling the Impact of HIV Prevention and Treatment for Men Who Have Sex with Men on HIV Epidemic Trajectories in Low- and Middle-Income Countries." *International Journal of STD & AIDS* 24 (1): 18–30.

World Bank. 2014. "Ukraine HIV Program Efficiency Study: Can Ukraine Improve Value for Money in HIV Service Delivery?" World Bank, Washington, DC. http://optimamodel.com/pubs/Ukraine%20HIV%20Program%20 Efficiency%20Report_final%20with%20Cover.pdf.

World Bank. 2015. "From Analysis to Action: A Case Study on How Allocative Efficiency Analysis Supported by Mathematical Modelling Changed HIV Investments in Sudan." World Bank, Washington, DC.

World Bank. 2016. "Optimizing Investments in Kazakhstan's HIV Response." World Bank, Washington, DC. https://openknowledge.worldbank.org/bitstream /handle/10986/24965/106814.pdf?sequence=5&isAllowed=y.

7

Kyrgyz Republic
Addressing the HIV Treatment Gap

*Meerim Sarybaeva, Andrew J. Shattock, Talgat Mambetov,
Larisa Bashmakova, Liutsiia Ianbukhtina, Manoela
Manova, Richard T. Gray, Clemens Benedikt,
and Katherine Ward*

Briefly

- Coverage for antiretroviral therapy (ART) has been particularly low in the Kyrgyz Republic, despite relatively high per capita spending on HIV.
- Management costs have accounted for a higher than average share of the HIV budget.
- The unit costs of some prevention programs have been high.
- Low ART coverage needs to be addressed.
- The implementation efficiency of all programs should be enhanced.

Introduction

One of the Central Asian countries that gained independence from the Soviet Union in 1991 and a nation with a proud heritage spanning many centuries, the Kyrgyz Republic has faced a number of challenges as the nation and its people have worked to chart a new course while dealing with the realities of limited resources and competing demands.

Human immunodeficiency virus (HIV) and acquired immune deficiency syndrome (AIDS) have been a significant and growing part of that portfolio of challenges. As both the challenge posed and the response to the epidemic grew, the Kyrgyz government recognized the importance of undertaking a systematic analysis of its response. To that end, in 2014–15, the World Bank was asked to conduct an allocative efficiency analysis of the national HIV response budget using the Optima HIV model. This analysis was particularly important in light of changes to the funding streams available—particularly the anticipated decline in support from the Global Fund to Fight AIDS, Tuberculosis and Malaria (the Global Fund), which had been the Kyrgyz Republic's major external funding partner for the HIV response.

The resulting allocative efficiency analysis highlighted a number of promising areas where improvement was important and possible (World Bank 2015).[1] Of particular note were findings concerning coverage and the high unit cost of HIV services. This analysis was continued within the framework of the mid-term evaluation of the government program in 2015 to revise the technical efficiency of the national response to HIV. The evaluation found that significant loss of clients was occurring at every stage of the treatment cascade, especially among people who inject drugs (PWID). This chapter reviews some of the main findings and recommendations from the allocative efficiency analysis, as well as steps taken to strengthen the government's HIV programming and funding allocations in light of those findings.

To ensure their consistency and relevance, and unless otherwise indicated, the data provided in this chapter relate to the situation in the Kyrgyz Republic at the time the analysis was conducted.

Overview of the Epidemic

Despite considerable efforts by the government, civil society, and international organizations, the HIV epidemic in the Kyrgyz Republic has continued to grow. From 2012 through 2016, the number of HIV infections in the country increased twofold from 3,317 to 7,108. HIV has continued to spread among men, women, and children; and it affects mainly people of working age (20–49 years).

The epidemic is transitioning from an early concentrated epidemic among PWID into an advanced concentrated HIV epidemic[2] with continued transmission among PWID, but with an increasing share of sexual transmission to female partners of PWID and among men who have sex with men (MSM). Newly diagnosed cases of HIV among PWID remain an issue, along with an increasing trend of sexual transmission and a growing number of women newly diagnosed with HIV. Since 2012, the number of HIV-positive women has increased by over 230 percent; among all newly diagnosed HIV cases, the percentage accounted for by women increased from 30 percent in 2012 to 42 percent in 2016. The prevailing mode of transmission for newly diagnosed women is sexual: as of the beginning of 2016, 84 percent of such newly diagnosed cases were attributed to sexual transmission, with 9 percent attributed to injections. In men, sexual and parenteral modes of transmission each accounted for 40 percent of all new cases, whereas MSM accounted for 8 percent according to self-reporting, which may be subject to reporting bias (figure 7.1).

At the same time, PWID constituted a smaller percentage of all newly registered cases—down to 24.6 percent from 59.6 percent in 2010. According to integrated biobehavioral surveillance in 2016, a risk remains that the epidemic could expand because of the high prevalence of antibodies to syphilis, the growth of viral hepatitis C, and the limited coverage of HIV prevention and testing.

New HIV diagnoses have been registered in all regions of the country, but the prevalence is unevenly distributed among the oblasts. In absolute numbers, the largest cumulative number of HIV infections is registered in Chui Oblast; HIV prevalence is highest in Osh (2.6 per 1,000), whereas prevalence in Chui Oblast is 1.5 per 1,000. Four regions

Figure 7.1   Self-Reported Modes of HIV Transmission in the Kyrgyz Republic, 2016

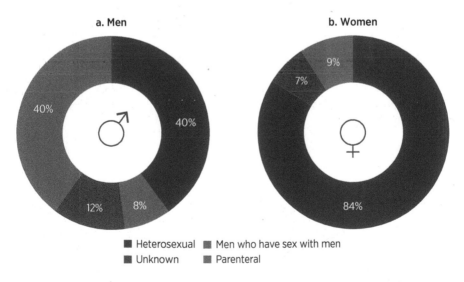

Source: World Bank based on Kyrgyz Republic National AIDS Center data from the integrated biobehavioral surveillance (IBBS).

Note: Data do not include children ages 0–15. HIV = human immunodeficiency virus.

Figure 7.2 Number of People Registered with HIV Infection in Oblasts, Cumulative Data, Kyrgyz Republic, 1996–2016

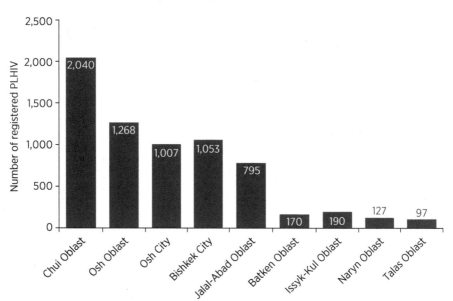

Source: World Bank based on National AIDS Center/ Kyrgyz Republic Ministry of Health 2017 program records.

Note: HIV = human immunodeficiency virus; PLHIV = people living with HIV.

(Batken, Issyk-Kul, Naryn, and Talas) have low observed levels of prevalence and low numbers of HIV cases (0.3 cases per 1,000 population) (figure 7.2). The trend of HIV infection in Issyk-Kul Oblast has been rising, however: in 2014, HIV prevalence increased by 19 percent. In the city of Osh and the Osh Oblast, where the epidemic first developed, the trend is now toward stabilization. In the other oblasts, the numbers of new HIV diagnoses continue to grow.

Funding for HIV Programming

In 2012, the proportion of government expenditure used for health was slightly above the global average of 11.7 percent, and 60 percent of the total health budget was covered by domestic government spending. In contrast, the HIV portion of the budget was more heavily reliant on foreign donors: international donors provided 71 percent of the HIV/AIDS budget in 2012, and the government financed the remaining 29 percent.

Figure 7.3 summarizes 2013 expenditures on HIV in the Kyrgyz Republic by program area according to data from the national Global AIDS Response Progress Reporting (GARPR) financial reporting tables.[3] Less than 10 percent of the country's HIV spending went to antiretroviral therapy (ART); thus, the proportion of expenditure going to treatment was lower than in most other countries in the Eastern Europe and Central Asia region. Conversely, costs classified as "management and other costs" accounted for 56 percent of spending. This proportion is high for the region and is explained in part by the country's classification of program-related human resource costs as management costs. As a result, the Kyrgyz Republic's overall HIV investment per capita and per person living with HIV appeared relatively high compared to regional averages.[4]

Figure 7.3   HIV Expenditure in the Kyrgyz Republic, by Program Area, 2013

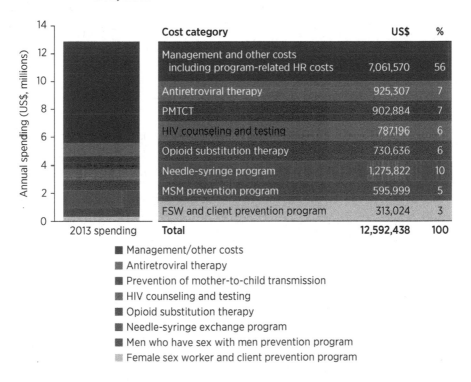

Cost category	US$	%
Management and other costs including program-related HR costs	7,061,570	56
Antiretroviral therapy	925,307	7
PMTCT	902,884	7
HIV counseling and testing	787,196	6
Opioid substitution therapy	730,636	6
Needle-syringe program	1,275,822	10
MSM prevention program	595,999	5
FSW and client prevention program	313,024	3
Total	**12,592,438**	**100**

2013 spending

■ Management/other costs
■ Antiretroviral therapy
■ Prevention of mother-to-child transmission
■ HIV counseling and testing
■ Opioid substitution therapy
■ Needle-syringe exchange program
■ Men who have sex with men prevention program
■ Female sex worker and client prevention program

Source: World Bank 2015.

Note: FSW = female sex worker; HIV = human immunodeficiency virus; HR = human resources; MSM = men who have sex with men; PMTCT = prevention of mother-to-child transmission; US$ = US dollar.

Figure 7.4 Breakdown of Management and Other Costs, Kyrgyz Republic, 2013

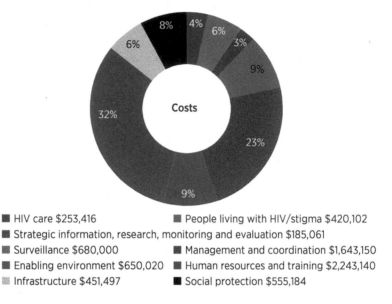

■ HIV care $253,416   ■ People living with HIV/stigma $420,102
■ Strategic information, research, monitoring and evaluation $185,061
■ Surveillance $680,000   ■ Management and coordination $1,643,150
■ Enabling environment $650,020 ■ Human resources and training $2,243,140
■ Infrastructure $451,497   ■ Social protection $555,184

Source: World Bank 2015.
Note: Costs are expressed in US dollars. HIV = human immunodeficiency virus.

The breakdown of management and other costs in the 2013 budget (figure 7.4) provides insights into the range of activities and costs that could not be included in the Optima mathematical optimization analysis of allocative efficiency. US$3.9 million—equal to more than 50 percent of all management and other costs and 31 percent of total HIV spending—was allocated for two categories: (1) management and coordination and (2) human resources and training.[5]

Reducing New Infections and Deaths

The Optima Analysis

In the context of developing a new national strategy, the Kyrgyz Republic faced the challenge of determining how to control a growing HIV epidemic with limited resources. This challenge was particularly daunting because of the large treatment gap in the Kyrgyz Republic. The Optima allocative efficiency analysis addressed a range of policy questions, particularly: What is the minimum spending required to meet the national targets? How should funds be allocated to achieve the targets? Table 7.1 shows the three key impact targets covered in the analysis.

The first analysis of what it would take to achieve national targets produced a somewhat sobering finding: the analysis concluded that, if costs and budgeting remained at the 2013 levels, meeting the targets would cost US$24 million, which would entail nearly doubling HIV spending over the 2013 levels. Resource constraints meant that such an increase was unlikely, so the model was used to explore ways to achieve efficiency gains. Figure 7.5 shows the total cost to achieve national targets by 2020 under two alternative scenarios. They combine allocative efficiency analysis with specific technical efficiency assumptions applied to the allocation to fully achieve national targets.

Allocation A shows actual 2013 allocations. Allocation E1 shows the optimized distribution of funding to achieve national targets, assuming that management and other costs are reduced by 20 percent.[6] A cost reduction of 20 percent was used as an estimate that could be achieved through technical efficiencies while maintaining core management functions and enablers. Allocation E2 represents the optimized allocation to achieve national targets (50 percent reduction in HIV incidence and deaths by 2020). Allocation E2 assumes technical efficiency gains in three programs that are needed to fully achieve national targets but that were not cost-effective in allocation scenarios using 2013 funding. These are programs for female sex workers (FSWs), MSM, and the prevention of mother-to-child transmission (PMTCT). For these programs, the costs per person in the Kyrgyz Republic were substantially above the median cost in other countries in the region; therefore, 50 percent reductions in costs for FSW and PMTCT programs were assumed, and a 75 percent reduction in cost per person was assumed in MSM programs. These reductions may appear very high, particularly for MSM programs;

Table 7.1 National Targets as Applied in Optimization Analysis

Targets	AIDS-related deaths	HIV infections	Mother-to-child transmission
National	50% reduction in annual deaths in 2020 compared to 2014 levels	50% reduction in annual new infections in 2020 compared to 2014 levels	Virtual elimination of mother-to-child transmission: fewer than 5% of infants born to HIV-positive mothers who breastfeed and fewer than 3% born to HIV-positive mothers who do not breastfeed are infected

Source: World Bank 2015.

Note: AIDS = acquired immune deficiency syndrome; HIV = human immunodeficiency virus.

Figure 7.5 Optimized Allocation to Achieve 2020 National Targets in the Kyrgyz Republic—Technical Efficiencies Can Further Reduce the Cost for Achieving National Targets

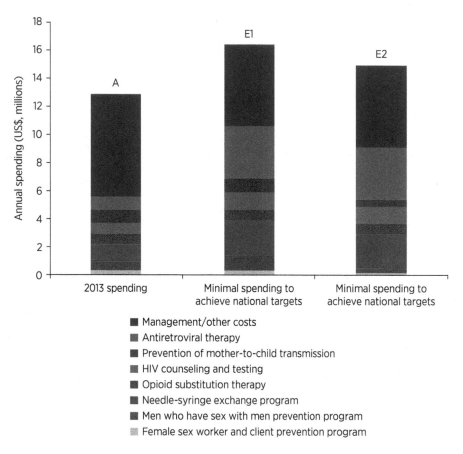

■ Management/other costs
■ Antiretroviral therapy
■ Prevention of mother-to-child transmission
■ HIV counseling and testing
■ Opioid substitution therapy
■ Needle-syringe exchange program
■ Men who have sex with men prevention program
▨ Female sex worker and client prevention program

Source: World Bank 2015.

Note: Column E1 assumes 20 percent efficiency in management cost. Column E2 assumes 20 percent efficiency in management costs and other technical efficiencies. HIV = human immunodeficiency virus; US$ = US dollar.

however, even with a 75 percent reduction, the cost per person in MSM programs (US$449 reduced to US$112) would remain above the median cost in the other countries included in the regional analysis.

With the assumed reductions in management and other costs, the Optima HIV model found that national targets could be achieved with approximately US$16 million in spending. The required amount could be reduced further to approximately US$15 million with the proposed reductions in unit costs for FSW, MSM, and PMTCT programs. By exploring technical efficiencies in other programs, it might be possible to reduce further the cost for achieving national targets.

Using Allocative Efficiency to Expand Coverage

Figure 7.6 shows the key epidemiological outcomes over time under each of the key allocation scenarios. In all four panels of figure 7.6, the maroon line represents outcomes for zero spending, and the dotted gray line shows results of maintaining the 2013 spending level (US$12.6 million) and distribution of resources among programs. The green line represents the key result: optimized allocations to achieve national targets (US$24 million at 2013 unit and management costs, US$16 million with reduced management costs, and US$15 million with specific additional technical efficiencies).

Figure 7.6 Outcomes under the Three Allocation Scenarios, Kyrgyz Republic, 2010–20

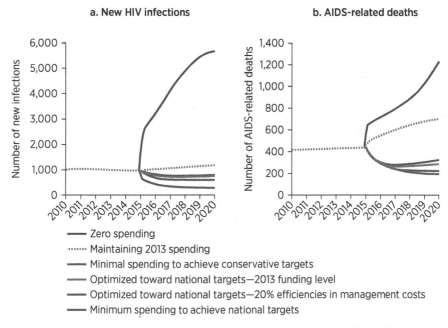

a. New HIV infections

b. AIDS-related deaths

——— Zero spending
·········· Maintaining 2013 spending
——— Minimal spending to achieve conservative targets
——— Optimized toward national targets—2013 funding level
——— Optimized toward national targets—20% efficiencies in management costs
——— Minimum spending to achieve national targets

continued next page

Figure 7.6 (*continued*)

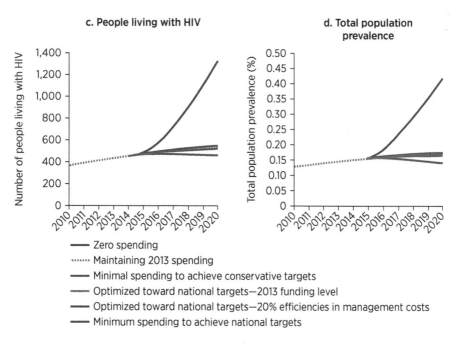

c. People living with HIV

d. Total population prevalence

—— Zero spending
•••••• Maintaining 2013 spending
—— Minimal spending to achieve conservative targets
—— Optimized toward national targets—2013 funding level
—— Optimized toward national targets—20% efficiencies in management costs
—— Minimum spending to achieve national targets

Source: World Bank 2015.
Note: AIDS =acquired immune deficiency syndrome; HIV = human immunodeficiency virus.

Table 7.2 shows the cost to achieve national targets with 20 percent efficiencies in management costs, the corresponding program coverage levels, and epidemic epidemiological outcomes, based on the Optima analysis. It shows that, with optimized allocations, coverage of key prevention and treatment interventions could be dramatically increased. In particular, treatment coverage could be increased more than fourfold. Achieving the national targets would translate to averting 4,200 (65 percent) new infections and 2,300 deaths (62 percent).[7]

Optima Analysis Findings

The Optima allocative efficiency analysis resulted in the following conclusions and recommendations:

1. HIV in the Kyrgyz Republic is transitioning from an early concentrated epidemic among PWID into an advanced concentrated epidemic

Table 7.2 Program Coverage Levels, Epidemiological Outcomes, and Cost-Effectiveness Calculations Relating to the Spending Scenarios Described for the Kyrgyz Republic

Analysis to the end of 2020	Maintaining 2013 spending		Minimal spending (average per year 2015–20) to achieve national targets with 20% efficiencies in management costs	
Annual allocations between 2015 and 2020 (average)	(US$)	(%)	(US$)	(%)
Allocation to FSW and client prevention program	313,024	2	261,129	2
Allocation to MSM prevention program	595,999	5	1.2 million	7
Allocation to NSP	1.3 million	10	2.5 million	15
Allocation to OST	730,636	6	730,636	5
Allocation to HIV counseling and testing	787,196	6	1.3 million	8
Allocation to PMTCT	902,884	7	966,953	6
Allocation to ART	925,307	7	3.7 million	23
Total annual direct program spending	5.5 million	44	10.6 million	65
Total for management and other costs	7.1 million	56	5.6 million	35
Total annual HIV spending	12.6 million	100	16.2 million	100
FSW and client prevention program coverage (%)	—	40	—	34
MSM prevention program coverage (%)	—	8	—	13
NSP coverage (%)	—	42	—	56
OST program coverage (%)	—	4	—	4
Annual allocations between 2015–20 (average)				
PLHIV who know their status (%)	—	63	—	83
PMTCT program coverage (%)	—	89	—	>90
ART coverage (eligibility: CD4 count <500 cells/µL) (%)	—	33	—	>90

continued next page

Table 7.2 *(continued)*

Analysis to the end of 2020	Maintaining 2013 spending		Minimal spending (average per year 2015–20) to achieve national targets with 20% efficiencies in management costs	
Annual allocations between 2015 and 2020 (average)	(US$)	(%)	(US$)	(%)
ART coverage (eligibility: CD4 count <350 cells/µL) (%)	—	43	—	>90
Those on treatment who are virally suppressed (%)	—	87	—	87
Number on first-line treatment	1,500	—	6,400	—
Number on second-line treatment	100	—	300	—
Number eligible for treatment (eligibility: CD4 count <500 cells/µL)	4,800	—	6,900	—
Number eligible for treatment (eligibility: CD4 count < 350 cells/µL)	3,800	—	6,800	—
Cumulative new infections, 2015–20	6,500	—	2,300	—
Cumulative AIDS-related deaths, 2015–20	3,800	—	1,400	—
Cumulative DALYs, 2015–20	52,300	—	42,300	—
Overall prevalence, 2020 (%)	—	0.17	—	0.14
Number of PLHIV, 2020	10,200	—	8,500	—
New infections averted, 2015–20	Baseline	—	4,200	—
AIDS-related deaths averted, 2015–20	Baseline	—	2,300	—
DALYs averted, 2015–20	Baseline	—	10,000	—

Source: World Bank 2015.

Note: AIDS = acquired immune deficiency syndrome; ART = antiretroviral therapy; DALY = disability-adjusted life year; FSW = female sex worker; HIV = human immunodeficiency virus; MSM = men who have sex with men; NSP = needle and syringe exchange program; OST = opioid substitution therapy; PLHIV = people living with HIV; PMTCT = prevention of mother-to-child transmission; µL = microliter; US$ = US dollar; — = not available.

characterized by continued transmission among PWID but an increasing share of sexual transmission to female partners of PWID and among MSM. There is continued need to scale up programs as specified in recommendations 3 through 8 below.

2. Investment in HIV programs in the Kyrgyz Republic has been substantial, and programs have been put in place to prevent a large expansion of the epidemic by 2020. With a total of US$12.6 million in 2013, HIV spending in the Kyrgyz Republic equated to approximately US$1,500 per PLHIV, one of the highest rates in the region. An analysis comparing the effect of existing programs under 2013 budget levels and allocations to a scenario of zero HIV spending revealed that the 2013 programming would avert 20,700 new infections and 1,800 deaths. This analysis clearly suggests that harm reduction focused on PWID in combination with other existing programs has prevented more rapid spread of HIV among PWID.

3. Optimizing allocations of resources at the 2013 spending levels would substantially reduce new HIV infections by 28 percent and deaths by 53 percent from 2015 to 2020. This additional impact would be achieved mainly by reallocating resources to two program areas: (1) a threefold increase in investment in ART accompanied by sustained HIV testing and counseling (HTC) and (2) a moderate increase in prevention programs for PWID, particularly needle exchange programs.

The following recommendations from the Optima analysis focus on the prioritization required to achieve national targets: reducing sexual transmission by 50 percent, reducing drug injection–related transmission by 50 percent, virtually eliminating mother-to-child transmission (MTCT) by 2020, and reducing AIDS-related deaths by 50 percent.

4. The top priority in the Kyrgyz Republic's HIV response is to substantially increase the allocation to and coverage of ART. In 2013, only 7 percent of total national HIV spending was allocated to ART. Coverage of 1,074 PLHIV on ART was achieved in 2013, which was approximately 13 percent of the total estimated PLHIV, or 43 percent of the PLHIV eligible for ART at the time. With optimized allocations to fully achieve national targets, investment in ART would increase from US$0.9 million to US$3.7 million, accompanied by increased investment in HTC from US$0.8 million to US$1.3 million. This level of spending would extend ART coverage to 6,700 PLHIV, or 79 percent of all PLHIV. With optimized allocations to achieve national targets, the projected number of PLHIV in 2020 would be 8,500.

5. The second priority in the Kyrgyz Republic's HIV epidemic is sustaining and expanding coverage of programs for PWID. The share of new infections due to needle sharing is declining; however, programs for this key

population remain critical because of the large potential for epidemic growth among PWID in the absence of such programs. With allocations optimized to achieve national targets, programs for PWID would receive 20 percent of all funding, or US$3.2 million (up from US$2.0 million), compared to 2013 allocations. In practical terms, it is critical to review unit costs of NSPs and OST programs. OST programs have multiple health and social benefits, and the 2013 coverage of 4 percent is insufficient to realize those benefits.

6. Although HIV transmission among MSM has been a small segment of the Kyrgyz Republic's HIV epidemic, it has also been the fastest-growing segment. Consequently, to achieve national targets, focused technically efficient programs for MSM should continue to be provided. At 2013 unit costs and based on projections from the Optima analysis, doubling coverage would require a budget increase from US$0.6 million to US$1.2 million. The exceptionally high cost per person reached (US$449), however, suggested that there may be extensive potential for technical efficiency gains of 65 percent to 85 percent in terms of unit cost reduction.

7. FSWs and their clients contributed to fewer than 1 in 20 new infections in the Kyrgyz Republic at the time of the Optima analysis. In this context, the technical efficiency of programs should be reviewed, unit costs reduced, and coverage expanded to enhance their cost-effectiveness.

8. MTCT, HTC, and ART should remain available to pregnant women, but at the lowest possible cost. MTCT accounts for approximately only 2 percent of new infections. Because the national strategy includes an exclusive MTCT target, the optimized allocation includes an amount of US$1.0 million for PMTCT, but additional technical efficiencies should be explored.

9. It is essential to critically study the large portion of HIV spending allocated to management and other costs (56 percent as of 2013), because reallocating 20 percent of these costs to core treatment and prevention programs would avert additional new infections and deaths. Even though blood safety and the management of sexually transmitted infections were excluded from the Optima analysis, management and other costs still accounted for 56 percent of HIV spending. Because this expenditure could not be reviewed in the optimization analysis, other methods of technical efficiency analysis should be applied to explore potential savings.

10. According to the Optima analysis, the minimum amount needed to achieve national targets with optimized allocations is US$24 million, which could be substantially reduced to US$16 million by reducing

management costs and further lowered by exploring technical efficiency gains. Achieving national targets in the Kyrgyz Republic would avert 2,300 deaths and 4,200 new infections. The amount needed to achieve these targets depends heavily on critical choices. With additional potential efficiency gains in FSW, MSM, and PMTCT programs, as identified by country experts (and described previously), the amount could be reduced to approximately US$15 million. The technical efficiency of core programs should be studied.

11. A robust national process to review technical efficiency, costing, and financing of the national HIV response in light of the Optima analysis could result in a detailed plan to close the financing gap and achieve national targets. This costed plan could outline how to realize allocative and technical efficiency gains and mobilize domestic resources for the response. Regional comparison of cost per person reached suggests that, in virtually all programs, there may be additional technical efficiencies in the range of 20 percent to 50 percent that would bring the estimated cost to achieve national targets closer to the US$12.6 million available in 2013.

Actions Taken and Next Steps

2017 Spectrum Analysis

In 2017, a Spectrum analysis was also conducted and provided additional updated information on the epidemic. The results of the Spectrum analysis indicate a trend toward stabilization of the epidemic (table 7.3). The analysis also shows that the number of new HIV diagnoses among women and among MSM is increasing, whereas the rate of new HIV diagnoses among PWID is decreasing, which matches the predictions from the earlier Optima allocative efficiency analysis.

It should be noted that the 2017 Spectrum findings differ from the Optima analysis as to the numbers of anticipated new HIV infections and deaths associated with HIV. The Optima model projected that, if 2013 spending levels were maintained, new infections would increase to approximately 1,100 per year and estimated deaths would increase to 600 deaths per year on average during the 2015–20 period. It also projected that the total number of PLHIV would increase from 8,400 in 2014 to 10,200 by 2020. The 2017 Spectrum analysis produced more optimistic predictions about the number of new HIV infections and deaths in the years ahead. Those findings from the Spectrum analysis suggest that, with the existing amount of funding and scale of the HIV

Table 7.3 Spectrum Analysis Forecast of Total Estimated Number of People Living with HIV, Kyrgyz Republic, 2010–21

Year	Estimated number of PLHIV (total)	Estimated number of new PLHIV infections	Estimated number of deaths among PLHIV
2010	5,200	900	—
2011	5,700	900	—
2012	6,300	900	—
2013	6,900	1,000	—
2014	7,400	1,000	300
2015	7,900	900	300
2016	8,300	800	300
2017	8,600	700	300
2018	8,800	600	300
2019	8,900	500	300
2020	8,900	500	300
2021	8,900	400	300

Sources: Data from Kyrgyz Republic 2017b, 2017c.

Note: HIV = human immunodeficiency virus; PLHIV = people living with HIV; — = not available.

response, the epidemic should stabilize and the number of new HIV infections per year after should average 500 new infections per year, as compared to the earlier Optima estimate of 1,100 per year. Similarly, the Spectrum analysis suggests that the yearly average number of HIV-related deaths will be 300 per year, versus the 600 per year estimate from the earlier Optima analysis.

Steps Taken to Strengthen the National Response to HIV

Since the Optima allocative efficiency analysis was conducted in 2014–15, the Kyrgyz Republic has continued to further strengthen its HIV programs in line with its commitment to the World Health Organization guidelines and the 90-90-90 goals of the Joint United Nations Programme on HIV/AIDS (UNAIDS). A significant factor for strengthening the national response to HIV was the high-level meeting that led to the Political Declaration on HIV and AIDS adopted by the United Nations General Assembly in 2016 and setting goals for 2030 (UNGASS 2016).

In the Kyrgyz Republic, the need to improve the effectiveness of HIV programming was recognized at the political level and formed the basis for a new national program on HIV for 2017–21 (the "State Program"; see Kyrgyz Republic 2017a). The program is based on priorities, taking into account the nature and trends in the epidemic and populations that are most affected by it. National measures have been set in two directions: (1) results-oriented along the cascade of services important to overcome the epidemic and (2) the distribution of responsibilities for achieving these results among partners. The State Program aims to enhance universal access to the services mainly for key populations in order to achieve the UNAIDS 90-90-90 strategy (UNAIDS 2014). It is built on the needs of the individual and complex services ranging from preventive services to diagnosis, treatment, and finally PLHIV achieving viral suppression.

Program objectives were revised with the goal of expanding HIV testing so as to identify 90 percent of PLHIV, to scale up treatment coverage to 90 percent of PLHIV and enhance the effectiveness of that treatment coverage to achieve viral suppression, and to increase coverage by targeting prevention programs to key populations. The revised national strategy highlights the importance of expanding public investment and includes a road map to increase public funding.

The new state strategy also included special actions to remove barriers to coverage and retention in the programs. Therefore, the strategy pays considerable attention to overcoming legislative barriers and abusive enforcement practices, as well as the stigma and discrimination associated with HIV.

Programs to meet the needs as reflected in the more optimistic epidemic forecasts generated by the Spectrum analysis can be implemented with appropriate investment. Despite the decline in the volume of international financial support, the country plans to expand the scope of activities to reach out to PLHIV and other people affected by the epidemic with a wide range of services for prevention, treatment, care, and support, by increasing the efficiency of how financial resources are used.

First, the budget of the program has been optimized. The overall costs for HIV programming were set at US$9.112 million in 2017, rising to US$10.673 million in 2021. These numbers reflect a substantial reduction in the unit cost per person living with HIV from US$1,500 per year in 2013 to US$1,058 in 2017 and US$1,199 in 2021. Moreover, ART coverage has already expanded—from 16 percent of the estimated number of PLHIV in 2013 (1,074/6,851) to 32 percent in 2016 (2,668/8,307). The State Program further plans to increase ART coverage to 90 percent of PLHIV with known HIV status before 2021, which will entail covering an estimated 7,211 PLHIV. The plan allows for substantially increasing the funding for prevention and treatment programs while reducing the budget—a plan that necessitates reallocating financial resources for priority activities. In line with the recommendations built on the Optima HIV model, resources are being allocated to two program areas: (1) a threefold increase in investment in ART including testing and counseling and (2) expanded prevention coverage with a focus on PWID and MSM.

As part of the institutionalization of the management of the State Program, measures are being put in place to increase the proportion of government funding of the HIV response—and particularly to expand the list of essential medicines and the state guarantees program, to improve procurement, to establish social contracting mechanisms through which government can fund civil society organizations, and to increase the share of government budgetary financing.

Progress on Budget Optimization

In 2015, the Optima analysis found that optimizing allocations of available resources at 2013 levels would lead to substantial reductions in new HIV infections by 28 percent and in deaths by 53 percent. Since that time, further analysis of the situation based on national statistics and estimates from the Spectrum analysis indicated that some progress has already been made through improvements in the efficiency of HIV programs and through expanding coverage of ART and prevention programs for key populations. The country could achieve even greater results, but external and domestic financing remains limited.

Despite the national objectives to reduce sexual transmission and transmission through needle use by 50 percent, sexual transmission has continued to grow to the point that it now accounts for twice as many new infections as needle sharing (with sexual transmission accounting for 50.8 percent of all new infections among newly registered PLHIV, versus 23.6 percent accounted for by needle transmission). On a more positive note, the country has made some progress in PMTCT but has not yet eliminated this mode of transmission. As of 2017, MTCT accounted for just under 1.6 percent of all new HIV infections. At the same time, AIDS mortality has continued to increase, mainly because of the late identification of individuals with HIV.

As recommended by the Optima allocative efficiency analysis, significantly increasing ART program funding and coverage is the main priority for the Kyrgyz Republic, and those efforts have already produced notable results. In 2013, only 7 percent of national HIV funding was allocated to ART and coverage amounted to 1,074 PLHIV— approximately 13 percent of the estimated number of all PLHIV or

43 percent of PLHIV who needed treatment at that time. Since then, by the end of 2016 ART coverage had increased 2.5 times and reached 2,668 people. The State Program for 2017–21 plans to further increase investment in this priority area and to expand ART coverage to 6.7 times the 2013 level. In the same time frame, investments in the expansion of ART will increase fourfold by 2021 compared to 2013 and will then constitute 37 percent of the total budget of the State Program on HIV (rising from US$0.9 million to US$3.9 million), as recommended in the Optima study (tables 7.4 and 7.5). To address the treatment gap, a combination of measures will be undertaken, including expanding HIV testing and enhancing treatment retention along with interventions to find lost clients. The latter is the priority for the country and ties into a relevant initiative under PEPFAR (the US President's Emergency Plan for AIDS Relief).

A reason for the reduced spending on HIV testing is the simplification of the testing algorithm, which has led to a reduction in the cost and time for diagnosis. Despite the reduction in the cost, however, HIV testing remains an important intervention for preventing morbidity, disability, and mortality from HIV. In terms of reallocated budgets, emphasis was given to testing of key populations and case management of newly identified PLHIV for treatment, care, and support—that is, to keep them in a continuous cascade of services. It is expected that by 2021, 90 percent of PLHIV will know their status. Since 2012, HIV testing provided by nongovernmental organizations has resulted in the expansion of the scope of key population testing, thus making the procedure available to clients. The new State Program includes self-testing for HIV, but the allocation for testing has been reduced from 6 to 5 percent of the total cost of HIV or US$0.79 to US$0.49 million (table 7.4).

Scaling up coverage of PWID so that prevention programs involve 90 percent of the estimated number of PWID is one of the main priorities of the State Program. Despite the significant decrease in the number of newly identified PWID who are living with HIV, they still represent about half of all PLHIV (49 percent) registered in the country and one-quarter of all new HIV diagnoses registered in 2016. It should be noted that integrated HIV biobehavioral surveillance (IBBS) conducted in 2016 indicates a national trend toward the stabilization of HIV prevalence among PWID (figure 7.7). Nevertheless, the growth of viral hepatitis C antibodies among PWID testifies to risky behaviors and, consequently, suggests the possibility of the further spread of HIV in this key population (figure 7.8). The analysis of the cascade of services showed significant losses of HIV-positive PWID along the cascade at all stages, especially at the stage of identifying HIV status and inclusion in treatment programs (UNAIDS 2015).

Table 7.4 Progress in Cost Optimization for Efficiency of the Kyrgyz National Response to the Epidemic by 2021

Program type	2020 costs if maintaining 2013 funding levels		Minimal costs for achieving national goals with 20% of the optimization of management costs		Planned total program costs in accordance with the State Program for 2017–21	
	(US$)	(% of total)	(US$)	(% of total)	(US$)	(% of total)
Prevention programs for sex workers and their clients	313,024	2	261,129	2	1.4 million	13
Prevention programs for MSM	595,999	5	1.2 million	7	—	—
NSP	1.3 million	10	2.5 million	15	2.3 million	22
OST	730,636	6	730,636	5	—	—
Testing and counseling	787,196	6	1.3 million	8	489,092	5
PMTCT	902,884	7	966,953	6	623,069	6
ART	925,307	7	3.7 million	23	4.0 million	37
Total annual direct program costs	5.5 million	44	10.6 million	65	8.7 million	82
Total management and other costs	7.1 million	56	5.6 million	35	2.0 million	18
Total annual spending for HIV	12.6 million	100	16.2 million	100	10.7 million	100

Source: Kyrgyz Republic National AIDS Center data.

Note: ART = antiretroviral therapy; HIV = human immunodeficiency virus; MSM = men who have sex with men; NSP = needle and syringe exchange program; OST = opioid substitution therapy; PMTCT = prevention of mother-to-child transmission; US$ = US dollar; — = not available.

The Kyrgyz Republic has seen some improvement in the coverage of services for PWID; however, more efforts should be taken. The flagship project launched in the country with support from Population Services International (PSI) and PEPFAR aims to increase the coverage of prevention and treatment programs for PWID. Despite considerable experience in

Table 7.5 HIV Programs in the Kyrgyz Republic: Coverage, Epidemiological Results, and Impact on the Epidemic by 2021

Program type	At 2013 spending levels (%)	Optimized spending per Optima, 2015 (%)	Actual progress as of 2016 (%) (number of individuals covered)	Expected results 2021 (%)
Coverage of prevention programs for sex workers and their clients	40	34	80 (5,643/7,100)	90
Coverage of prevention programs for MSM	8	13	20 (4,376/22,000)	75
Coverage of NSPs	42	56	69 (17,08/25,000)	90
Coverage of OST	4	4	5	10
PLHIV who know their status	63	83	62	90
PMTCT coverage	89	>90	91	95
ART coverage (CD4 count <500 cells/μL)	33	>90	32	81
Viral suppression	87	87	62	90
The number of people on first-line treatment	1,500	6,400	—	—
The number of people on second-line treatment	100	300	—	—
PLHIV in need of treatment (when: CD4 count <500 cells/μL)	4,800	6,900	6,470	7,211
Cumulative new infections (2015–20)	6,500	2,300	—	3,878
Cumulative AIDS-related deaths (2015–20)	3,800	1,400	—	1,534
Cumulative DALYs (2015–20)	52,300	42,300	—	—
Overall prevalence by 2020	0.17	0.14	0.13	0.06

continued next page

Table 7.5 *(continued)*

Program type	At 2013 spending levels (%)	Optimized spending per Optima, 2015 (%)	Actual progress as of 2016 (%) (number of individuals covered)	Expected results 2021 (%)
Number of PLHIV, 2020	10,200	8,500	8,307	8,903
New infections averted (2015–20)	Baseline 4,200	—	—	—
AIDS-related deaths averted (2015–20)	Baseline 2,300	—	—	—
DALYs averted (2015–20)	Baseline 10,000	—	—	—

Source: Kyrgyz Republic National AIDS Center data.

Note: Data provided reflect available information at time of writing; information related to blank boxes may subsequently become available. AIDS = acquired immune deficiency syndrome; ART = antiretroviral therapy; DALY = disability-adjusted life year; HIV = human immunodeficiency virus; MSM = men who have sex with men; NSP = needle and syringe exchange program; OST = opioid substitution therapy; PLHIV = people living with HIV; PMTCT = prevention of mother-to-child transmission; μL = microliter; — = not available.

Figure 7.7 HIV Prevalence among Key Populations according to IBBS for 2008–16, Kyrgyz Republic

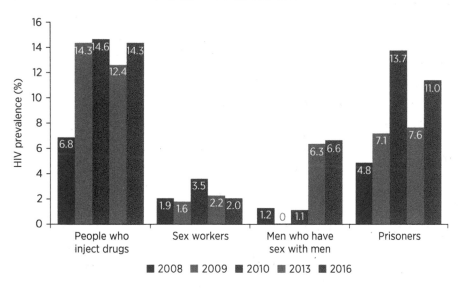

Source: World Bank based on Kyrgyz Republic National AIDS Center data from the integrated biobehavioral surveillance (IBBS) 2008–16.

Note: HIV = human immunodeficiency virus.

Figure 7.8 Hepatitis C Prevalence among Key Populations, Kyrgyz Republic, 2008–16

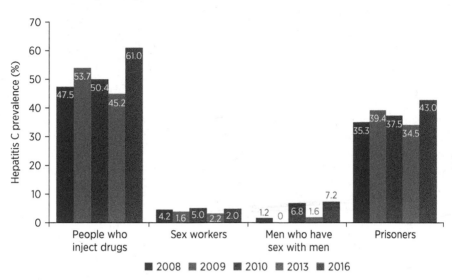

Source: World Bank based on Kyrgyz Republic National AIDS Center data from the integrated biobehavioral surveillance (IBBS) 2008–16.

implementing OST programs, there is still low coverage of therapy and a large loss of clients throughout the treatment cascade.

As recommended in the Optima analysis, investments to scale up programs for PWID have increased—from 16 percent to 22 percent of the total HIV budget—but the total dollar amount remains less than the recommended level (US$2.3 million instead of US$3.2 million) (tables 7.4 and 7.5). Expanding program coverage to reach 90 percent of PWID is intended to include scaling up OST to cover 10 percent of PWID. This scale-up will require reducing the unit cost of NSPs and OST programs to enhance cost-effectiveness. To this end, a pilot project has been launched with the support of ICAP at the Columbia University Mailman School of Public Health, the US Centers for Disease Control and Prevention, and PEPFAR involving a mandatory health insurance fund to manage and finance OST programs run using national budget financing.

Reported HIV transmission among MSM remains low but is showing a tendency to increase. Despite the fact that MSM accounted for 4 percent of the newly diagnosed PLHIV in 2016, the number of registered persons has continued to increase annually since 2011. This trend is evidenced by the biobehavioral surveillance (IBBS) of MSM conducted in 2016.

Viral hepatitis C antibodies have risen (figure 7.8), indicating the existence of dangerous sexual and injecting practices among MSM, the IBBS showed. In general, programs for MSM—together with programs for sex workers and transgender people—target the reduction of sexual HIV transmission. The cost of programming for these three key populations grew from 7 percent to 13 percent of the total cost of the State Program (from US$0.9 million to US$1.35 million per year). Implementing prevention programs for key populations is made more complex by high levels of stigma and discrimination, as well as law enforcement practices in relation to these groups. Recognizing these challenges, the State Program includes in its budget activities to create a supportive environment for the implementation of the national response to HIV.

PMTCT program costs have been cut because of a reduction of HIV testing in pregnant women from 6 percent to 5 percent of the total HIV budget (a decrease from US$0.9 million to US$0.6 million) (table 7.5). This important area requires further action, taking into consideration the need to improve the technical effectiveness of the programs and to ensure the access of pregnant women with high-risk behavior to programs for diagnosis, treatment, care, and support.

Conclusions

Taking into account the recommendations of the allocative efficiency study, the State Program significantly reduces administrative and other costs associated with HIV from 56 percent to 18 percent of the total cost of the State Program (a decrease from US$5.5 million to US$1.95 million). Because of significant redistributions of financial resources to priority areas, the government has managed to implement the Optima analysis recommendations to optimize investments. As shown by statistical and epidemiological data, as well as Spectrum estimates for the period of 2013 through 2016, the Kyrgyz Republic has made progress in terms of prevention and treatment coverage. Nevertheless, it must continue to make great efforts to further improve the cost-effectiveness of the national response to HIV—as well as to find additional resources—because not all planned resources are covered by actual secured financing. The Optima estimates found that US$24 million was the minimum amount of funding needed to achieve the national goals. The findings of the 2017 Spectrum analysis, which takes into account more recent reforms, indicates that the amount needed can be significantly reduced to US$16 million through optimization of administrative costs and further revision of certain programs. The budget for the State Program is US$10.7 million, which is less than half (44.5 percent) of the minimum budget recommended by the Optima analysis and only two-thirds (66.8 percent) of the Spectrum analysis recommendation. In view of the existing financing gap and reduction of Global Fund financing, allocative and technical efficiency remain critical to ensure that funds continue to be allocated to the highest-impact interventions. The country has also established benchmarks for unit costs in the budget of the State Program, which, in combination with effective allocation, will remain essential for achieving program targets with available resources.

Notes

1. Note that much of this chapter reviews the process and findings of the modeling exercise documented in the report produced for that analysis; as such, the material herein draws significantly on that report.
2. "Advanced concentrated HIV epidemic" as used herein refers to an epidemic in which HIV transmission remains related to key populations but in which shifts in the mode of transmission within key populations have occurred. In several countries in the region encompassing Eastern Europe and Central Asia, the largest mode of HIV transmission among PWID was initially needle sharing. More recently, sexual transmission has grown as a transmission method in this population. Because sexual transmission remains concentrated among members of key populations and their sexual partners, however, these epidemics are not generalized.
3. Optima data spreadsheet based on the National AIDS Spending Assessment [NASA] report (Kyrgyz Republic 2014).
4. Calculation based on national HIV estimates and total HIV expenditure per the Optima data spreadsheet, which was derived from the NASA report.
5. Although they were part of national reporting, expenditures for management of sexually transmitted infections (US$2.5 million in 2013) and blood safety/universal precautions (US$3.4 million in 2013) are not included here within the management and other costs because those expenses are considered part of wider health services rather than primarily HIV-related services.
6. Twenty percent was used as the estimate for a reduction in costs excluded from optimization, which could be achieved through efficiencies without putting at risk major management functions and synergies. The 20 percent reduction is roughly equivalent to the level of allocative efficiency gains for programs included in the mathematical optimization because, at 80 percent of 2013 funding, results would not be compromised if resources are allocated optimally. Optimization was able to compensate for a 20 percent reduction in program resources.
7. Achieving all three targets (reducing new sexual infections by 50 percent, new injecting infections by 50 percent, and virtually eliminating MTCT) cumulatively leads to higher overall reductions in new infections and deaths. The reason is that the effects of individual interventions such as ART required to achieve one target have additional effects on other target areas.

References

Kyrgyz Republic. 2014. "National AIDS Spending Assessment (NASA) Report for the Kyrgyz Republic for 2012–13." Russian version, Government of the Kyrgyz Republic, Bishkek.

Kyrgyz Republic, Ministry of Health. 2017a. "State Programme on HIV in the Kyrgyz Republic for 2017–2021." Ministry of Health, Bishkek.

Kyrgyz Republic, National AIDS Center. 2017b. "Global AIDS Monitoring Report 2017." National AIDS Center, Bishkek.

Kyrgyz Republic, National AIDS Center. 2017c. "Spectrum Analysis 2017." Unpublished document, National AIDS Center, Bishkek.

UNAIDS (Joint United Nations Programme on HIV/AIDS). 2014. "90-90-90: An Ambitious Treatment Target to Help End the AIDS Epidemic." UNAIDS, Geneva.

UNAIDS (Joint United Nations Programme on HIV/AIDS). 2015. "A Study of the Area of HIV in the Kyrgyz Republic." UNAIDS, Geneva.

UNGASS (United Nations General Assembly Special Session). 2016. "Political Declaration on HIV and AIDS: On the Fast Track to Accelerating the Fight against HIV and to Ending the AIDS Epidemic by 2030." Resolution 70/266 adopted by the General Assembly on June 8, United Nations, New York.

World Bank. 2015. "Optimizing Investments in the Kyrgyz Republic's HIV Response." World Bank, Washington, DC.

8

Moldova
Designing Efficient HIV Programs for Subnational HIV Epidemics

Svetlana Plamadeala, Richard T. Gray, Iulian Oltu, Lucia Pirtina, Svetlana Popovici, Lilia Gantea, David P. Wilson, Alona Goroshko, and Clemens Benedikt

Briefly

- The human immunodeficiency virus (HIV) epidemic in Moldova is different in the two main regions of the country, which made it important to consider subnational allocative efficiency analysis and prioritization.
- Moldova's HIV epidemic is most severe in the breakaway left bank region (Transnistria) with people who inject drugs (PWID) experiencing the highest levels of HIV prevalence; in the right bank region, transmission among men who have sex with men (MSM) is becoming more important.
- The findings of the allocative efficiency study recommend increased investment, in particular for scaling up treatment nationally as well as HIV prevention programs for key populations (PWID, MSM, and female sex workers), especially on the left bank.
- Funds allocated to programs for the general population should be reinvested in the previously mentioned priority programs.
- Unit cost and technical efficiency of antiretroviral therapy and opioid substitution therapy programs as well as response management costs should be reviewed.

Introduction

Country Basics

Moldova is a landlocked, lower-middle-income country in transition, situated in Eastern Europe. With a population of 3.5 million people, Moldova is undergoing significant demographic changes, characterized by low fertility rates, an aging population, and relatively low life expectancy— all of which have economic and social implications in areas such as social security. Migration from Moldova has been steadily increasing, with an estimated one-third of the working-age population abroad (Moldova 2016).

Political instability and slow economic development have contributed to high poverty rates, placing Moldova among countries with the lowest income levels in Europe, despite the national poverty rate having decreased from 26 percent in 2007 to 11.4 percent in 2014. Economic growth reached a high of 12.9 percent in the third quarter of 2013 but contracted to −3.7 percent in the third quarter of 2015 when the economy fell into recession. Sustaining growth has been a challenge because gross domestic product (GDP) gains have been fueled by remittances and export growth through increased access to external markets, both of which were affected by the global financial crisis and the trade sanctions imposed by the Russian Federation. GDP picked up in 2016, however, registering a growth rate of 4.1 percent (World Bank 2016).

Despite political instability, the government of Moldova succeeded in concluding a visa-liberalization agreement and an Association Agreement (AA) with the European Union (EU) in 2014. The AA reaffirms mutual commitment to support Moldova in strengthening the rule of law, democracy, and human rights standards and principles. In addition, the Deep and Comprehensive Free Trade Area (DCFTA) stimulates trade integration between Moldova and the EU. Nevertheless, Moldova's future path is not certain, with diverging views on Moldova's integration into the EU. Social cohesion is weak, and the society remains divided, primarily along geopolitical and ethnolinguistic fault lines. Following independence in 1991 and the armed conflict of 1992, Chisinau lost control of the eastern region, the self-proclaimed Transnistrian Republic.

HIV Challenges

Historical, political, and economic factors—combined with punitive regulations applied in the eastern region—have meant that communicable diseases have had a more severe epidemiological impact in the eastern region (on the left bank of the Nistru River) than in the region on the right bank.

Data on new cases suggest that the HIV and tuberculosis burdens are approximately three times higher in the eastern region, placing them among the most severe HIV and tuberculosis epidemics in Europe.

Moldova made substantial progress on several Millennium Development Goals (MDGs) before the target date of 2015 (Moldova 2013). Poverty incidence decreased from 34.5 percent in 2006 to 20.8 percent in 2012. Moldova also met the 2015 MDG targets set for mortality rates among infants and children under 5 years old. HIV, however, remained a challenge. Moldova's 2013 MDG report described MDG 6 on combatting HIV/AIDS (acquired immune deficiency syndrome), tuberculosis, and other diseases as the most troubling area: "None of the targets under this goal was achieved, and it will not be possible to reach them by 2015" (Moldova 2013, 11). A critical review of national strategies, plans, and investments was needed.

Moldova continues to experience a concentrated HIV epidemic, in which the largest portion of new infections occurs among three key populations: people who inject drugs (PWID); men who have sex with men (MSM); and female sex workers (FSWs), their clients, and their sexual partners.

To ensure their consistency and relevance, and unless otherwise indicated, the data provided in this chapter relate to the situation in Moldova at the time the analysis was conducted.

Geographic Variations in the HIV Epidemic

Within Moldova, there is a large variation in the HIV epidemic between the areas west of the Nistru River (the "right bank") and the areas east of the Nistru River (the "left bank"). Available evidence suggests that the HIV epidemic is more severe on the left bank. In 2013, in the left bank areas, the rate of new HIV diagnoses was 47 per 100,000 people, compared to 13 per 100,000 on the right bank. Moldova's HIV disease burden is among the highest in Europe, accounting for 9.4 percent of years of life lost (YLL) in the 15–49 age group.[1]

The general burden of disease in Moldova is characterized by prevailing noncommunicable diseases. Among people aged 45 and above, cardiovascular disease, cancer, and cirrhosis are predominant causes of total YLL. In the working-age population, the main causes of YLL are noncommunicable diseases and injuries, as well as HIV/AIDS and tuberculosis. In the 15–49 age group, HIV is the second-largest cause of YLL accounting for 9.4 percent of all YLL, exceeded only by cirrhosis of the liver. The HIV disease burden in Moldova is among the highest in Europe, and the second-highest after Ukraine among the countries covered in this book.

HIV Allocative Efficiency Analysis

Reliance on International Aid

In 2014–15, Moldova used the Optima model to conduct an HIV allocative efficiency analysis to inform its strategic decisions on investments in its HIV response (World Bank 2015).[2] This analysis was part of a regional initiative in which similar studies were conducted in Armenia, Belarus, Georgia, Kazakhstan, the Kyrgyz Republic, Ukraine, and a number of other countries (see, for example, Duric et al. 2014; Fraser et al. 2014). Figure 8.1 illustrates that, although HIV accounted for 3.0 percent of YLL and 2.1 percent of disability-adjusted life years (DALYs) overall at the time of the analysis, it received only 0.8 percent of total health expenditure. In most other countries that conducted similar studies as part of this regional effort, the level of HIV disease burden and the percentage of health spending allocated to HIV were similar to each other.[3] This finding suggests that total HIV spending in Moldova has been relatively low compared to disease burden and—considering the large disease burden—low compared to most other countries in this region.

Although the government spent a considerable share of its total expenditure on health (13.3 percent in 2012), the Moldova HIV response budget has been moderate compared to other countries in the region. Moreover, the HIV response has been heavily dependent on international support. In 2013

Figure 8.1 Levels of HIV Disease Burden, Compared to Levels of HIV Spending, Moldova

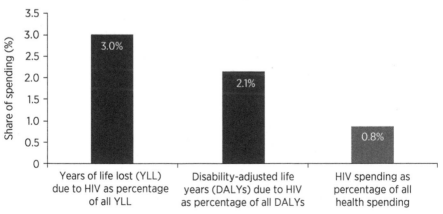

Sources: World Health Organization (WHO) Global Health Expenditure Database, http://apps.who.int/nha/database; UNAIDS 2014; University of Washington 2014.

Note: HIV = human immunodeficiency virus.

government expenditure on HIV was slightly less than US$2.46 million (30 percent of total HIV spending). At the same time, international resources topped US$5.50 million (68 percent), and funds from private domestic sources accounted for US$173,357 (2 percent). From 2012 to 2013, public financial resources increased by 7.6 percent—rising from approximately US$2.38 million to just under US$2.46 million. Conversely, compared to 2012, overall 2013 expenditures for the HIV response decreased by 8.6 percent to slightly less than US$8.14 million because of a 14.8 percent drop in funding from international sources. As of 2013, HIV spending represented 0.8 percent of Moldova's total health expenditures (US$8.1 million out of US$937 million). This situation suggested that deciding how to invest HIV resources in Moldova needs to consider several dimensions: the low existing investment levels, the country's high dependence on international funding, a growing epidemic, and high epidemic diversity.

Regional Comparisons

With these factors in mind, as part of the allocative efficiency analysis mentioned above, a special analytical framework was applied in Moldova, which was designed specifically to address the epidemic dynamics in the regions on the right bank and left bank of Nistru River. Table 8.1 shows the

Table 8.1 Modeling Parameterization Designed for the Moldova Analysis

Category	Parameterization in Optima model	
Populations defined in model	**Right bank**	**Left bank**
	• Females aged 15–49	• Females aged 15–49
	• Males aged 15–49	• Males aged 15–49
	• FSW	• FSW
	• CSW	• CSW
	• MSM	• MSM
	• PWID	• PWID
Expenditure areas defined in model and included in optimization analysis	• FSW and client programs	• FSW and client programs
	• MSM programs	• MSM programs
	• NSPs	• NSPs
	• OST	• OST
	Right and left banks	
	• PMTCT	
	• HIV testing and counseling	
	• Antiretroviral therapy	
	• Behavior change communication and condom programs	

continued next page

Table 8.1 *(continued)*

Category	Parameterization in Optima model
Expenditure areas not included in optimization	• Stigma reduction • Strategic information, research, monitoring and evaluation • Management • Control of sexually transmitted diseases • Blood safety; post-exposure prophylaxis; precautions • Enabling environment • Training • Infrastructure • Social protection
Time frames	• Baseline: 2013 • Modeling periods: 2015–20, 2015–30
Baseline scenario funding	As per National AIDS Spending Assessment for 2013

Source: World Bank 2015.

Note: AIDS = acquired immune deficiency syndrome; CSW = client of female sex worker; FSW = female sex worker; HIV = human immunodeficiency virus; MSM = men who have sex with men; NSP = needle and syringe exchange program; OST = opioid substitution therapy; PMTCT = prevention of mother-to-child transmission; PWID = people who inject drugs.

Table 8.2 Unit Costs Established in the Analysis

Cost per person reached	Moldova (%)		Regional comparison (6 countries including Moldova right bank) (%)			
	Right bank	Left bank	Lowest	Highest	Average	Median
FSW programs	41.66	—	41.66	166.24	102.94	105.35
MSM programs	23.67	—	23.67	449.13	159.45	71.25
PWID/NSP programs	40.90	42.04	40.90	129.25	109.73	84.11
OST	935.15	—	31.41	1,645.24	747.36	790.23
PMTCT[a]	738.08	544.18	738.08	8,905.27	4,616.80	4,267.59
ART[b]	1,264.12	826.64	576.48	2,278.52	1,203.26	1,127.29

Source: World Bank 2015.

Note: ART = antiretroviral therapy; FSW = female sex worker; MSM = men who have sex with men; NSP = needle and syringe exchange program; OST = opioid substitution therapy; PMTCT = prevention of mother-to-child transmission; PWID = people who inject drugs; — = not available.

a. Total program cost divided by the number of HIV-positive pregnant women receiving ART prophylaxis/ART.

b. Average cost per person on ART (including first and subsequent lines of treatment and clinical visits, which explains differences in costs between the two subregions despite the fact that commodity costs are the same).

analytical framework and populations used in the allocative efficiency analysis. There were some gaps in the data, particularly for MSM and FSW and sex worker client populations on the left bank of the Nistru River. As in other models, estimates of HIV prevalence in the general population were derived from data for pregnant women as a proxy for prevalence in the general population.

Table 8.2 presents costs per person reached at the time of the analysis. These costs per person were derived from coverage information and total spending on programs. The numbers reflect differences in the two regions, but the overall cost data suggest that cost of prevention programs for FSWs, MSM, PWID, and prevention of mother-to-child transmission (PMTCT) was particularly low in Moldova by regional standards, whereas the cost of clinical treatment (antiretroviral therapy [ART] and opioid substitution therapy [OST]) was above average.

Understanding the HIV Epidemic

Between 1987 and the end of 2013, over 8,500 HIV diagnoses were registered in Moldova. In 2013, the country had 706 newly registered diagnoses of HIV after a rapid increase in HIV incidence in the 2000s. The number of newly registered diagnoses of HIV peaked in 2008, with some stabilization at the beginning of the 2010s. The total number of people living with HIV (PLHIV) receiving ART by the end of 2013 was 2,493, which represents fewer than 20 percent of PLHIV covered. The epidemic in Moldova remains concentrated among key populations—mostly PWID, but with an increasing incidence among FSWs and MSM. Between 2008 and 2013, sexual transmission became the most common self-reported mode of HIV acquisition. In 2013, 92 percent of people who were newly diagnosed with HIV self-reported sexual transmission as the most probable route. Figure 8.2 shows the annual rates of newly diagnosed PLHIV per 100,000 population on the right bank and left bank of the Nistru River, as well as the national rate. The data suggest that, between 2004 and 2013, new diagnosis rates on the left bank were consistently more than three times higher than the rates on the right bank.

The allocative efficiency estimates suggest that, in 2014, there were 13,200 PLHIV in Moldova. This number is consistent with the registered number of PLHIV and moderately lower than the estimated number of PLHIV in the Spectrum model, which was used by the Joint United Nations Programme on HIV/AIDS (UNAIDS) to produce national and global HIV estimates (UNAIDS 2015). The analysis predicted that, assuming that 2013 conditions (behaviors and program coverage) are maintained, the PLHIV population would grow to 17,700 by 2020. The estimated number of new

Figure 8.2 Newly Diagnosed People Living with HIV per 100,000 Population, Moldova, 2003–13

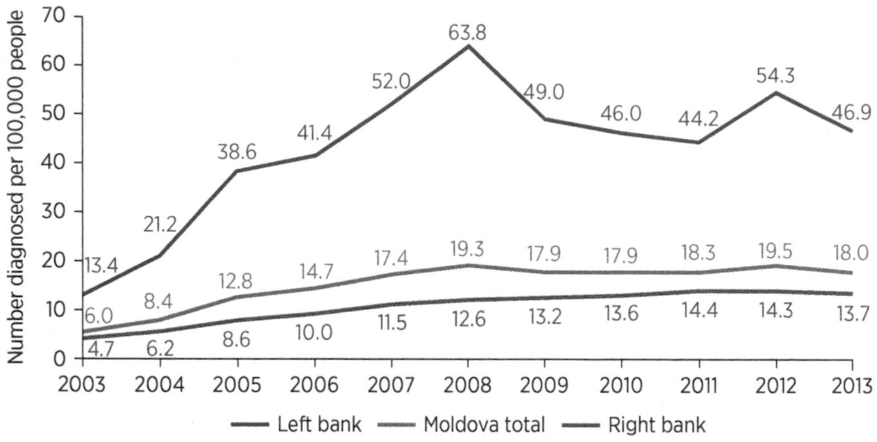

Source: World Bank 2015.

Note: HIV = human immunodeficiency virus.

infections in 2014 was 1,400, and, assuming that 2014 conditions continue to apply, this number is projected to grow to 1,700 by 2020. Estimated AIDS-related deaths were approximately 580 in 2014 and are projected to grow to 680 by 2020.

Trends If 2013 Conditions Are Maintained

The model-predicted evolution of new HIV infections in different populations is presented in figure 8.3. The projections assume that all programs receive funding at the 2013 levels through 2030, and they suggest that the epidemic would grow continuously, with the annual number of new infections growing by over 67 percent by 2030 (from 1,400 new infections in 2015 to approximately 2,500 new infections in 2030). On the right bank, the HIV epidemic among MSM is projected to be the fastest-growing segment of the epidemic because annual new infections will triple by 2030. HIV incidence among other key populations is likely to be stable in the medium term. On the left bank also, the model suggests an increase in new infections among MSM and a moderate increase in new infections among FSWs, their clients, and PWID.

The results show that, at the time of the study, new infections among the general population represented approximately one-third of the total

Figure 8.3 Model-Predicted Evolution of Annual HIV Incidence, Moldova, 2000–30

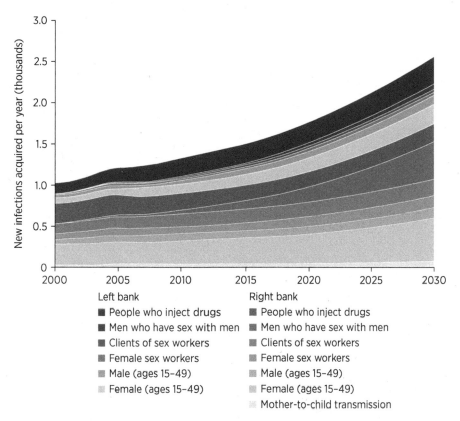

Left bank
- People who inject drugs
- Men who have sex with men
- Clients of sex workers
- Female sex workers
- Male (ages 15–49)
- Female (ages 15–49)

Right bank
- People who inject drugs
- Men who have sex with men
- Clients of sex workers
- Female sex workers
- Male (ages 15–49)
- Female (ages 15–49)
- Mother-to-child transmission

Source: World Bank 2015.
Note: HIV = human immunodeficiency virus.

annual incidence on both banks, and a large portion of these infections were among female sexual partners of PWID, MSM, and FSW clients. The number of infections was projected to increase among both female and male adults on the left bank, and in female adults on the right bank.

Optimizing Allocations under the 2013 Funding Level

Using the Optima model, the research team carried out optimization analyses for different levels of funding and different policy questions. The results show some variations for different policy questions, but also indicate some overarching trends. When interpreting the results, it is important to note that all management costs and other costs for related health services were kept stable and were not included in the mathematical optimization. All optimization analyses conducted for the study suggested room for substantial improvement of the 2013 allocations among the program areas, as detailed below.

The first optimization presented here describes optimized allocations if HIV funding remains constant at the 2013 levels up to 2020.

The analysis suggests that optimized allocation of 2013-level resources could avert 20 percent of deaths and 16 percent of new infections. The largest proposed reallocation if total funding remains constant at 2013 levels would be to prioritize ART by increasing its funding from approximately US$2.7 million to US$4.1 million. This would result in an increase of coverage from 23 percent to 35 percent (figure 8.4). A rough comparison of ART unit costs in the region shows that Moldova implements its treatment program at costs that run slightly above average and median costs, which suggests that there could be some efficiency gains within the program to increase value for money. On the left bank, the annual treatment cost per person in 2013 was US$826, compared to US$1,264 on the right bank, suggesting the potential for unit cost reduction on the right bank.

Akin to recommendations for other countries with concentrated epidemics, in Moldova the model suggests discontinuing provision of services for the general population. HIV testing and counseling (HTC), as well as behavior change communication (BCC) and condom programs for the general population, are not part of the optimized allocation at the 2013 level of spending. These interventions accounted for over 20 percent of the actual investment in 2013, or US$1.8 million—a substantial amount to be reallocated. HTC is part of programs for key populations and would also receive increased allocations. This finding should not be seen as calling for stopping HTC; instead it calls for strengthening the targeting of HTC. In short, the model indicates that, with limited resources and given unit costs, it will be most cost-effective to initiate already diagnosed PLHIV on ART and provide HTC to key populations.

Optimized allocations at the 2013 funding level would also provide funds to scale up three prevention interventions on the left bank, and to scale up prevention for key populations on the right bank. Prevention services for PWID, FSWs, and MSM should receive significantly more funding on both banks, with needle and syringe exchange programs (NSPs) receiving the biggest share of funds in both. Although OST was not available on the left bank at the time of the study, the model suggests introducing OST to the left bank by providing US$31,000 of annual funding to this program. On the right bank, the modeling results would call for slightly smaller budget allocations for OST—which should not be seen, however, as a

Figure 8.4 Actual versus Optimized Allocation of 2013 Funding to Minimize HIV Incidence and Deaths, Moldova

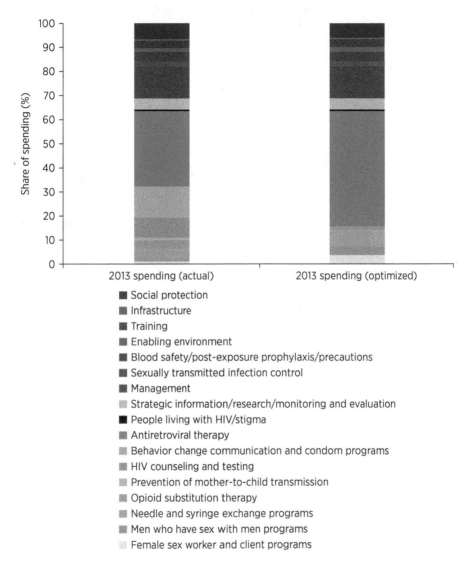

Legend:
- Social protection
- Infrastructure
- Training
- Enabling environment
- Blood safety/post-exposure prophylaxis/precautions
- Sexually transmitted infection control
- Management
- Strategic information/research/monitoring and evaluation
- People living with HIV/stigma
- Antiretroviral therapy
- Behavior change communication and condom programs
- HIV counseling and testing
- Prevention of mother-to-child transmission
- Opioid substitution therapy
- Needle and syringe exchange programs
- Men who have sex with men programs
- Female sex worker and client programs

Source: World Bank 2015.

Note: HIV = human immunodeficiency virus.

recommendation to decrease OST coverage. This finding is due to the fact that this optimization seeks to minimize both new infections and deaths. Because there is no alternative to ART for reducing death in the medium term, high allocations are given to ART despite the relatively high unit cost. For reducing new infections, the model allocated limited resources to the most cost-effective programs, which for PWID in this context were NSPs. Moldova has relatively low unit costs for other prevention programs, but it has—according to a big-picture comparison of costs per person reached—a relatively high OST unit cost compared to other countries in the region. In the six countries included in the analysis, OST unit cost averages US$747; in Moldova, OST is provided at a unit cost of US$935 (INSERM and UNAIDS 2015). This large difference suggests that possible technical efficiency gains in the OST program could be explored.

Optimizing Allocations under Different Levels of Funding

The results in this section present the findings of the allocative efficiency study concerning optimized allocations for different levels of funding available ranging from 0 percent to 200 percent of 2013 spending on direct programs with the goal to minimize both HIV incidence and deaths. In this optimization, the level of spending on management, enablers, and other costs was kept stable.

At all levels of funding, provision of ART for PLHIV requires the largest funding allocations. In case of budget reductions compared to the 2013 level of spending, the key interventions would be ART and prevention for key populations including PWID, MSM, and FSWs and their clients. If, instead, additional funds are available, the funds should be invested in continuous increase of ART and prevention programs for key populations. At the 2013 level of budget availability, the model suggests stopping all prevention services for the general population. With 200 percent of budget availability, HTC should receive approximately 7 percent of the budget (US$0.8 million). This allocation is required because, to increase ART coverage further, HIV testing must be provided beyond key populations.

The optimization analysis was carried out for two different time frames (2015–20 and 2015–30) to test whether substantial differences in allocations exist; however, the overall trend remained the same. Because the contextual analysis established that HIV funding in Moldova has been relatively low and that the treatment gap is substantial, the results presented in figure 8.5 focus on possible scenarios to increase HIV funding.

The level of available funding and the focus of allocations would have a substantial effect on the number of new infections in Moldova. The modeling results found that, assuming there was no funding starting from 2015,

Figure 8.5 Optimized Allocations to Minimize HIV Infections and HIV-Attributable Deaths at Different Budget Levels, Moldova, 2015–20

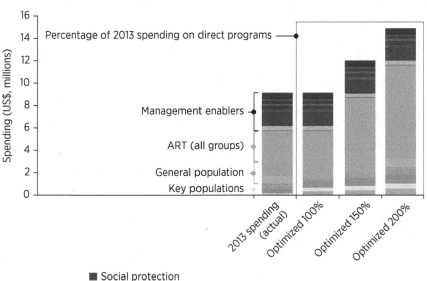

- ■ Social protection
- ■ Infastructure
- ■ Training
- ■ Enabling environment
- ■ Blood safety/post-exposure prophylaxis/precautions
- ■ Sexually transmitted infection control
- ■ Management
- ▒ Strategic information/research/monitoring and evaluation
- ■ People living with HIV/stigma
- ▒ Antiretroviral therapy
- ▒ Behavior change communication and condom programs
- ▒ HIV counseling and testing
- ▒ Prevention of mother-to-child transmission
- ▒ Opioid substitution therapy
- ■ Needle and syringe exchange programs
- ▒ Men who have sex with men programs
- ▒ Female sex worker and client programs

Source: World Bank 2015.
Note: ART = antiretroviral therapy; HIV = human immunodeficiency virus; US$ = US dollar.

by 2020 there would be cumulatively approximately 18,000 new infections. With the 2013 level of funding and 2013 allocations, there would be approximately 11,000 new infections in six years (figure 8.6). In contrast, optimizing the 2013 budget would reduce the cumulative number of new infections to 9,200 cases in five years—a decrease in incidence of 16 percent. Doubling the 2013 budget for direct programs and allocating it optimally would decrease new infections to 7,000 during the same period—a decrease in incidence of 36 percent compared to the baseline scenario.

Levels of HIV funding would also affect the number of AIDS-related deaths. The modeling results indicated that, if starting from 2015 there was no funding for the HIV response, there would be approximately 7,000 AIDS-related deaths by 2020. With the 2013 spending levels and allocations, the estimated number of cumulative AIDS-related deaths would be approximately 5,000 by 2020 (figure 8.7). Optimization of 2013 spending could reduce the cumulative number of deaths by 1,000 (to 4,000 deaths in five years, or a 20 percent reduction). The availability of

Figure 8.6 Cumulative New Infections at Different Levels of Budget Availability, Moldova, 2015–20

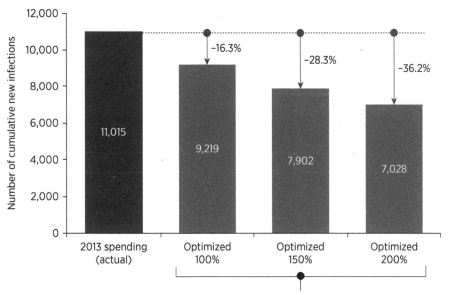

Source: World Bank 2015.

Note: Negative numbers = percentage reduction compared to the baseline scenario.

200 percent of the 2013 budget for direct programs could reduce AIDS-related deaths to approximately 2,600 (a 48 percent reduction compared to the baseline scenario). Table 8.3 presents the actual levels of funding for different programs and corresponding impacts.[4]

The large increase and relatively large share of spending allocated to ART is caused by a combination of factors. As mentioned previously, ART is without an alternative for reducing death in the short and medium terms and for reducing new infections. In addition, the ART unit cost in Moldova, particularly for the right bank, is above average among the six countries included in the regional comparison discussed earlier. If the ART unit cost could be reduced, substantially more funding could be allocated to HIV prevention—even if less than 200 percent of the 2013 spending on direct programs is available. Programs for PMTCT were not part of the optimized mix of interventions. Purely from a cost-effectiveness perspective, low value for money is common in concentrated epidemics because a large number of pregnant women must be tested to identify one HIV-positive woman, which leads to a

Figure 8.7 Cumulative Number of AIDS-Related Deaths at Different Levels of Budget Availability, Moldova, 2015–20

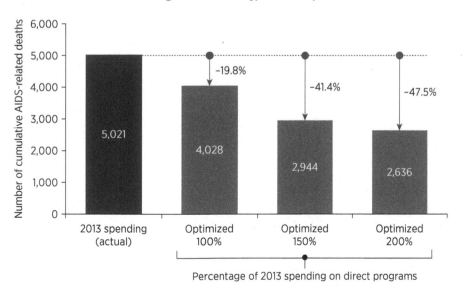

Source: World Bank 2015.

Note: Negative numbers = percentage reduction compared to the baseline scenario. AIDS = acquired immune deficiency syndrome.

high cost per HIV infection averted. This reality does not mean that funding for PMTCT should be discontinued; it means that HTC and ART for pregnant women should be provided at minimal cost by including and prioritizing pregnant women within the allocations for ART and HTC. Within the scenario for 200 percent of 2013 spending on direct programs (US$14.2 million), the increased allocations for these two programs could be partially used for continued HTC and ART access for pregnant women.

The allocative efficiency analysis suggests substantial increases in programs for key populations, particularly OST and NSP on the left bank; it also suggests substantial increases in programs for FSWs, MSM, and NSP on the right bank (table 8.3 and figure 8.8). Working within the levels of funding available, the analysis also proposes a moderate increase in funding for OST on the right bank, which is limited because of existing cost assumptions. The relatively high unit cost for OST in Moldova has the opposite effect from ART in the model allocations. The model—using the unit cost assumptions based on 2013 expenditure data—prioritizes NSPs and other prevention programs for key populations because of their lower cost. As has been shown in other countries in the region where OST costs are relatively lower, OST can be cost-effective with lower unit costs. To be able to expand OST, the unit costs for ART (which absorbs the bulk of funding) and OST should be reviewed. As mentioned, scaling up OST is justified because of the

Table 8.3 Distribution of HIV Prevention and Treatment Spending to Reduce New Infections and AIDS-Related Deaths, Moldova, 2015–20

Program/indicator	2013 allocations	Optimized 100% of 2013 program spending	Optimized 150% of 2013 program spending	Optimized 200% of 2013 program spending
Direct programs (US$)				
FSW and client programs (RB)	113,000	300,000	380,000	463,000
MSM programs (RB)	40,000	253,000	304,000	354,000
NSP (RB)	362,000	541,000	646,000	759,000
OST (RB)	315,000	84,000	234,000	350,000
FSW and client programs (LB)	0	14,000	48,000	71,000

continued next page

Table 8.3 *(continued)*

Program/indicator	2013 allocations	Optimized 100% of 2013 program spending	Optimized 150% of 2013 program spending	Optimized 200% of 2013 program spending
MSM programs (LB)	0	42,000	59,000	74,000
NSP (LB)	36,000	86,000	90,000	97,000
OST (LB)	0	31,000	167,000	241,000
PMTCT	96,000	0	0	0
HIV testing and counseling	703,000	0	0	770,000
Antiretroviral therapy	2.7 million	4.1 million	6.3 million	7.8 million
BCC and condom programs	1.1 million	0	0	0
Subtotal direct programs	5.5 million	5.5 million	8.2 million	11.0 million
Indirect programs (US$)				
PLHIV/stigma	15,000	15,000	15,000	15,000
Strategic information/ research/M&E	403,000	403,000	403,000	403,000
Management	1.2 million	1.2 million	1.2 million	1.2 million
STI control	165,000	165,000	165,000	165,000
Blood safety/PEP/ precautions	363,000	363,000	363,000	363,000
Enabling environment	168,000	168,000	168,000	168,000
Training	243,000	243,000	243,000	243,000
Infrastructure	33,000	33,000	33,000	33,000
Social protection	622,000	622,000	622,000	622,000
Subtotal indirect programs	3.2 million	3.2 million	3.2 million	3.2 million
Total spending (US$)	8.7 million	8.7 million	11.4 million	14.2 million
Total 2013 spending (%)	100	100	132	163
Epidemiological outcomes				
Cumulative new infections	11,000	9,200	7,900	7,000
Cumulative AIDS-related deaths	5,000	4,000	2,900	2,600

continued next page

Table 8.3 *(continued)*

Program/indicator	2013 allocations	Optimized 100% of 2013 program spending	Optimized 150% of 2013 program spending	Optimized 200% of 2013 program spending
Programs for key populations (RB)	**Coverage (%)**			
FSW and client programs (RB)	29	61	69	75
MSM programs (RB)	21	82	85	87
NSP (RB)	41	52	56	58
OST (RB)	3	1	3	3
Programs for key populations (LB)	**Coverage (%)**			
FSW and client programs (LB)	0	15	44	56
MSM programs (LB)	0	62	75	81
NSP (LB)	60	70	70	70
OST (LB)	0	1	3	4
Programs for all populations (RB and LB)	**Coverage (%)**			
PMTCT	84	0[a]	0	0
HIV testing and counselling	23	0[b]	0	25
Antiretroviral therapy	2,996 (23% of all PLHIV)	4,549 (35% of all PLHIV)	6,932 (53% of all PLHIV)	8,576 (65% of all PLHIV)
BCC and condom programs	58	0	0	0

Source: World Bank 2015.

Note: AIDS = acquired immune deficiency syndrome; BCC = behavior change communication; FSW = female sex worker; HIV = human immunodeficiency virus; LB = left bank; M&E = monitoring and evaluation; MSM = men who have sex with men; NSP = needle and syringe exchange program; OST = opioid substitution therapy; PEP = post-exposure prophylaxis; PLHIV = people living with HIV; PMTCT = prevention of mother-to-child transmission; RB = right bank; STI = sexually transmitted infection; US$ = US dollar.

a. Pregnant women should continue to be covered with antiretroviral therapy (ART) as part of the increased ART budget; in practice, this would also require continued HIV testing and counseling for pregnant women, which could be financed from maternal health budgets.

b. HIV testing and counseling would continue to be provided as part of programs for key populations.

Figure 8.8 Allocations for Prevention Programs among Key Populations in Moldova's Two Geographic Subregions, the Right Bank and the Left Bank, under Different Spending Scenarios

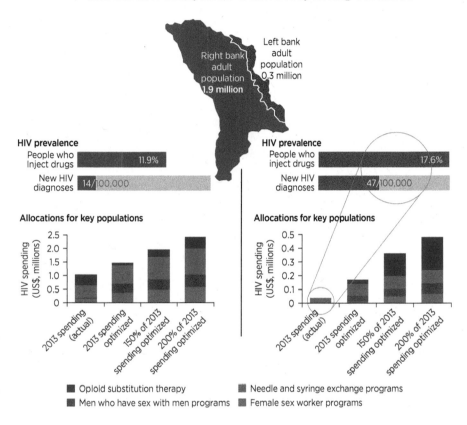

Source: World Bank 2015.

Note: HIV = human immunodeficiency virus; US$ = US dollar.

number of health and social benefits (beyond HIV) that it provides; this scale-up should be pursued with cofinancing from different health and social sectors.

Figure 8.8 details the optimized allocations for prevention among key populations on the right bank and the left bank at different levels of available funding. As noted earlier, new HIV diagnoses per 100,000 people are three times higher on the left bank, as is HIV prevalence among both PWID and women in the general population. Nevertheless, investment in HIV prevention for key populations on the left bank is limited. Regardless of the spending level, the analysis suggests substantially increasing prevention allocations for key populations on both the left bank and the right bank, but the increases are more pronounced for the left bank.

Allocative Efficiency Analysis Recommendations

The allocative efficiency modeling study produced the following eight key recommendations (World Bank 2015):

1. Moldova's HIV epidemic remains concentrated among key populations (PWID, FSWs, and MSM) and their sexual partners. Available data at the time of the modeling study suggested that the epidemic had transitioned from an early concentrated epidemic, in which the highest rates of transmission were among PWID, to an advanced concentrated epidemic, in which onward transmission to sexual partners of PWID and other key populations had become a large source of new infections. Data gaps on HIV prevalence among key populations such as FSWs and MSM, particularly on the left bank, should be filled by including sites on the left bank in biobehavioral surveillance studies for these groups.

2. Moldova should continue to prioritize ART scale-up, which is essential to minimize both HIV incidence and AIDS-related deaths. Depending on the amount of funding available, ART spending should account for between 50 percent and 70 percent of all HIV spending. If total HIV spending could be increased from US$8.7 million to over US$14.0 million between 2015 and 2020, a threefold increase in ART spending and coverage was recommended. This increase would permit ART coverage of 65 percent of all PLHIV and avert 48 percent of AIDS-related deaths, compared to the rates associated with business as usual with 2013 funding. Scaling up a test-and-treat approach (in which individuals are tested and offered early treatment if HIV-positive) would reduce new infections by 36 percent, compared to the business as usual rate. Overall, however, it would be less effective than a combined scale-up of ART plus prevention for key populations. This finding is consistent with a cost-effectiveness analysis carried out in the region, which showed that the combined scale-up of ART and harm reduction programs would have the largest impact on HIV and hepatitis C in Moldova (INSERM and UNAIDS 2015).

3. HTC is a critical component of programs for key populations at all levels of spending as an entry point for ART. At the 2013 funding levels, HTC for the general population is not cost-effective. With increased availability of funding, achieving high ART coverage will require expanding HTC beyond key populations. Nevertheless, HTC would remain focused on

the geographic locations in which members of key populations and their partners are likely to be found. As noted previously, PMTCT should be provided at minimal cost and focus on ensuring that diagnosis of HIV in pregnant women is integrated into comprehensive maternal health services.

4. The study indicates a need to focus prevention interventions on key populations and reallocate funding from general population prevention programs such as BCC to interventions that reach key populations. At all levels of funding up to 200 percent of 2013 program spending, prevention for the general population (BCC and condom programs) should be replaced with targeted programs for PWID, MSM, and FSWs and their clients and partners. Particular attention should be paid to the following two key populations: (1) MSM on the right bank, because HIV prevalence is projected to increase from 4 percent in 2014 to 11 percent in 2020; and (2) PWID on the left bank, among whom HIV prevalence already stood at an estimated 18 percent and has been projected to increase to 21 percent by 2020.

5. Given the severe HIV epidemic on the left bank, prevention programs should be scaled up as soon as possible, including through further increases in the coverage of NSPs, while also introducing services for MSM and FSWs, as well as OST. These key prevention programs are not in place on the left bank, a region in which general adult HIV prevalence has been projected to increase beyond 1 percent according to allocative efficiency modeling and to even higher levels according to the 2015 Spectrum estimates.

6. Rapid assessments of technical efficiency of ART and OST programs should be conducted because the costs for these programs in Moldova are above the regional average. Cost differences between regions within the country should also be explored in search of specific areas for unit cost reductions, particularly for ART, which will absorb most of the funding if programs are scaled up.

7. Given the multiple health benefits of OST, additional cofinancing for OST should be sought from other social and health budget lines. Management, enablers, and other costs that are considered part of national HIV spending include a number of areas whose scope goes beyond HIV programming. Examples are OST, blood safety, control of sexually transmitted infections, and social protection. A technical efficiency analysis of these costs and a review of funding sources would reveal whether the potential exists to reallocate funding to the high-impact programs prioritized in optimized allocation scenarios. Over the long term, in the context of transitioning to full national ownership and program sustainability, HIV programs should be integrated with the wider health response. Within that, HIV components of the budget would complement, rather than pay for, these services.

8. By increasing investments in the HIV response, including domestic financing, Moldova could realize high returns in reducing deaths and improving lives by averting new HIV infections. HIV made up approximately 3.0 percent of the disease burden in YLL, but it accounted for only 0.8 percent of total health expenditures in 2013; and 67.0 percent of HIV funding was provided by international partners. This vast gap suggests the necessity for a substantial increase in domestic financing of the HIV response. Increasing total HIV spending from the 2013 level of US$8.7 million to US$14.2 million and optimally allocating resources would decrease incidence by 36 percent and AIDS-related deaths by 48 percent. In the long term, these effects would have not only health benefits but also financial benefits in reduced health care costs for PLHIV.

Making Use of the Findings

National Plans

In 2015, building on the findings from the allocative efficiency modeling, a series of meetings and workshops were held to discuss the findings and way forward. The evidence and resulting discussions became key contributors to the development of the National HIV/AIDS/STI Prophylaxis Program (NAP) for 2016 through 2020. The NAP sets clear priorities, focusing on key epidemic drivers, key populations, and the interventions demonstrated to have an impact on the epidemic, with special attention to the left bank, the most affected region of the country. In addition, building on these efforts and participation in a key regional workshop in Vienna, Moldova developed a national action plan for 2016–17 based on the investment approach of UNAIDS (2013).

The results of the allocative efficiency study also informed the June 2016 high-level national dialogue on successful transition to national funding of harm reduction in Moldova. The dialogue discussed the status of harm reduction programs in the framework of the NAP, volumes of planned government and donor funding, and government measures to ensure sustainability of harm reduction programs, as well as different mechanisms of state funding for nongovernmental organizations for implementation of nonmedical harm reduction services for key populations.

The allocative efficiency study confirmed that Moldova continues to experience a concentrated epidemic among key populations. With that in mind, the NAP focused on and prioritized the identified populations most affected by HIV. As a result, the NAP was designed around three key strategies:

1. Prevention of HIV and STI within the PWID, sex workers, MSM, and prisoner populations through providing access to harm reduction programs and testing for at least 60 percent of the estimated number of PWID and sex workers and 40 percent of MSM by 2020
2. Universal access to treatment, care, and support to PLHIV covering 60 percent from estimated PLHIV with ART by 2020 (tripled from the baseline of 17 percent)
3. NAP management on efficiency, management, coordination, resilient and sustainable systems for health, human rights, financial sustainability, evidence generation, and systems for monitoring and evaluation

The NAP sets much more ambitious targets to ensure the reversal of the epidemic. It also strengthens the interventions in key populations for the eastern (left bank) region, because it was demonstrated that more efforts and investments should be provided for that work.

Left Bank Funding and Procurement Strategies

The results of the investment approach also served as the basis of the transition and sustainability plan for the regional HIV program on the left bank of the river, which was created after several meetings with nongovernmental organizations and health and finance specialists at the beginning of 2017. For the first time, the left bank region is receiving increased financial commitments for its HIV programming: rising from 3 percent in 2016 up to 20 percent in 2020. The investments are being provided in a holistic way and cover prevention, treatment, care, and support programs.

Attention to prevention programming has also been strengthened. In 2014, Moldova's NFM (new funding model) application to the Global Fund to Fight AIDS, Tuberculosis and Malaria succeeded in doubling the resources for prevention programs. The allocative efficiency analysis showed that such an increase will support an efficient HIV response. Building on these factors, the NAP takes this emphasis further by ensuring sufficient budgeting for prevention programs—up to 30 percent of the total budget.

In addition, in January 2017, the Ministry of Health and the United Nations Development Programme signed a memorandum of understanding related to procurement of medicines for the national programs, including ART drugs, in order to optimize the budget and to ensure procurement of affordable and accessible drugs for HIV patients. The first analyses of the procurement showed an estimated 30 percent savings.

Notes

1. Based on Institute for Health Metrics and Evaluation's 2010 Global Burden of Disease Study Data Visualizations (University of Washington 2014). For more information, see http://www.healthdata.org/gbd/data-visualizations.
2. Much of this chapter reviews the process and findings of the modeling exercise documented in the report produced for that analysis; as such, the material herein draws significantly on that report. For more detail, see World Bank 2015 in the reference list for this chapter.
3. As part of the allocative efficiency analysis efforts, the research team gathered data from six countries in the region to better understand specific costs across those nations and to facilitate regional comparisons. For purposes of this chapter, references to regional cost comparisons refer to this group of countries.
4. In practice, this coverage also would require continued HTC for pregnant women, which could be financed from maternal health budgets; HTC would continue to be provided as part of programs for key populations. People requesting HIV testing should continue to receive the service even if they are not part of key populations. What the model suggests is that, from a cost-effectiveness perspective, expanded testing for the general population is not among the most cost-effective programs when no additional resources are available.

References

Duric, P., C. Hamelmann, D. P. Wilson, and C. Kerr. 2014. "Modelling an Optimised Investment Approach for Tajikistan: Sustainable Financing of National HIV Responses." Government of Tajikistan, Dushanbe.

Fraser, N., C. Benedikt, M. Obst, E. Masaki, M. Görgens, R. Stuart, A. Shattock, R. Gray, and D. P. Wilson. 2014. "Sudan's HIV Response: Value for Money in a Low-Level HIV Epidemic. Findings from the HIV Allocative Efficiency Study." World Bank, Washington, DC.

INSERM (Institut national de la santé et de la recherche médicale) and UNAIDS (Joint United Nations Programme on HIV/AIDS). 2015. "Intervention Packages against HIV and HCV Infections among People Who Inject Drugs in Eastern Europe and Central Asia: A Modeling and Cost-Effectiveness Study. Preliminary Report on Cost-Effectiveness, Belarus." INSERM and UNAIDS, Paris/Geneva.

Moldova. 2013. "The Third Millennium Development Goals Report. Republic of Moldova." Government of Moldova, Chisinau.

Moldova, National Bureau of Statistics. 2016. "Labour Force Survey Report 2016." National Bureau of Statistics, Chisinau.

UNAIDS (Joint United Nations Programme on HIV/AIDS). 2013. "Smart Investments." UNAIDS, Geneva.

UNAIDS (Joint United Nations Programme on HIV/AIDS). 2014. AIDSinfo database. Geneva. http://www.unaids.org/en/dataanalysis/datatools/aidsinfo.

UNAIDS (Joint United Nations Programme on HIV/AIDS) 2015. "HIV Estimates with Uncertainty Bounds 1990–2014." UNAIDS, Geneva.

University of Washington. 2014. 2010 Global Burden of Disease Study. Data Visualizations. IHME (Institute for Health Metrics and Evaluation), Seattle. http://vizhub.healthdata.org/gbd-cause-patterns/; http://www.healthdata.org/results/data-visualizations.

World Bank. 2015. "Optimizing Investments in Moldova's HIV Response." World Bank, Washington, DC.

World Bank. 2016. "Moldova Economic Update October 5, 2016." World Bank, Washington, DC.

9

North Macedonia
Tackling a Small but Rapidly
Growing Epidemic

Vladimir Mikik, Laura Grobicki, Lidija Kirandjiska,
Natasha Nikolovska Stankovikj, Jasmina Panovska-Griffiths,
Feng Zhao, and Katherine Ward

Briefly

- North Macedonia has one of the region's smallest epidemics, but the epidemic is growing fast.
- New infections among men who have sex with men started at a low level but have increased rapidly.
- The end of support from the Global Fund to Fight AIDS, Tuberculosis and Malaria means there is a need to reprioritize human immunodeficiency virus (HIV) spending, while sustaining key services.
- The transition to significantly greater reliance on domestic funding for HIV programming is taking place during a time of epidemic growth.

Introduction

Governance, Demographics, and the Economy

North Macedonia is located in the Balkan peninsula in Southeast Europe. It declared independence from the former Yugoslavia in 1991. The constitution has defined North Macedonia as a parliamentary democracy.

The parliament is the legislative body of the country and elects the government, which has the executive power. Since 2004, when the process of decentralization was initiated, 84 municipalities have been established throughout the country, 10 of which constitute the capital city of Skopje. In 2014, the country's total population was 2,075,625 inhabitants. According to the data from the most recent census (2002), 64.2 percent of that population are of Macedonian nationality, 25.2 percent are Albanians, 3.9 percent are Turks, 2.7 percent are Roma, and 1.8 percent are of Serbian nationality.

The 1990s were characterized by high inflation, a decreasing gross domestic product (GDP), and continuous political instability. In 2001, North Macedonia faced an internal conflict that further impaired the overall development of the economy, including the political and social structures. In recent years, however, major economic reform processes have substantially contributed to the stabilization of the inflation rate and to an increase in GDP. Currently, North Macedonia is considered an upper-middle-income country according to World Bank data.[1] The unemployment rate decreased from 37.2 percent in 2005 to 22.1 percent in late 2017.[2]

To ensure their consistency and relevance, and unless otherwise indicated, the data provided in this chapter relate to the situation in North Macedonia at the time the analysis was conducted.

Contours of the HIV Epidemic

North Macedonia has a low-level HIV epidemic. Between the detection of the first case of HIV in 1987 and December 2014, 236 people were diagnosed with HIV (North Macedonia 2015b) and 75 registered acquired immune deficiency syndrome (AIDS) deaths were recorded (North Macedonia 2015a). The number of people diagnosed has increased more recently, however, with 39 of the 236 registered people living with HIV (PLHIV) diagnosed in 2014 alone (figure 9.1). The HIV epidemic in this context is concentrated among males (80 percent), and 64 percent of newly diagnosed PLHIV in 2014 were men who have sex with men (MSM) (North Macedonia 2015b). There have also been small numbers of new diagnoses among other key populations, including male sex workers (MSWs) and people who inject drugs (PWID). New HIV diagnoses among the general population are low in number.

A significant proportion of PLHIV are not aware of their status, as indicated by the late diagnoses in 2014 where 41 percent of newly diagnosed PLHIV already had AIDS (North Macedonia 2015b). Poor detection leads to late presentation for treatment, which in turn adversely

Figure 9.1   Number of Registered HIV Cases, North Macedonia, 2000–14

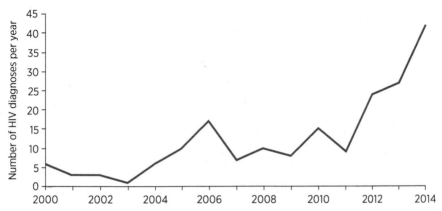

Source: World Bank 2015.
Note: HIV = human immunodeficiency virus.

affects treatment outcomes, significantly increases short-term mortality risk, and reduces the cost-effectiveness of treatment. The introduction of antiretroviral therapy (ART) has reduced mortality among PLHIV over recent years, but the data suggest that earlier detection could significantly improve the effectiveness of ART.

Dependence on Donor Contributions

Total HIV spending in North Macedonia increased by nearly 80 percent between 2008 and 2013, and most of this increase was due to substantial growth in international funding (North Macedonia 2014b). The Global Fund to Fight AIDS, Tuberculosis and Malaria (the Global Fund) has been the country's major international donor, contributing about 90 percent of all donor funds in 2013. Domestic funding (combined state and private spending) in 2013 was marginally higher than international funding (with 53 percent). Domestic funding has increased about 70 percent since 2008, almost entirely due to the substantial growth in public HIV funding. It should be noted that private spending in this context includes only contributions made by charitable organizations; it does not include household (out-of-pocket) spending and is therefore likely to be underestimated.

Reliance on international donors for a significant portion of HIV financing and the substantial expected reduction in international assistance in the short term are key challenges to the sustainability of HIV program-ming in North Macedonia. These challenges will be compounded if HIV incidence continues to rise. Further reducing North Macedonia's depen-dence on external donor funding may require the establishment of tran-sitional funding mechanisms to supplement and redirect public funding sources.

Domestic Spending and Allocative Efficiency

According to World Health Organization (WHO) estimates for 2013, total health expenditure as a percentage of GDP in North Macedonia was 6.4 percent, showing a reduction of about 30 percent since 2000.[3] This figure is lower than the WHO Europe regional average (8.0 percent) and significantly lower than most other former Yugoslav countries such as Serbia (10.6 percent), Bosnia and Herzegovina (9.6 percent), and Slovenia (9.2 percent). In 2013, per capita health care expenditure was US$312, and nearly 70 percent of health expenditure was funded from public sources. Expenditure from public sources increased by almost 20 percent since 2000, whereas out-of-pocket payments decreased from 42 percent to 31 percent of total health expenditure.

An allocative efficiency analysis using the Optima model was carried out in 2015 when a new national strategic plan for 2017–21 was being developed in a new funding climate, amid concern for the sustainability of North Macedonia's HIV response as available donor funding declines (World Bank 2015).[4] In response, a sustainability and transition plan was developed and adopted by the Country Coordinating Mechanism in December 2016 to identify transitional funding mechanisms and facili-tate the shift from international to domestic financing of HIV programs.

To support North Macedonia in the context of sustainability planning, the study addressed two questions: What is the trajectory of the epidemic under different scenarios, in comparison to the predicted epidemic trends under the existing HIV response? How can North Macedonia optimize the allocation of HIV funding if 2013 funding or less or more funding is available?

Projections from the Allocative Efficiency Analysis

Trends If the 2013 Spending Level Is Maintained

The HIV epidemic in North Macedonia is a concentrated epidemic with 236 people diagnosed with HIV and 75 registered AIDS deaths cumulatively recorded by December 1, 2014 (North Macedonia 2015b). MSM accounted for 64 percent of newly diagnosed HIV infections in 2014. Input data on population size and HIV prevalence for key populations at higher risk of HIV exposure are outlined in table 9.1. With 2013 levels of funding and 2013 allocations to HIV intervention programs maintained, the model projects that the epidemic will remain at a low level; however, the total number of PLHIV is projected to increase from a model-estimated 307 in 2014, to 438 by 2020, and to 846 by 2030. This increase is primarily a consequence of the expected increase in HIV incidence. As figure 9.2 shows, MSM are projected to account for 73 percent of PLHIV in 2020 and 78 percent in 2030. The same figure shows that PWID are likely to constitute 5 percent of all PLHIV in 2020 and 2 percent in 2030; MSWs are expected to constitute 5.1 percent of PLHIV in 2020 and 4.6 percent in 2030. Females in the general population are projected to represent 11 percent of PLHIV in 2020 and 10 percent of PLHIV in 2030.

Overall HIV prevalence is projected to increase from a low base—from modeled estimates of 0.018 percent in 2014, to 0.026 percent in 2020, and to 0.050 percent by 2030. The largest increases in HIV prevalence are projected to occur among MSWs and MSM. In the MSW population, the model projects a steady increase in HIV prevalence from an estimated 3 percent in 2014, to 4 percent by 2020, and to approximately 7 percent by 2030. On a similar trajectory, HIV prevalence among MSM is expected to increase from almost 2 percent in 2014, to just less than 3 percent by 2020, and to approximately 6 percent by 2030. These projected figures are indicative only because changes in risk behaviors, mobility, or interactions with epidemics

Table 9.1   Population Size and Prevalence among Key Populations, North Macedonia, 2014

Population	Population size (most recent value)	HIV prevalence (%, most recent value)
FSW	2,136 (CI: 1,181–5,588)	0.05 (estimate)
FSW clients	52,614 (estimate)	0.01 (estimate)
MSM	19,300 (CI: 11,300–36,350)	1.90
MSW	1,466 (CI: 810–3,835)	3.43
PWID	11,532 (CI 9,782–14,632)	0.12

Source: World Bank 2015.

Note: The FSW population size estimation is based on Kuzmanovska, Mikik, and Memeti 2012. The percentage of sex workers who are female (59.3 percent) is based on Mikik et al. 2014a. Concerning FSW HIV prevalence, Mikik et al. 2014a estimated a 0 percent prevalence based on no diagnosed cases of HIV among FSW; however, it is plausible to assume that there is one case of HIV among this population, which would equal 0.05 percent. The MSW population size estimation is based on Kuzmanovska, Mikik, and Memeti 2012. The percentage of sex workers who are male (40.7 percent) is based on Mikik et al. 2014a. The PWID HIV prevalence is based on nongovermental organization testing data from 2014; one diagnosed person living with HIV out of 815 PWID tested. CI = confidence interval; FSW = female sex worker; HIV = human immunodeficiency virus; MSM = men who have sex with men; MSW = male sex worker; PWID = people who inject drugs.

Figure 9.2 Estimated Number of People Living with HIV, according to the Model Calibration

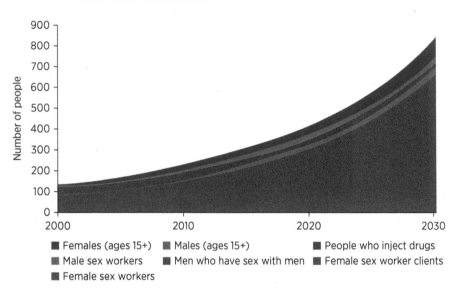

Source: World Bank 2015.
Note: HIV = human immunodeficiency virus.

in neighboring countries may influence future HIV prevalence trends. Projections within small populations such as those in this context will always be more sensitive to small changes in risk factors than projections calculated for larger-scale epidemics.

HIV prevalence among FSWs is projected to remain stable at about 0.06 percent, and HIV prevalence among PWID is projected to decline slightly from an estimated prevalence of 0.24 percent in 2014, to 0.19 percent in 2020, and to 0.16 percent by 2030. Using available data on HIV prevalence and behavior, the allocative efficiency modeling has projected further reductions in HIV prevalence and incidence among PWID. This projection suggests that the country's epidemic among PWID is under control, but the model does not account for changes in behavior or interactions with HIV epidemics among PWID in neighboring countries, which may negatively influence the epidemic trajectory.

Underpinning the small increase in HIV prevalence described earlier is a predicted increase in HIV incidence (figure 9.3). Most new HIV infections are predicted to be among MSM—from 64 percent of registered new cases

Figure 9.3 Number of New HIV Infections per Year in North Macedonia, per Model Calibration

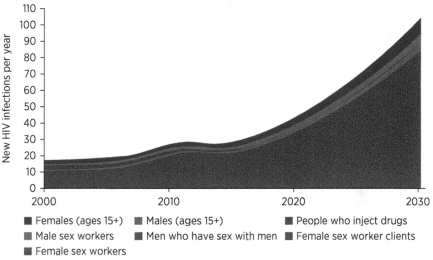

Source: World Bank 2015.
Note: HIV = human immunodeficiency virus.

In 2014, to a model-estimated 78 percent of new infections in 2020, and to 80 percent by 2030. Much of the expected increase in HIV incidence is driven by the share of transmission attributed to unprotected sex between MSM and their partners. Low condom use (46.8 percent) among MSM and casual partners (Mikik et al. 2014c) is a particular concern, as is relatively low condom use with commercial partners (that is, 84 percent for MSWs, compared with 93 percent for FSWs) (Mikik et. al. 2014a); therefore, interactions between MSWs and MSM remain important. Furthermore, 77 percent of MSM in the 2010 integrated biobehavioral surveillance (IBBS) survey and 64.9 percent of MSM in the 2014 IBBS survey (Mikik 2012; Mikik et al. 2014b) reported having sex with a female in the past 12 months. The high probability of sex with female partners raises concerns about the potential role of MSM in bridging HIV transmission to their sexual partners within the female adult population.

Until 2014, the number of AIDS-related deaths was estimated to have been relatively stable at 10 per year across all populations, reflecting the low-level epidemic of the 1990s. Overall, however, the number of deaths attributable to HIV is predicted to increase to 17 in 2020 and to 36 by 2030 if PLHIV are not diagnosed promptly and put on treatment.[5]

At the end of 2014, 96 people were receiving HIV treatment. With the predicted increase in new infections, however, demand for treatment will rise. Furthermore, at the time of the model analysis, North Macedonia provided treatment only when the CD4 count was less than 350 cells/mm³; however, WHO (2015) guidance recommended commencing treatment for adults at any CD4 count. If North Macedonia was to adhere to international guidelines for HIV treatment, additional registered PLHIV would require treatment and more PLHIV might be newly diagnosed.

The Impact of Spending before and as of 2013

Prevention has been the largest component of HIV spending in North Macedonia, at an average of 77 percent of total spending between 2008 and 2013 (figure 9.4). Within prevention, the largest share of spending has been on interventions targeting PWID, including opioid substitution therapy (OST), needle and syringe exchange programs (NSPs), and hepatitis C prevention. Between 2008 and 2013, interventions targeting PWID made up on average 61 percent of prevention spending. In 2013, 63 percent of prevention spending and 51 percent of total HIV spending were allocated to harm reduction programs. In contrast to PWID interventions, investment in other preventive programs targeting the general population or other key populations, such as MSM and sex workers, has been relatively low. Program management, the main indirect cost category in this context, constituted an average of 14 percent of total HIV spending between 2008 and 2013. Although this proportion was reduced to 9 percent in 2013, it remains higher than spending on HIV care and treatment.

These investments in HIV prevention and treatment may not be benefitting the people most in need (figure 9.5). Model-based estimates suggest that incidence and prevalence are increasing among key high-risk populations, with the exception of PWID, and among MSM in particular. These estimates therefore suggest that prevention could be better targeted. If the potential role of MSM in bridging the epidemic between MSWs and general population women is further considered, the case for better-targeted prevention is even more compelling because it is likely to yield benefits for both high-risk and low-risk populations.

Examination of the unit costs per person suggests other areas of the 2013 baseline spending that may merit further attention. Using cost-coverage relationships, the analysis estimated the costs per person reached at 2013 spending levels. This basic analysis demonstrated that costs for many programs, in particular ART and OST, have been high when compared with data for other comparable countries in the region (table 9.2).

Figure 9.4 HIV Expenditure in North Macedonia, by Type of Spending

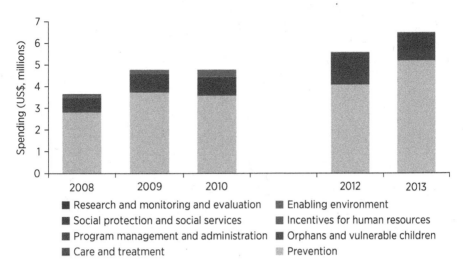

Source: World Bank 2015.
Note: HIV = human immunodeficiency virus; US$ = US dollar.

Figure 9.5 Trends in Spending across Key Priority Prevention and Treatment Programs, North Macedonia

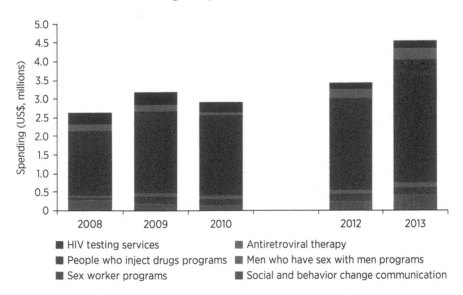

Source: World Bank 2015.
Note: HIV = human immunodeficiency virus; US$ = US dollar.

Table 9.2 Comparing Cost per Person Reached in North Macedonia with Other Countries in the Eastern Europe and Central Asia Region

US dollars

Cost per person reached	2013	Comparison to other countries			
		Lowest	Highest	Average	Median
SW programs	203.39	41.66	203.39	117.29	107.05
MSM programs	48.96	23.67	449.13	133.66	48.96
PWID-NSP	174.51	40.90	174.51	99.09	101.36
OST	1054.26	431.41	1,645.24	880.19	935.15
ART	3835.43	576.48	3,835.43	1,509.50	1,195.70

Source: World Bank 2015.

Note: The table reflects how costs were categorized by countries for this analysis. The method is not based on detailed matching of classification of inputs but on how countries had actually classified expenses using the detailed available guidance for National AIDS Spending Assessment (NASA) and Global AIDS Response Progress Reporting (GARPR) reports. Although this guidance is detailed and specific, differences cannot be ruled out, particularly regarding cross-cutting costs such as human resources. In addition, even if costs are classified consistently, the comprehensiveness of service packages may differ. The completed Optima data matrixes for seven Eastern Europe and Central Asian countries (Armenia, Belarus, Georgia, Kazakhstan, the Kyrgyz Republic, Moldova, and Ukraine) were compiled by the study team from a range of country-specific data sources during 2014–15. These data are based primarily on coverage data from program records for 2013–14 and total HIV spending for a program area per 2013–14 GARPR and NASA reports. ART = antiretroviral therapy; MSM = men who have sex with men; NSP = needle and syringe exchange program; OST = opioid substitution therapy; PWID = people who inject drugs; SW = sex worker.

Comparing HIV Response Scenarios

The allocative efficiency analysis considered whether reaching prespecified targets regardless of the budget required could potentially further reduce HIV prevalence, new infections, and AIDS-related mortality. It did so by comparing the trajectory of the HIV epidemic by 2030 in North Macedonia under the 2013 HIV response against the following three alternative response scenarios that are not constrained by a budget and are instead determined solely by targets:

1. Test and offer treatment: In this scenario, it is assumed that, by 2020, 90 percent of PLHIV would be aware of their status and 90 percent of diagnosed PLHIV would be on ART (with treatment efficacy in reducing new infections for PLHIV on ART assumed to be 70 percent).
2. Attaining global targets for all key populations: In this scenario, the country aims to reach global goals for all key populations.

3. Defunding all preventive programs: In this scenario, the possible impact of defunding all prevention programs for key populations, including HIV testing and counseling (HTC), is explored.

The resulting analyses predicted that the scenario offering testing and treatment (scenario 1 above) would substantially reduce new infections and deaths compared with the 2013 strategy. The test and offer treatment scenario is estimated to result in a 72 percent decrease, or 636 fewer infections, and an 80 percent decline, or 246 fewer deaths by 2030, compared with the baseline scenario assuming that 2013 treatment coverage and other epidemic conditions remain unchanged (figures 9.6 and 9.7).

The findings also show, however, that reaching global treatment and prevention targets for all key populations (scenario 2) is even more effective in reducing the number of new infections and deaths than only testing and offering treatment. This scenario is projected to achieve an estimated 86 percent reduction in both new infections and deaths, with an estimated 757 fewer infections and 264 fewer deaths by 2030. Findings from these analyses show that defunding all prevention programs is expected to increase overall prevalence, the number of new

Figure 9.6 Model-Predicted Evolution of Annual HIV Prevalence under Different Scenarios, North Macedonia, 2000–30

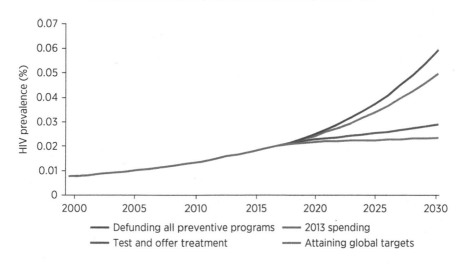

Source: World Bank 2015.

Note: HIV = human immunodeficiency virus.

Figure 9.7 Model-Predicted Evolution of Annual New Infections under Different Scenarios, North Macedonia, 2000–30

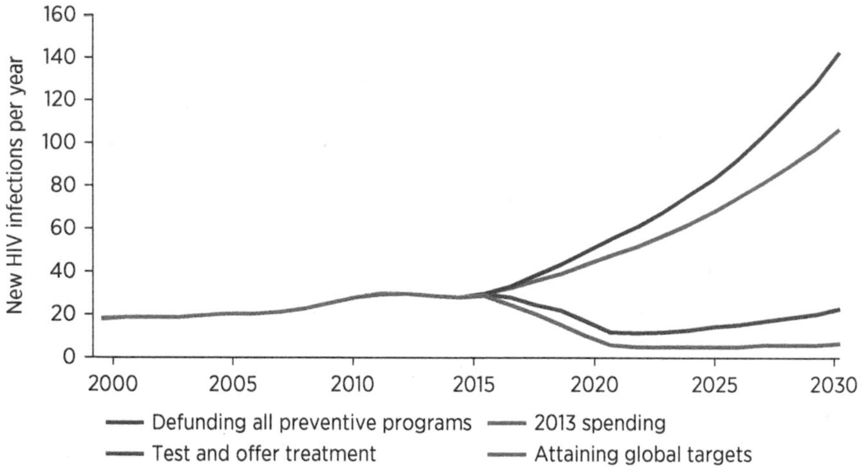

Source: World Bank 2015.
Note: HIV = human immunodeficiency virus.

infections, and the number of deaths—by 9 percent, 19 percent, and 5 percent, respectively—compared with the rates expected with the HIV response plan as of 2013.

Effects of Optimizing the Allocation of Funding

An optimization analysis was conducted comparing the allocation of the 2013 budget of US$5,154,743[6] and an optimized allocation of the same budget for the time period 2015–30. The findings suggest differences between the actual 2013 distribution of funding and the model-optimized allocation of the 2013 budget that would seek to minimize both new infections and deaths (figure 9.8). The optimized allocation of the 2013 budget would avert an estimated 856 additional HIV infections (85 percent), predominantly among MSM, and 294 additional deaths (87 percent) between 2016 and 2030.

Optimized allocations to programs and the corresponding impact were also estimated and compared for different levels of funding. Specifically, the analysis considered what could be gained by increasing HIV spending from 2013 levels. Conversely, the analysis also considered which programs would have the largest impact on the epidemic if less funding was available and the response needed to be further rationalized.

Figure 9.8 Comparison of Actual and Optimized Allocation of the 2013 Budget to Minimize Both New Infections and Deaths in North Macedonia for the Period 2015–30

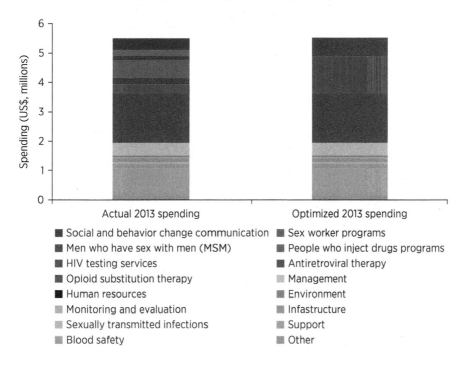

Source: World Bank based on Optima model.
Note: HIV = human immunodeficiency virus; US$ = US dollar.

The optimization analysis suggests that, if 75 percent to 90 percent of 2013 funding is available, ART, OST, and MSM programs should be given priority (figure 9.9). This finding results from a combination of factors. ART is essential to minimize deaths, and it also helps reduce incidence. For further prevention, increasing condom use among MSM is an important behavioral strategy in the context of North Macedonia. The model protects OST funding at 100 percent because of its substantial benefits beyond HIV prevention and also because of the rationale that no one on OST should stop receiving treatment. (Similarly, no one on antiretroviral treatment would have treatment withdrawn.) At the same time, efforts should be made to ensure the high unit costs of OST are reduced as far as possible—without compromising the quality of care. Savings achieved through OST efficiency gains could be used to sustain other programs for PWID, in particular NSPs.

Figure 9.9 Optimized Allocations to Minimize HIV Incidence and Deaths in North Macedonia by 2030 at Different Budget Levels, 2013 Spending

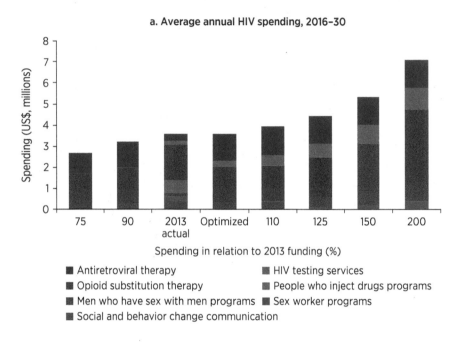

a. Average annual HIV spending, 2016–30

- Antiretroviral therapy
- Opioid substitution therapy
- Men who have sex with men programs
- Social and behavior change communication
- HIV testing services
- People who inject drugs programs
- Sex worker programs

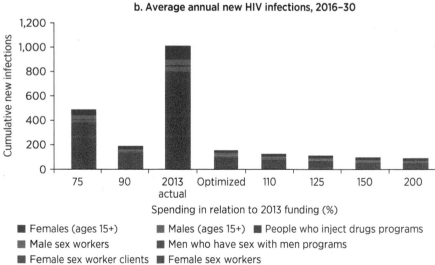

b. Average annual new HIV infections, 2016–30

- Females (ages 15+)
- Male sex workers
- Female sex worker clients
- Males (ages 15+)
- Men who have sex with men programs
- Female sex workers
- People who inject drugs programs

continued next page

Figure 9.9 *(continued)*

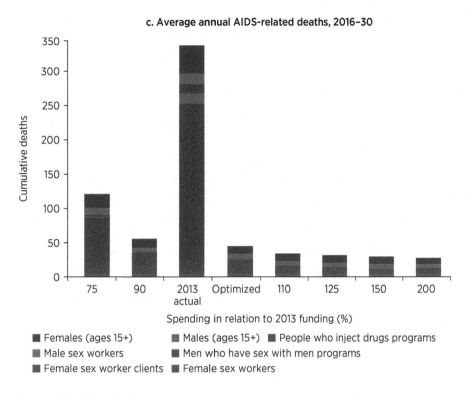

c. Average annual AIDS-related deaths, 2016–30

Spending in relation to 2013 funding (%)

- Females (ages 15+)
- Males (ages 15+)
- People who inject drugs programs
- Male sex workers
- Men who have sex with men programs
- Female sex worker clients
- Female sex workers

Source: World Bank 2015.

Note: AIDS = acquired immune deficiency syndrome; HIV = human immunodeficiency virus; US$ = US dollar.

The optimization analysis suggests that, if 100 percent to 200 percent of 2013 funding is available, investment should continue to focus on ART and OST. Funding for MSM programs should also increase in this scenario. This analysis suggests that, with a larger budget, a significant share of funding should be allocated to HTC programs for key populations. Spending on programs for the low-risk, general population (such as social and behavior change communication [SBCC]) is recommended only at higher multiples of the 2013 budget—that is, when the optimized spending budget is approximately 200 percent of 2013 spending.

This analysis shows that increased and optimally allocated spending on HIV programs may continue to yield some gains in terms of infections and deaths averted (figure 9.9). The most substantial gains, however, can be made in optimizing the allocation of the 2013 budget, with proportionately smaller gains made by further increasing spending over the 2013 level.

Sustaining Effectiveness through Efficiency Gains

Historically, the Global Fund was the primary source of funding for prevention and treatment programs in North Macedonia. More recently, the National Ministry of Health has taken over responsibility for the funding of some programs previously funded by the Global Fund, including the provision of methadone for OST since 2008, and ART and supportive treatment for PLHIV since 2010 (North Macedonia 2014a, 2018). As North Macedonia prepared for the full withdrawal of Global Fund support during 2017, however, the process highlighted a substantial funding gap—particularly in prevention programming—that must be met if the existing HIV response is to be sustained.[7] Using the analyses discussed earlier, this section highlights the specific challenges and recommendations for successful transition to national ownership of a sustained and effective HIV response.

Using Allocative Efficiency to Do More with Less

The allocative efficiency gains described previously should enable the Ministry of Health to achieve greater health impact with a sustained or slightly smaller HIV budget. Allocative efficiency gains in this context will primarily be achieved by increasing funding to programs that target prevention in key populations, reducing spending on prevention in the general population where the risk of new infections is low, and increasing spending on ART. Key populations to target include MSM and MSWs. Scaling up ART delivery will benefit both key populations and the general population.

The Ministry of Health finances ART and associated treatment from the Health Insurance Fund and other Ministry of Health resources. As coverage expands, so too will the funding needs of this program. Because the Health Insurance Fund currently only partly funds ART provision, the ministry may seek to expand contributions from this source to meet or reduce the funding gap.

Exploring Efficiency Gains in Future Work

As mentioned previously, the unit costs of programs such as ART and OST are higher in North Macedonia than in other comparable countries in the region. A thorough review of potential strategies to reduce costs, while maintaining the quantity and quality of service provision, should therefore be considered.

On a positive note, drug prices for antiretrovirals have been declining since 2014. Further savings may also be achieved by exploring opportunities to switch from branded to generic drugs, moving toward single drug regimens where appropriate, engaging with pooled procurement schemes, changing the drugs prescribed to cheaper, equally effective alternatives, or some combination of these actions.

As of the time of writing, no comparable reduction in OST costs has been observed. It may be important to note that 16 percent of those on OST treatment in 2014 were on buprenorphine. Buprenorphine is substantially more expensive then methadone, and studies from other settings found no difference in effectiveness (Gowing, Ali, and White 2006; Mattick et al. 2004). As such, Buprenorphine may be less cost-effective than methadone (Mattick et al. 2004), and a change in the drug used may yield significant technical efficiency savings. Aside from any changing drug regimens, achieving further technical efficiency gains in drug pricing may be difficult for North Macedonia because of low economies of scale. With increasing coverage, however, enhanced price negotiations could be explored. Pooled procurement processes may warrant further exploration in this context.

Technical efficiency gains could also be considered for other prevention programs targeting key populations. These gains may require further collaboration between nongovernmental organizations (NGOs) for providing preventive care, or further integration of HIV testing with other elements of the existing basic care package. To improve technical efficiency, there may also be scope for further collaboration with NGOs that support different key populations.

Sex worker (SW) and MSM programs have been funded almost entirely by the Global Fund. Sourcing alternative funding for these programs remains critical. With the transition to national ownership, programs serving these populations may need to explore new cofunding opportunities and possible income-generating activities. Service models may need to be reviewed when considering how to meet the needs of the epidemic after the transition from international to domestic funding. Mechanisms for the government to contract and manage NGOs need to be decided upon and developed.

Program management and administration, the main indirect cost category in this context, constituted 9 percent of total HIV spending in 2013. This proportion is lower than in some other countries in the region, but it is higher than HIV care and treatment spending, which constituted 7 percent of total HIV spending in 2013. Although these indirect costs were fixed in the allocative efficiency modeling analyses, future work could explore opportunities to rationalize program management and administration costs, with the savings then allocated to the direct costs of the HIV response.

Finally, further analysis could explore whether HIV services could be further integrated into other existing health services, including those for sexually transmitted infections, reproductive health, tuberculosis, and others. One of the strengths of North Macedonia's HIV response is the coordination of its services across service delivery modalities. This strength could potentially be harnessed further with better integration of services.

Allocative Efficiency Analysis Recommendations

The allocative efficiency modeling study produced the following key recommmendations (World Bank 2015):

1. The government of North Macedonia has implemented an effective HIV response, maintaining a very low-level HIV epidemic. The government could allocate future HIV spending optimally to further minimize HIV incidence, prevalence, and HIV-related deaths.
2. Allocative efficiency analysis modeling highlights a strong risk that prevalence and incidence will increase overall in North Macedonia, mainly among MSM, in spite of existing efforts to contain the epidemic.
3. The expected overall increase in the epidemic appears to be driven by increasing incidence and prevalence among MSM, a key population that receives only a small portion of HIV funding. High-risk behavior in this population, including low condom use, calls for significant strengthening of interventions targeting MSM. Increasing the use of condoms with casual and commercial partners is likely to be an effective preventive measure. Additional programs such as pre-exposure prophylaxis (PrEP) may also be considered for MSM and MSWs at highest risk; however, rates of HIV incidence are still substantially below 3 per 100 person years, which WHO has suggested as an indicative level for PrEP to be cost-effective. Hence, PrEP might be a useful tool for specific individuals at highest risk, but not for entire subpopulations of MSM and MSWs.
4. Funding allocations that prioritize improved condom use, higher HIV testing rates among MSM and MSWs, and scale-up of ART to all populations in need will be most effective in containing the epidemic overall. An optimized allocation of the 2013 level of funding may increase longer-term financial commitments to the HIV response by increasing

uptake of ART, but it will substantially decrease financial commitments needed because of new infections, which would decline with optimized allocations.

5. Presentation for testing and treatment is delayed for some PLHIV, thus increasing costs and reducing positive outcomes of treatment. These delays are likely caused by multiple factors, including possible fear of stigmatization and discrimination among MSM and MSWs. These deterrents to effective care-seeking may add the additional risk of weak adherence to treatment. Risk factors such as these are best addressed with a rights-based approach to care.

6. The allocative efficiency analysis suggests that reallocating funding toward prevention among MSM and MSWs would improve efficiency at the 2013 spending level. The estimations from the allocative efficiency analysis and contextual data suggest that the HIV epidemic among PWID and FSWs is relatively well contained because of significant and prolonged efforts to target these populations. Because of the risk of rising HIV infection among PWID in the future (as experienced in other countries in the region) and also the risk of transmission of other, more prevalent infectious diseases such as hepatitis C, it is essential that coverage levels of NSP and OST are sustained. It is also an important public health priority that the wider sexual and reproductive health needs of FSWs continue to be met.

7. The allocative efficiency study found that comparing the unit costs of care in North Macedonia with data from other countries in the region suggested that greater efficiency in spending might be achieved through strategies to reduce the average spend per person reached. These strategies should not intentionally or unintentionally compromise the existing quantity, quality, or scope of prevention or treatment programs. Further analyses of technical efficiency are needed before more robust conclusions can be reached.

8. If optimally allocated, annual spending at the 2013 level should be sufficient to achieve potential national HIV strategic plan and international targets. By describing the likely trajectories of the HIV epidemic under different conditions, highlighting areas of particular risk in the short to medium term, and suggesting ways to incrementally improve the efficiency of spending at the 2013 level, these suggestions should assist North Macedonia in optimizing its HIV response. Modeling the epidemic in the absence of HIV program spending highlighted the significant gains already achieved from spending at the 2013 level in the form of new infections and deaths averted. Analyses of what is needed to achieve possible targets set by the National HIV Strategic Plan,

however, have identified the need for continued investment in an optimized HIV response.

9. Mapping of key populations will be essential in planning for scaling up recommended programs, particularly in the case of MSM and MSW populations. The findings show that the number of new infections is increasing among the MSM population, so it is important to increase coverage of MSM programs. The MSM population is hard to reach for a number of reasons, with a large proportion of the MSM population remaining "hidden." Fear of stigmatization and discrimination may prevent affected individuals from accessing health services and undergoing testing—demonstrated by the fact that only 19 percent of MSM had an HIV test in 2014 (Mikik et al. 2014b). The MSM population is also not homogeneous: many MSM have female partners, and a significant proportion pay for commercial sex. Condom use also varies significantly among MSM (46.8 percent with a casual partner and 83.7 percent with a paid partner in 2014). The ability to meet male partners over the internet adds an extra challenge to measuring and reaching this population. Existing service models could potentially be reviewed in light of the role of internet dating in moving MSM out of existing key locations, and all these factors will need to be taken into account when considering scale-up of these programs.

10. MSWs remain a challenging population to reach. MSWs can face stigmatization and discrimination both for having sex with men and for having commercial sex, and they are at a high risk of contracting HIV because of biological, behavioral, and structural reasons (Baral et al. 2015). MSM should be a central focus of the HIV response. Programs for sex workers may need to consider innovative ways to better map and scale up programs targeted at the MSW population. Further research specifically among this population would be beneficial, and ongoing work to change the structural determinants of discrimination and stigma needs to be a core focus.

11. Additional domestic resources are needed to sustain the HIV response after the withdrawal of Global Fund support. Although funding for HIV in North Macedonia has increased since 2008, international donors financed much of this increase. Preventive programs and programs targeted at key populations are primarily funded by international donors. As such, the withdrawal of international funding without a concurrent increase in domestic funding will have a significant negative impact on the HIV epidemic in North Macedonia. Transitional funding mechanisms need to be explored with the aim of raising domestic funding to at least the level of the total 2013 budget for the HIV response. International donor funding must be replaced with alternate funding.

Actions Taken and Next Steps

North Macedonia has been implementing the final stage of its HIV grant from the Global Fund, which was extended for a final period that ended in December of 2017 to cofinance the preventive activities funded from the national budget. Taking into account that the country was no longer eligible for additional Global Fund grants, the country started to prepare itself for successful transition from international to domestic financing of the preventive activities among key populations. The preparations have also been addressing the need to adequately respond to the new challenges related to a rapid increase in the number of new HIV infections, mainly among the MSM population.

The Ministry of Health, in close collaboration with the HIV program implementation unit and civil society including NGOs, has moved forward considerably toward finalizing several crucial stages of the transition process. To this end, the Country Coordinating Mechanism prepared and adopted the Transition Plan at the end of December 2016.

With joint efforts by all concerned stakeholders, the HIV Strategy for 2017–21 was developed. Most of the activities in the strategy rely on findings from the allocative efficiency analysis report, especially in terms of prioritizing key populations—with MSM and MSWs defined as the primary focus. At the same time, the main strategic goal in terms of financing is to ensure a stable and continuous source of financing from the national budget while also stimulating new and innovative financing mechanisms aimed toward interventions with greater efficiency.

In 2016, through a consultative process, the Ministry of Health adopted criteria for establishing a social contracting mechanism, and it has committed to have this financing mechanism put into practice and made fully operational.

In 2017, the Ministry of Health announced a public call for cofinancing of NGOs as implementing partners in the annual HIV prevention program and gradually supported the NGOs' prevention activities in the total amount of MKD 5.9 million, which was disbursed to the NGOs and implemented by the end of 2017. Most important, in 2018, the Ministry of Health significantly increased the budget of the program to MKD 95 million (approximately €1.5 million). Out of this amount, MKD 47 million (approximately €800,000) is designated for NGOs' prevention activities for key populations—especially for those activities that have been identified as crucial priorities: (1) MSM, both facility-based and outreach programs; (2) maintaining and increasing the stationary and outreach HTC among key affected populations; (3) continued financing of the two key population youth-friendly services for sexually transmitted infection diagnosis and treatment; and (4) maintaining the existing services for NSPs for PWID, as well as existing SW programs. The contracted amount of MKD 47 million is very close to the annual funding provided by the Global Fund in previous years. Challenges still exist, however, especially in terms of developing and putting into place functional financing mechanisms concerning NGOs within the prevention program.

For 2018, the optimization of resources for delivery areas also lowered the cost of care per person reached. The absolute number (US$ per person reached) might not be the best metric for measuring success when comparing the situation in North Macedonia to other countries in the region; the context is different in different countries (for example, GDP, costs of services and goods, potential for economies of scale, and the cost of generic versus branded ART), and the cost per PLHIV can appear higher if an HIV response is very successful in preventing HIV (because there are fewer PLHIV). Assessments should also take into account how successful the activities are in containing the HIV epidemic.

Notes

1. See the World Bank's country classification data at http://data.worldbank.org /income-level/upper-middle-income.
2. See North Macedonia's State Statistical Office labor market web page at http:// www.stat.gov.mk/PrikaziSoopstenie_en.aspx?rbrtxt=98.
3. Data from the World Health Organization's National Health Accounts Database. For more information, see http://www.who.int/health-accounts/en/.
4. Note that much of this chapter reviews the process and findings of the modeling exercise documented in the report produced for that analysis; as such, the material herein draws significantly on that report. For more detail see World Bank 2015 in the reference list for this chapter.
5. In calibration, the allocative efficiency model assumes that the number of PLHIV on ART remains constant.
6. This figure does not include spending on hepatitis C (about US$1 million). Moreover, only direct programs such as key population programs (FSWs, MSM, PWID), ART, SBCC (social and behavior change communication), and HTC programs are included in the optimization analysis. The indirect programs or cost items—such as program management, enabling environment, blood safety, and so on—were not included.
7. Actions taken by the government to address the end of Global Fund funding are discussed further in the final section of this chapter.

References

Baral, S. D., M. R. Friedman, S. Geibel, K. Rebe, B. Bozhinov, D. Diouf, D., K. Sabin, C. E. Holland, R. Chan, and C. Caceres. 2015. "Male Sex Workers: Practices, Contexts, and Vulnerabilities for HIV Acquisition and Transmission." *Lancet* 385 (9964): 260–73.

Gowing, L., R. Ali, and J. White. 2006. "Buprenorphine for the Management of Opioid Withdrawal." *Cochrane Database of Systematic Reviews* 8 (3): CD002025.

Kuzmanovska, G., V. Mikik, and S. Memeti. 2012. "Report from the Bio-Behavioural Survey and Assessment of Population Size of Sex Workers in Macedonia, 2010." Institute for Public Health of the Republic of North Macedonia, Skopje.

Mattick, R., J. Kimber, C. Breen, and M. Davoli. 2004. "Buprenorphine Maintenance versus Placebo or Methadone Maintenance for Opioid Dependence." *Cochrane Database Systematic Reviews* 2004 (3): CD002207.

Mikik, V. 2012. "Report on the Bio-Behavioral Study and Assessment of Population Size of Men Having Sex with Men in Macedonia, 2010." Institute for Public Health of the Republic of North Macedonia, Skopje.

Mikik, V., et al. 2014a. "Report on the Bio-Behavioral Study among Male and Female Sex Workers in Macedonia." Institute for Public Health of the Republic of North Macedonia, Skopje.

Mikik, V., et al. 2014b. "Report on the Bio-Behavioral Study among the Men Having Sex with Men Population in Skopje, Macedonia, 2013–2014." Institute for Public Health of the Republic of North Macedonia, Skopje.

Mikik, V., et al. 2014c. "Report on the Bio-Behavioral Study among People Who Inject Drugs in Macedonia, 2014." Institute for Public Health of the Republic of North Macedonia, Skopje.

North Macedonia, Country Coordinating Mechanism. 2014a. "Request for Renewal from the Global Fund to Fight AIDS, Tuberculosis and Malaria, May 2014." Unpublished document, Ministry of Health, Skopje.

North Macedonia, Ministry of Health. 2014b. "National HIV/AIDS Spending Report 2008–2013." Ministry of Health, Skopje.

North Macedonia, IPH (Institute for Public Health of the Republic of North Macedonia). 2015a. "Annual Report for 2014 on HIV." IPH, Skopje.

North Macedonia, IPH (Institute for Public Health of the Republic of North Macedonia). 2015b. "Facts about HIV/AIDS in the Republic of Macedonia for 2014." Fact sheet, IPH, Skopje. http://lph.mk/en/facts-about-hiv-aids-in-the-republic-of-Macedonia-for-2014/.

North Macedonia. 2018. Official Gazette. No. 17, dated January 26 (including Program for Health Protection of People with Drug Addiction Illnesses, in RM for 2018, 36, and Program for Protection of the Population in RM from HIV infection, in 2018, 49). Government of North Macedonia, Skopje.

WHO (World Health Organization). 2015. *Guideline on When to Start Antiretroviral Therapy and on Pre-Exposure Prophylaxis for HIV.* Geneva: WHO.

World Bank. 2015. "Optimizing Investments in Former Yugoslav Republic of Macedonia's HIV Response." World Bank, Washington, DC.

10

Tajikistan
Toward a Rights-Based Response for Key Populations

Predrag Duric, Christoph Hamelmann, and John Macauley

Briefly

- The human immunodeficiency virus (HIV) epidemic in Tajikistan remains concentrated among key populations.
- Analysis indicates that a rights-based approach, including "test and treat" and focusing on key populations, would avert the greatest number of deaths and new infections.
- It is crucial that the government of Tajikistan seek opportunities for partial funding of key HIV program interventions from domestic resources.

Introduction

Tajikistan is a mountainous, landlocked nation with more than half the country above 3,000 meters, and the Pamir and Alay Mountains

The mathematical model discussed in this chapter was developed and run by David Wilson and Cliff Kerr, University of New South Wales. Bakhtiyor Mirzoev, advocacy and communication officer for United Nations Development Programme (UNDP) Tajikistan, and Sabir Kurbanov, health specialist, national consultant for UNDP Tajikistan, provided an overview of the implementation of the resulting dominating the landscape. It is also the smallest nation in Central Asia. After independence in 1991, the country endured a civil war lasting five years, which caused tens of thousands of deaths and forced hundreds of thousands to become internally displaced or migrate abroad. The civil war also devastated Tajikistan's economy. More than 20 years after that war, Tajikistan is still the poorest country in Eastern Europe and Central Asia and is also among the poorest countries in Asia. Most of the population (74.6 percent) lives in rural areas. Tajikistan also has a young population: every third person is younger than 15 years old.

To ensure their consistency and relevance, and unless otherwise indicated, the data provided in this chapter relate to the situation in Tajikistan at the time the analysis was conducted.

The HIV Epidemic

The first HIV infection in Tajikistan was diagnosed in 1991, and until 2000 only 14 people living with HIV (PLHIV) were diagnosed. Since 2005, more than 150 new HIV infections have been diagnosed in Tajikistan each year, with a new high reached in 2015 (1,151 new infections reported) (Republican AIDS Center data).[1] The HIV situation in Tajikistan was similar to that in other former republics of the Soviet Union, with HIV infection mainly diagnosed among people who inject drugs (PWID). With increased availability of HIV testing for over 12 years, however, HIV infections have been diagnosed more often and sexual transmission has become the predominant mode of transmission.

report, verified epidemiological data, and reviewed this chapter. Rosemary Kumwenda (UNDP's Team Leader for Regional HIV, Health and Development in Europe and the Commonwealth of Independent States [CIS]) also reviewed the chapter. The chapter was based on the report that built on the inputs and reviews of the Tajikistan country team working on the development of an HIV investment case for Tajikistan: Tatjana Majitova, Zuhra Nurlyaminova, Murodali Mehmondustovich Ruziev, Safarhon Sattorov, and Alijon Soliev (Republican AIDS Center); Muratboki Beknazarovich Beknazarov (Country Coordinating Mechanism [CCM] Secretariat); Ulugbek Aminov (Joint United Nations Programme on HIV/AIDS [UNAIDS] Tajikistan); Mavzuna Burkhanova, Saodat Kasymova, Zarina Iskhanova, and Tedla Mezemir (UNDP Tajikistan); and in coordination with Roman Gailevich, Jean-Elie Malkin, and Manoela Manova from the regional UNAIDS office in Moscow. Many others have participated in reviews of drafts, data verification, and translations, including Lusine Aydinyan, Victoria Froltsova, Alisher Juraev, Alisher Latypov, Alexandra de Olazarra, Julia Whitman, and Karen Zhang. The study would not have been possible without the valuable comments and support from Boyan Konstantinov (from the regional UNDP HIV, Health and Development Team, Regional Bureau for Europe and the CIS).

The HIV epidemic in Tajikistan has other important dimensions. For instance, the number of HIV infections diagnosed among women and children has been increasing. The proportion of women among new cases of HIV infection increased from 12 percent in 2003 to 43 percent in 2014 and 40 percent in 2016. Also, like in some other countries in the region, particularly those with struggling economies, a significant proportion (14 percent) of the new HIV infections was diagnosed among international labor migrants.

Among the many challenges for the HIV response in Tajikistan and for achieving the 90–90–90 strategy of the Joint United Nations Programme on HIV/AIDS (UNAIDS), the most important are the limited access to counseling, testing, and treatment (UNAIDS 2014a).[2] Of the estimated 16,000 PLHIV in Tajikistan, 42 percent had been diagnosed. Only 25 percent of the estimated number of PLHIV were on treatment in 2015.

Three Scenarios

In response to a clear need for data analysis to inform decision-making on how to spend the limited funds available for HIV programming, a research team was assembled to take on the project. The team developed three scenarios the government of Tajikistan could use to make the right investment decisions for its national HIV response. The analysis had to be done keeping in mind that Tajikistan has been highly dependent on international support and is affected by a weak economy and overall low access to essential services. The team considered the following three scenarios, with 2013 used as the reference year:

* *Scenario 1*: Continue with the 2013 investment allocations and the 2013 budget ceiling.
* *Scenario 2*: Continue with optimized investment allocations and the 2013 budget ceiling.
* *Scenario 3*: Continue by scaling up to universal coverage for essential HIV prevention and treatment services.

The analysis had the following objectives:

* To provide model estimates of future epidemic trajectories in the context of the development of an HIV investment case and sustainable financing strategies for the national response for Tajikistan under the three scenarios.
* To estimate and compare the program costs and the impact (that is, the return on investment expressed in new HIV infections averted and disability-adjusted life years [DALYs] averted) of the three scenarios in

the medium term (2020) and long term (2030). These estimations and comparisons had to be done while keeping in mind short-term objectives such as the development of a Concept Note for the Global Fund to Fight AIDS, Tuberculosis and Malaria (the Global Fund) using the new funding model (NFM), and long-term objectives such as the UNAIDS "Getting to Zero" goals, the "Together We Will End AIDS" campaign, and the "End of HIV/AIDS Epidemic" target by 2030 proposed for the Sustainable Development Goals (SDGs) (UNAIDS 2010, 2014b; United Nations General Assembly 2015).[3]

The findings from this analysis were assembled in a modeling report published by the United Nations Development Programme (UNDP) (Duric et al. 2014).[4]

Key Populations in a Rights-Based Approach

A shift in the two main modes of HIV transmission has been observed in Tajikistan; similar shifts have also been noted in other countries in the Commonwealth of Independent States (CIS). Since 2011, sexual transmission has been the dominant mode of HIV transmission in Tajikistan (figure 10.1). Mother-to-child transmission was reported in 0.4 percent of the new HIV infections in 2006. Since then, the percentage first increased (reaching 5.7 percent in 2014) and subsequently dropped to 4.9 percent in 2016.

Figure 10.1   Modes of Transmission for HIV Infection in Tajikistan, 2005–16

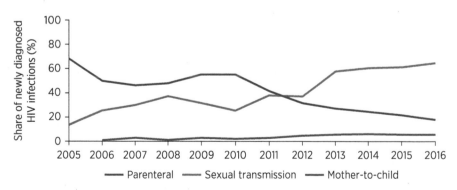

Source: Republican AIDS Center.
Note: HIV =human immunodeficiency virus.

The shift between the two leading modes of HIV transmission should be interpreted in the context of the 11-fold increase in HIV testing between 2005 and 2015 (figure 10.2). The possible effects of the Global Fund programs implemented in Tajikistan since 2003 should also be considered. It is possible that, in the early years of the HIV epidemic, HIV testing and counseling (HTC) was limited to PWID and a small number of others and that, with broader availability and promotion of HTC, a higher proportion of HIV infections was diagnosed.

HIV prevalence among PWID has remained very high (for example, 13.5 percent in 2014). HIV prevalence has been stable among sex workers but has been uncertain among men who have sex with men (MSM) because of limitations in the samples used in the relevant bio-behavioral surveys (figure 10.3). In some regions, injecting drug use is still the most common mode of transmission. For example, 48.2 percent of all HIV infections reported in Gorno-Badakhshan Autonomous Oblast were diagnosed among PWID, compared to 13.9 percent in Khatlon Oblast.

In recent years, men have accounted for approximately 60 percent of all newly diagnosed HIV infections. In the 15–29 age group, however, women account for most newly diagnosed cases (figure 10.4). Table 10.1 presents a summary of key national HIV indicators.

Figure 10.2   New HIV Infections and HIV Tests Performed in Tajikistan, 2000–16

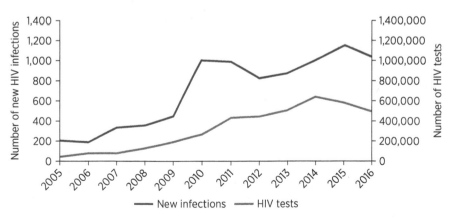

Source: Republican AIDS Center.

Note: HIV =human immunodeficiency virus.

Figure 10.3 HIV Prevalence in Key Populations and Prison Inmates

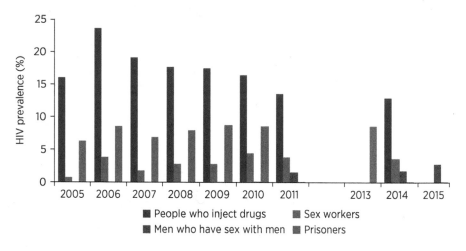

Source: Republican AIDS Center.
Note: HIV =human immunodeficiency virus.

Figure 10.4 Proportion of Women among Newly Diagnosed HIV Infections, Tajikistan

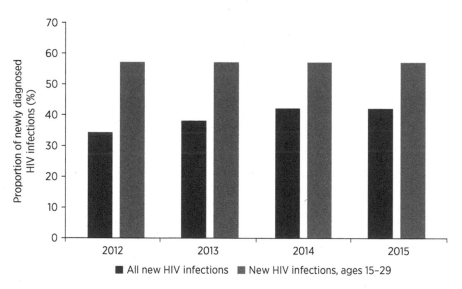

Source: Republican AIDS Center.
Note: HIV =human immunodeficiency virus.

Table 10.1 Summary of Key National HIV Data, Tajikistan, 2000–16

	2000	2005	2010	2014	2015	2016	Source
HIV diagnoses							
Cumulative number of people diagnosed with HIV, total	32	505	2,857	6,519	7,709	8,750	Republican AIDS Center
Cumulative registered number of people diagnosed with HIV and alive, total	–	–	2,203	5,241	6,117	6,782	Republican AIDS Center
Estimated number of PLHIV, total	<1,000	7,979	11,786	16,000	15,721	16,321	Republican AIDS Center, UNAIDS
New diagnoses							
Number of people newly diagnosed with HIV, total	18	217	1,004	1,008	1,151	1,041	Republican AIDS Center
Number of people newly diagnosed with HIV (ages 15 and older)	18	216	989	–	1,020	918	Republican AIDS Center
Number of people newly diagnosed with HIV (ages 0–14)	0	1	15	–	131	123	Republican AIDS Center
Number of people newly diagnosed with HIV, women	0	22	215	430	463	415	Republican AIDS Center
Number of people newly diagnosed with HIV, men	18	195	789	578	688	626	Republican AIDS Center
Deaths among PLHIV							
Annual registered number of deaths among PLHIV	–	–	118	309	344	160	Republican AIDS Center
Cumulative registered number of deaths due to AIDS, total	–	–	365	1,278	1,592	1,968	Republican AIDS Center

continued next page

Table 10.1 (continued)

	2000	2005	2010	2014	2015	2016	Source
HIV prevalence among key populations (%)							
Sex workers	—	0.7	4.4	3.5	—	—	CCM Tajikistan, Government of the Republic of Tajikistan
Men who have sex with men	—	—	—	1.7	2.7	—	CCM Tajikistan, Government of the Republic of Tajikistan
People who inject drugs (PWID)	—	16.0	16.3	12.9	—	—	CCM Tajikistan, Government of the Republic of Tajikistan
Prison inmates	—	6.2	8.4	—	—	—	CCM Tajikistan, Government of the Republic of Tajikistan
Service coverage and utilization							
Number of HIV tests performed	—	58,899	280,281	647,978	597,426	510,138	Republican AIDS Center
Number of people receiving ART	—	—	483	2,167	3,139	4,002	Republican AIDS Center
Number of syringes distributed per estimated PWID	—	27.2	88.3	214	—	345	UNDP Tajikistan
Share of PWID receiving OST (%)	—	—	0.2	—	—	2.4	UNDP Tajikistan

continued next page

Table 10.1 *(continued)*

	2000	2005	2010	2014	2015	2016	Source
Self-reported modes of HIV transmission (% of newly diagnosed with HIV)							
Sexual transmission	16.6	13.2	25.0	60.6	61.7	65.0	Republican AIDS Center
HIV transmission through IDU	83.3	68.3	55.6	24.2	21.4	17.7	Republican AIDS Center
Mother-to-child transmission	0	0	1.4	5.7	4.8	4.9	Republican AIDS Center

Sources: Combined data from government ministry reports (Tajikistan 2014a, 2014b, 2015, 2016), personal communication with Republican AIDS Center (RAC), government sources including the CCM/Coordination Committee (National Coordination Committee for Prevention and Control of AIDS, Tuberculosis and Malaria 2014), and unpublished RAC data.

Note: Analysis based on historical data available at the time of analysis (up to 2013) and updated with available data in 2017. Please note that the number of PLHIV registered and number of new infections include reported cases only; they do not necessarily reflect the HIV incidence presented in the analysis. HIV prevalence in key populations should be interpreted according to the methodology used in integrated biobehavioral surveys. AIDS = acquired immune deficiency syndrome; ART = antiretroviral therapy; CCM = Country Coordinating Mechanism; HIV =human immunodeficiency virus; IDU = injecting drug use; OST = opioid substitution therapy; PLHIV = people living with HIV; PWID = people who inject drugs; UNDP = United Nations Development Programme; — = not available.

Projections of the Optima HIV Modeling Analysis

Maintaining 2013 Conditions

Assuming that 2013 conditions (behaviors and program coverage) remain stable, the Optima HIV modeling analysis for Scenario 1 (maintaining the 2013 investment allocations and budget level) in Tajikistan resulted in the following six main findings (see figure 10.5):

1. For future projection, the model-estimated annual HIV incidence[5] would show a moderate decline from approximately 1,450 in 2013 to about 1,150 in 2020.
2. The projected declining incidence is mainly driven by key populations at higher risk of HIV exposure. Among sex workers (SWs) incidence is projected to decline by 28 percent, in PWID by 27 percent, in prison inmates by 27 percent, in MSM by 20 percent, and in labor migrants by 20 percent. The model also projects spillover effects for women and men, with incidences declining by 13 percent and 6 percent, respectively.

Figure 10.5 Estimated Numbers of PLHIV, ART-Eligible PLHIV, and PLHIV on ART under Scenario 1, Tajikistan

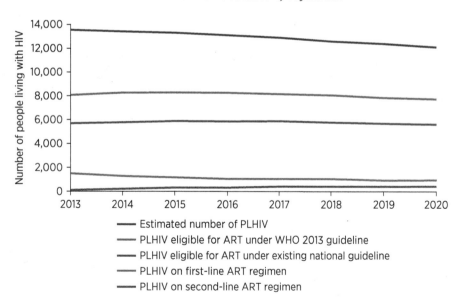

Source: Duric et al. 2014.

Note: See WHO (2013) for guidelines on ART. ART = antiretroviral therapy; HIV =human immunodeficiency virus; PLHIV = people living with HIV; WHO = World Health Organization.

3. HIV will continue to be transmitted among PWID in Tajikistan, but the trend toward a larger share of sexual transmission will progress.
4. Proceeding with the existing investment allocations at the 2013 budget level, the estimated number of PLHIV was projected to slightly decrease from approximately 13,000 in 2013 to 12,000 in 2020.
5. If testing rates do not increase, only 3,300 of the estimated 12,000 PLHIV will know their HIV status.
6. Because the total number of PLHIV on antiretroviral therapy (ART) would slightly decrease because of budget constraints (if budget constraints continue without domestic funding, especially after Global Fund financing ends) and the increasing number of second-line ART, and because the model predicts the number of PLHIV will only slightly decrease, ART coverage in 2020 would remain low. Coverage will shift from 11 percent of the estimated total number of PLHIV (1,350 out of 12,000) to 41 percent of the total PLHIV registered (1,350 out of 3,300).

Resource allocation in Tajikistan must take into account the disease burden, the distribution among subpopulations, and the potential for impact. There is an important opportunity to further improve the resource allocation to program components and subpopulations in such a way that those resources can achieve the greatest impact.

Optimizing Allocations at the 2013 Budget Level

For Scenario 2 (optimizing the investment allocations at the 2013 budget level), the analysis considered two alternative options:[6]

1. Option A: Improving allocative efficiency for the prevention and the care and treatment program components (which together made up about 60 percent of the total budget in 2013), leaving the program management and human resources (HR) components constant.
2. Option B: Improving allocative efficiency for the prevention and the care and treatment program components but reducing allocations for program management and HR by 20 percent (approximately US$1 million) and using the savings to further improve the allocative efficiency for the prevention and the care and treatment components. (Note that overall management and administration costs in Tajikistan appeared to be high compared with direct program costs and compared to other countries in the region.)

The analysis identified that, overall, the 2013 budget envelope was insufficient to scale up all essential and effective standard interventions to universal coverage. Therefore, the results for an optimized allocative efficiency under the 2013 budget ceiling (that is, for the programming underfunded at the time) must be interpreted with caution in the context of service rationalization. This caution is especially important when considering the competing effectiveness of essential key interventions to reduce infections, disease burden, and death.

With these constraints in mind, the model suggested an optimized resource allocation under the 2013 budget constraints by shifting resources from behavior change communication (BCC), community mobilization, and prevention for vulnerable and accessible populations and youth toward key populations at higher risk for HIV infection. It also suggested shifting resources from HTC toward treatment because the low treatment rates mean, under the model assumptions, that the benefits from diagnosing additional people are relatively limited (figure 10.6).

The modeling suggested that the following allocative efficiency results are possible by 2020 (figure 10.7):

- An estimated 11,500 PLHIV
- An estimated 6,000 PLHIV eligible for ART in 2020 based on the national ART guidelines at that time, and 7,900 if the WHO (2013) guidelines were adopted in 2015
- Approximately 1,800 PLHIV on first-line ART regimens and 500 PLHIV on second-line regimens in 2020
- An increase in estimated ART coverage from 20 percent of the total estimated number of PLHIV (2,300 out of 11,500) in 2014 to 96 percent of all registered PLHIV in 2020 (2,300 out of 2,400)

The modeling results for Scenarios 1 and 2 clearly demonstrate the limitations of 2013 budget levels. Under these scenarios, too many PLHIV will remain undiagnosed and without essential services—even under optimized allocative efficiency and reduced program management and HR costs; and the impact on HIV incidence and DALYs will remain limited.

Rights-Based Investment and Universal Coverage

The objective of a rights-based investment approach is to reach universal coverage of essential HIV prevention services and ART by 2020. The analysis therefore considered Scenario 3 (scaling up to universal coverage by 2020). Starting at the 2013 estimated service coverage levels for HTC, ART, prevention of mother-to-child transmission (PMTCT), and special interventions for key populations, the model assumed an approximately linear increase over time to reach universal coverage for the key prevention and

Figure 10.6 Comparison of Tajikistan's Budget Allocations under the 2013 Budget Envelope

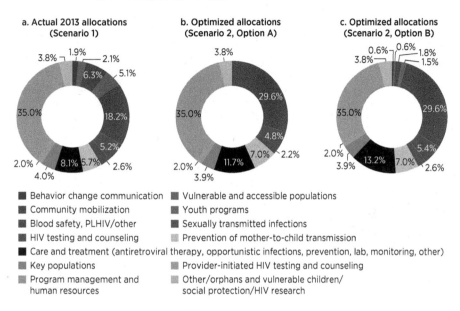

a. Actual 2013 allocations
(Scenario 1)

b. Optimized allocations
(Scenario 2, Option A)

c. Optimized allocations
(Scenario 2, Option B)

■ Behavior change communication   ■ Vulnerable and accessible populations
■ Community mobilization   ■ Youth programs
■ Blood safety, PLHIV/other   ■ Sexually transmitted infections
■ HIV testing and counseling   ■ Prevention of mother-to-child transmission
■ Care and treatment (antiretroviral therapy, opportunistic infections, prevention, lab, monitoring, other)
■ Key populations   ■ Provider-initiated HIV testing and counseling
■ Program management and   ■ Other/orphans and vulnerable children/
  human resources   social protection/HIV research

Source: Duric et al. 2014.

Note: Scenario 1 is to maintain the 2013 investment allocations and budget level; Scenario 2 is to optimize the investment allocations at the 2013 budget level, leaving the program management and human resources components constant (Option A) or reducing allocations for program management and human resources by 20 percent (approximately US$1 million) and using the savings to further improve the allocative efficiency for the prevention and the care and treatment components (Option B). Optimized allocations in panel b are based on National AIDS Spending Assessment (NASA) report classification. Vulnerable and accessible populations category includes specific vulnerable populations such as indigenous groups, conscripts, truck drivers, prisoners, and migrants. HIV =human immunodeficiency virus; PLHIV = people living with HIV.

ART services by 2020. For ART services, the model investigated alternatively the following three options to determine universal coverage under Scenario 3:

1. Option A: Coverage for 95 percent of diagnosed PLHIV and eligible for ART under the national ART guidelines as of 2013
2. Option B: Coverage for 95 percent of diagnosed PLHIV and eligible for ART under WHO 2013 guidelines
3. Option C: Coverage for 95 percent of all diagnosed PLHIV in accordance with the "test-and-treat" concept, in which individuals are offered treatment as soon as they test positive for HIV (see Dodd, Garnett, and Hallett 2010)

Figure 10.7 Estimated Numbers of PLHIV, ART-Eligible PLHIV, and PLHIV on ART in Tajikistan under Scenario 2, Option B

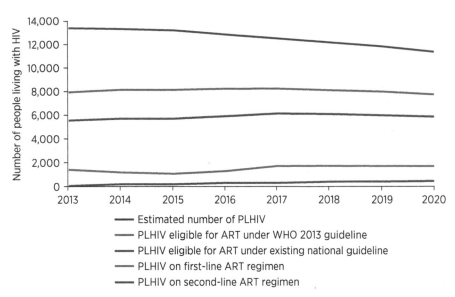

Source: Duric et al. 2014.

Note: Scenario 2 (Option B) is to optimize the investment allocations at the 2013 budget level, reducing allocations for program management and human resources by 20 percent (approximately US$1 million) and using the savings to further improve the allocative efficiency for the prevention and the care and treatment components. See WHO (2013) for guidelines on ART. ART = antiretroviral therapy; HIV =human immunodeficiency virus; PLHIV = people living with HIV; WHO = World Health Organization.

For PMTCT, the objective of the modeling was to achieve 95 percent coverage; 80 percent coverage of estimated need was used for harm reduction specific to PWID and special preventive services for other key populations. For HTC, the objective was to have 80 percent of key populations at higher risk know their status.

To achieve universal treatment access under Scenario 3, Option C (test and treat), the number of PLHIV on ART would need to reach about 9,700; for Option B (WHO 2013 guidelines) the number would be approximately 9,000; and for Option A (national guidelines as of 2013) it would be about 8,200 by 2020. These numbers reflect a five- to sixfold increase over the 2013 ART figures.

The number of people who received HIV testing in the last 12 months will be 9 percent higher in 2020 than in 2013 (Option C).

Table 10.2 Projected Estimated Epidemiological Impact and Program Costs Using Three Options for Antiretroviral Therapy Eligibility Criteria in Scenario 3, Tajikistan

Point estimates

By 2020	Universal ART coverage		
	Option A[a]	Option B[b]	Option C[c]
Estimated PLHIV	13,670	13,660	12,700
Estimated new HIV infections averted	7,000	7,150	8,360
Estimated DALYs averted	95,400	100,000	101,700
Total program costs 2014–20 (US$)	120.0 million	122.4 million	123.6 million

Source: Duric et al. 2014.

Note: ART = antiretroviral therapy; DALYs = disability-adjusted life years; HIV =human immunodeficiency virus; PLHIV = people living with HIV; US$ = US dollar.

a. Coverage of 95 percent of diagnosed and eligible PLHIV by 2020 (2013 national guidelines).

b. Coverage of 95 percent of diagnosed and eligible PLHIV by 2020 (WHO 2013 guidelines).

c. Coverage of 95 percent of all diagnosed PLHIV by 2020 ("test and treat").

Because the coverage rate for PMTCT is already high, it would see only a modest increase by 2020. PWID coverage in needle and syringe exchange programs/opioid substitution therapy (NSP/OST) will increase substantially to reach at least 20,000 PWID by 2020 (Option C). Table 10.2 summarizes the comparisons of projected impacts and costs.

Comparing Impacts of the Three Scenarios

Compared to the counterfactual scenario of no HIV programs at all, Scenario 1 (maintaining the 2013 investment allocations and budget level) would avert approximately 3,100 new HIV infections and 5,100 DALYs by 2020 at a total program cost of US$98.5 million, not accounting for inflation (table 10.3). Compared to the counterfactual scenario of no HIV programs, Scenario 2 (optimizing the investment allocations under the current (2013) budget level) would avert approximately 4,400 new HIV infections and 15,600 DALYs by 2020 at a total program cost of US$98.5 million. The model predictions showed the highest impact for Scenario 3 (scaling up to universal coverage) in terms of averting new HIV infections and DALYs by 2020. Table 10.3 summarizes the comparisons of projected impact and costs.

The long-term impact of Scenario 3 until 2030 is even more impressive (figure 10.8 shows comparisons of all of the scenarios). Under Scenario 3 (scaling up to universal coverage), the estimated number of PLHIV would be about 13,500 by 2030 using the 2013 national treatment guidelines, approximately 13,700 using the WHO 2013 treatment guidelines, and about 12,300 using the "test and treat" approach. These numbers compare to an estimated 9,000 PLHIV for Scenario 2[7] and 10,700 for Scenario 1 (figure 10.8, panel a). The variations can be explained by the long-term dynamics of differences in averted HIV infections and averted AIDS-related deaths.

An estimated cumulative total of 29,000 new HIV infections would be averted between 2014 and 2030 under Scenario 3 using the "test and treat" approach—compared to about 27,000 using the WHO 2013 guidelines, and about 26,000 using the 2013 national guidelines. Scenarios 2 and 1 also achieve significantly lower numbers of averted new HIV infections: approximately 20,000 and 16,000 respectively (figure 10.8, panel b).

Between 2014 and 2030, nearly 323,000 DALYs would be averted under Scenario 3 using the "test and treat" approach (versus 314,000 using the WHO 2013 guidelines and 302,000 using the 2013 national guidelines). Less than half as many DALYs would be averted under Scenario 2 (119,000) and Scenario 1 (78,000).

Table 10.3 Point Estimates of Cumulative New HIV Infections Averted, Cumulative Disability-Adjusted Life Years Averted, and Total Program Costs under the Three Scenarios, Tajikistan, 2014–20

	Scenario 1	Scenario 2	Scenario 3 Option A[a]	Scenario 3 Option B[b]	Scenario 3 Option C[c]
New HIV infections averted	3,100	4,400	7,000	7,150	8,360
DALYs averted	5,100	15,600	95,400	100,000	101,700
Total program costs (US$)	98.5 million	98.5 million	123.3 million	126.6 million	129.0 million

Source: Duric et al. 2014.

Note: DALYs = disability-adjusted life years; HIV =human immunodeficiency virus; PLHIV = people living with HIV; US$ = US dollar.

a. Coverage of 95 percent of diagnosed and eligible PLHIV by 2020 (2013 national guidelines).

b. Coverage of 95 percent of diagnosed and eligible PLHIV by 2020 (WHO 2013 guidelines).

c. Coverage of 95 percent of all diagnosed PLHIV by 2020 ("test and treat").

Figure 10.8 Long-Term Comparisons of the Epidemiological Impact of Scenarios 1, 2, and 3, Tajikistan, 2013–30

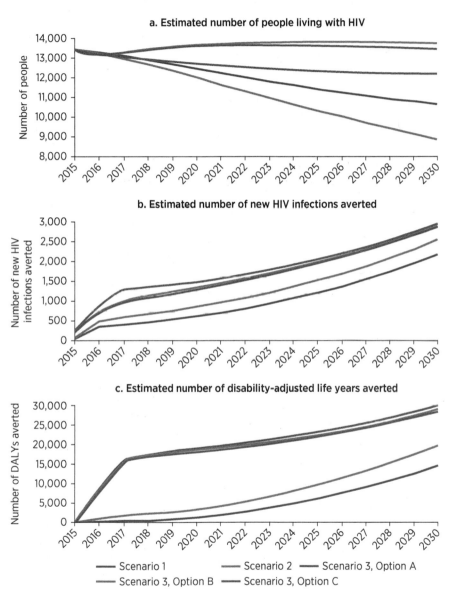

a. Estimated number of people living with HIV

b. Estimated number of new HIV infections averted

c. Estimated number of disability-adjusted life years averted

——— Scenario 1 ——— Scenario 2 ——— Scenario 3, Option A
——— Scenario 3, Option B ——— Scenario 3, Option C

Source: Duric et al. 2014.

Note: For Scenario 2, Option B was used. For explanations of the scenarios and options within them, see the main chapter text. For panel b and panel c, the analyzed figures reflect the 12-month period before each year. DALYs = disability-adjusted life years; HIV = human immunodeficiency virus.

Allocative Efficiency Analysis Recommendations

The model results suggested the following:

1. The 2013 budget ceiling was too low to achieve universal coverage of essential HIV services.
2. To end the HIV epidemic and particularly to fulfill the basic right for access to essential HIV services (Scenario 3), the overall investment until 2020 would need to be increased by 25 percent.
3. About 30,000 new HIV infections would be averted between 2014 and 2030 under Scenario 3 using the "test and treat" approach. Scenarios 2 and 1 avert significantly fewer HIV infections: approximately 21,000 and 17,000, respectively.
4. Despite the significantly higher number of HIV-related deaths averted under Scenario 3, the model predicted that the "test and treat" option under Scenario 3 would result in the lowest number of PLHIV by 2030 (approximately 11,000).
5. The modeling work triggered discussion on the three recommended scenarios, with the aim to allow for effective transition between international and other financial sources. Scenario 2 (continue with optimized investment allocations and current (2013) budget ceiling) was initially chosen for further consideration. The modeling analysis showed, however, that Scenario 3 would be necessary to fulfill commitments and end the AIDS epidemic by 2030.
6. Taking into account the limited financial resources available for achieving universal coverage of essential HIV services, it is crucial that the government of Tajikistan seek opportunities for partial funding of key HIV program interventions (prevention and provision of antiretroviral medicine) from domestic resources.

Actions Taken and Next Steps

On May 22, 2015, the United Nations Joint Advocacy Project on HIV/AIDS (involving UNAIDS, UNDP, the United Nations Population Fund [UNFPA], and the United Nations Children's Fund [UNICEF]) in Tajikistan, with technical support from the US Agency for International Development (USAID) and in cooperation with the Republican Center for AIDS under the Ministry of Health and Social Protection of the Population of Tajikistan (MHSP), and other international and local partners, organized a roundtable meeting dedicated to the results of the modeling report. The event brought together approximately 60 representatives from the Regional Centers for HIV and AIDS of Tajikistan, government agencies, networks of PLHIV, civil society, and international organizations, as well as decision-makers. On the basis of a comprehensive analysis of the funding situation and HIV prevalence in the country, the report suggested three key scenarios to be adopted by and agreed to with MHSP authorities, taking into consideration the existing and projected financial contributions of the government. Following the discussion with key stakeholders, the MHSP preliminarily agreed to consider Scenario 2.

For further advocacy concerning the modeling report recommendations, UNDP, in close coordination with the National Coordination Committee (NCC), organized a second national roundtable meeting, "Steps to Sustainable Financing of the HIV Response Plan in Tajikistan," on October 28, 2015. The participants included key stakeholders (representatives from the MHSP, the Ministry of Finance, the Ministry of Economic Development and Trade, the Youth Committee, and the Women's Affairs Committee), international donor agencies, and local nongovernmental organizations (NGOs) involved in the implementation of components of the National Program. The main aim of the roundtable was to discuss the opportunities for leveraging funds from various domestic sources. It also included discussion of the three scenarios from the modeling report. A commitment was obtained to determine which of the scenarios is applicable to the Tajik situation and to determine next steps in implementation:

1. To present results of the National AIDS Spending Assessment (NASA) and investment modeling at the annual health summit within the implementation framework of the National Health Strategy of the Republic of Tajikistan 2010–2020 (Tajikistan 2010)
2. To advocate for future increases in funding by the government of Tajikistan for the HIV response plan
3. To ensure the implementation of country commitments to increase national funding for the HIV response, including for harm reduction services (OST and NSP in particular) and as reflected in the Tajikistan country position and announced at the Tbilisi Regional Dialogue[8]
4. To continue regular mapping of existing HIV resources, to follow up with in-depth analysis, and to identify existing gaps

In 2016, UNDP published a social contracting factsheet for Tajikistan (Abdullaev et al. 2016). This document provides an overview of NGOs engaged in the national HIV response and emphasizes the importance of NGOs in ensuring access to prevention, treatment, care, and support for key populations at higher risk for HIV exposure and PLHIV.

Notes

1. Note that the information in this section draws extensively on data from the Republican AIDS Center.
2. The 90-90-90 initiative involves the following goals: by 2020, 90 percent of all people living with HIV will know their HIV status, 90 percent of them will receive sustained antiretroviral therapy, and 90 percent of those on therapy will have viral suppression (UNAIDS 2014a).
3. For more information on the "Together We Will End AIDS" campaign, see http://www.unaids.org/en/resources/campaigns/togetherwewillendaids. For more information on "Sustainable Development Goal 3: Targets and Indicators," visit https://sustainabledevelopment.un.org/sdg3.
4. Note that much of this chapter reviews the process and findings of the modeling exercise documented in Duric et al. 2014; as such, the material herein draws significantly on that report.
5. Note that HIV incidence is not equal to the number of new cases. The former includes HIV infections that happen in an actual year, whereas the latter includes HIV infections diagnosed in that year (both HIV infections that happened in that year and those from previous years), and some incident cases will remain undiagnosed, unregistered, or both.
6. For both options, prevention of HIV transmission aimed at PLHIV, blood safety, and "other prevention" (prevention of HIV transmission at the workplace, post-exposure prophylaxis), provider-initiated HIV testing, and "other" program components (orphans and vulnerable children, social protection, enabling environment, and HIV-related research) were kept constant. For Option B, savings in program management/human resources (HR) were partially used to continue services that are essential components of the national HIV program but that were set to zero or substantially reduced under Option A because of their assumed lower effectiveness in the overall context of service rationalization.
7. Using the optimized budget allocation with 20 percent reduction of program management and HR allocations (Option B).
8. The Tbilisi Regional Dialogue was an event hosted by the Ministry of Labor, Health and Social Affairs of Georgia and organized together with the Eurasian Harm Reduction Network. Held in 2015 in Tbilisi, the event gathered 318 delegates from 31 countries to participate in the Regional High-Level Dialogue on Successful Transition to Domestic Funding of HIV and TB [Tuberculosis] Response in Eastern Europe and Central Asia "Road to Success."

References

Abdullaev, T., P. Duric, B. Konstantinov, and C. Hamelmann. 2016. "NGO Social Contracting: Factsheet Tajikistan." Eastern Europe and Central Asia Series on Sustainable Financing of National HIV Responses, UNDP.

Dodd P. J., G. P. Garnett, and T. B. Hallett. 2010. "Examining the Promise of HIV Elimination by 'Test and Treat' in Hyperendemic Settings." *AIDS* 24 (5): 729–35.

Duric, P., C. Hamelmann, D. P. Wilson, and C. Kerr. 2014. "Modelling an Optimised Investment Approach for Tajikistan." A joint publication of the United Nations Development Programme Regional Hub for Europe and the Commonwealth of Independent States and the Ministry of Health and Social Protection. The Government of Tajikistan, Dushanbe.

National Coordination Committee for Prevention and Control of AIDS, Tuberculosis and Malaria. 2014. "National HIV/AIDS Strategic Plan (2015–2017)." National Coordination Committee for Prevention and Control of AIDS, Tuberculosis and Malaria, Dushanbe.

Tajikistan, Ministry of Health. 2010. "National Health Strategy of the Republic of Tajikistan 2010–2020." Ministry of Health, Dushanbe.

Tajikistan, Ministry of Health and Social Protection. 2014a. "Report with Data Analysis of Sentinel Surveillance among People Who Inject Drugs in the Republic of Tajikistan in 2014." Republican AIDS Center, Dushanbe.

Tajikistan, Ministry of Health and Social Protection. 2014b. "Report with Data Analysis of Sentinel Surveillance among Sex Workers in the Republic of Tajikistan." Republican AIDS Center, Dushanbe.

Tajikistan, Ministry of Health and Social Protection. 2015. "Analytical Report of the Results of the Second Generation HIV Sentinel Surveillance 'Men Who Have Sex with Men in the Republic of Tajikistan.'" Republican AIDS Center, Dushanbe.

Tajikistan, Ministry of Health and Social Protection. 2016. "Country Progress Report." Republican AIDS Center, Dushanbe.

UNAIDS (Joint United Nations Programme on HIV/AIDS). 2010. *Getting to Zero: 2011–2015 Strategy*. Geneva: UNAIDS.

UNAIDS (Joint United Nations Programme on HIV/AIDS). 2014a. "90-90-90: An Ambitious Treatment Target to Help End the AIDS Epidemic." UNAIDS, Geneva.

UNAIDS (Joint United Nations Programme on HIV/AIDS). 2014b. *Fast-Track: Ending the AIDS Epidemic by 2030*. Geneva: UNAIDS.

United Nations General Assembly. 2015. "Transforming Our World: The 2030 Agenda for Sustainable Development." United Nations document A/Res/70/1, October 21, United Nations, New York.

WHO (World Health Organization). 2013. *Consolidated Guidelines on the Use of Antiretroviral Drugs for Treating and Preventing HIV Infection: Recommendations for a Public Health Approach*. Geneva: World Health Organization.

11

Ukraine
HIV Treatment in a Time of Crisis

Igor Kuzin, Katerina Sharapka, Eleonora Hvazdziova, Cliff C. Kerr, Robyn M. Stuart, Feng Zhao, and Emiko Masaki

Briefly

- Ukraine has the second-largest human immunodeficiency virus (HIV) epidemic in the region in absolute terms, with an estimated 223,000 people living with HIV (at the time of the analysis discussed in this chapter) and a particularly large contribution of HIV to total disease burden nationally.
- The epidemic has stabilized as a result of a large-scale response, but the risk of the epidemic resurfacing remains because of the ongoing political crisis, limited antiretroviral therapy coverage, and the unclear future of funding of programs for key populations.
- Increasing HIV investment at reduced unit cost to maximize impact could make a real difference. Greater impact could be achieved by using more efficient and innovative types of service delivery.
- Reduced procurement costs for drugs and laboratory equipment over the period covered by the analysis could save US\$47 million annually (out of a projected budget of US\$160 million) to meet the national strategic plan targets of reducing new infections and deaths by more than 45 percent.

Introduction

Ukraine has the second-largest HIV epidemic in the Eastern Europe and Central Asia region and, at the time of the analysis discussed in this chapter, was home to 15–20 percent of all of the region's people living with HIV (PLHIV).[1] The epidemic has remained concentrated among key populations, with 0.9 percent HIV prevalence in the adult population (those aged between 15 and 49) at the time of the analysis (Ukraine 2016). It is geographically concentrated in the south and east of the country, with six regions accounting for approximately 50 percent of estimated cases but only 31 percent of the total population. Self-reporting of sexual transmission has been growing since 2008 and accounted for 73.3 percent of the newly registered cases in 2016 (IEID 2017).

Since 2010, the Ministry of Health, with support of international partners and donors, has been analyzing fiscal opportunities to allocate more resources to HIV to scale up the response. In 2013, the baseline year for the allocative efficiency analysis discussed in this chapter, total expenditure on health in Ukraine was US$311 per capita,[2] of which only 0.6 percent was allocated to HIV (World Bank 2015). To ensure their consistency and relevance, and unless otherwise indicated, the data provided in this chapter relate to the situation in Ukraine at the time the analysis was conducted.

The need to make better use of existing resources in the HIV response was brought to the top of the government's agenda in the midst of the political, financial, and economic crisis after the Maidan Dignity Revolution (2013–14), the annexation of the Crimea by the Russian Federation, and the continued armed conflict in the East of Ukraine—all of which fueled a concern that the epidemic might grow. The task of establishing effective allocation of domestic and donor resources for health reform in light of the changing funding environment for HIV and tuberculosis was further set out in a series of international agreements and policies.[3]

Against the epidemiological and funding background outlined above, the government of Ukraine decided to carry out an HIV allocative efficiency analysis to establish different options for optimizing investment in HIV programs in Ukraine. The study was carried out over 2014 and 2015 by the Ukrainian Center for Socially Dangerous Disease Control (UCDC) together with the Joint United Nations Programme on HIV/AIDS (UNAIDS), the World Bank, and the University of New South Wales Australia, using the Optima HIV model, an allocative efficiency analysis tool used to inform HIV investment choices. The analysis focused on the following key policy questions:

- How should HIV spending be allocated to ensure maximum impact and to consolidate the epidemic gains already made?

- Which programmatic areas should be prioritized in a situation of limited resources?
- What resources and programs would be necessary to achieve the targets outlined in the National AIDS Program 2014–18?
- Ukraine partially depends on external funding, particularly for prevention programs for key populations. What should be done to ensure the transition to domestic funding for those programs and their continuity after the phasing out of support from the Global Fund to Fight AIDS, Tuberculosis and Malaria (the Global Fund)?
- The efficiency gains required for a sustainable HIV response must be realized against the backdrop of not only the political and economic crisis but also the process of a comprehensive reform of the wider health sector. What could be the first steps under these circumstances?

The results of this analysis are the focus of this chapter. The analysis was very much informed by the epidemiological, programmatic, fiscal, and political context within Ukraine at the time. The next section of this chapter describes this context in more detail, before the results are presented in the following section.

The Funding Challenge

In 2013 (the latest year for which HIV spending data were available when the study was conducted), US$79.6 million was available for Ukraine's HIV response. Approximately 60 percent of the HIV expenditures were financed from domestic sources, whereas the rest was from external funding—primarily from the Global Fund.

Domestic funding of the HIV response had been growing steadily but then declined because of economic hardship and national currency devaluation. The phasing out of Global Fund support to the country was initially expected to take place in 2017 and is still anticipated in the coming years (with an ongoing 2018–20 grant and US$120 million allocated for 2020–22).

The level of funding made available in 2013 for Ukraine's HIV response was relatively low compared to other countries in the region, especially when considering the scale of the epidemic and burden of disease. Figure 11.1 shows years of life lost due to HIV as a percentage of all years of life lost in 2013, alongside total HIV spending in the same year as a percent of total health spending in seven countries in the region. Of the US$14.1 billion spent on health in Ukraine in 2013, US$79.6 million was spent on HIV, representing 0.6 percent of all health spending. Even after taking into account the contributions of other local budget allocations to acquired immune deficiency syndrome (AIDS)

Figure 11.1   HIV Disease Burden and HIV Spending in Seven Countries in the Eastern Europe and Central Asia Region, 2013

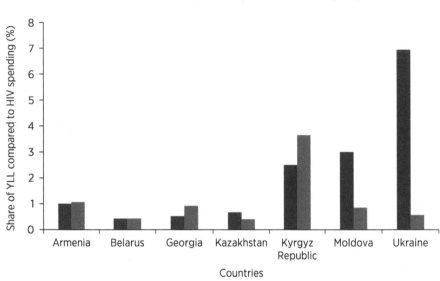

Source: World Bank 2015.

Note: HIV = human immunodeficiency virus; YLL = years of life lost.

centers or community centers, as well as the contributions of allocations to the health system more broadly, the level of HIV spending in Ukraine was low relative to the level of disease burden, which is very high in comparison to other countries in the region.

As shown in table 11.1, HIV prevalence has remained high among key populations, particularly people who inject drugs (PWID)—among whom the HIV prevalence was 18.8 percent for males and 22.4 percent for females. According to estimates from the Optima HIV model, PWID were expected to account for one-third of new adult HIV infections over the 2015–20 period, but the epidemic was also shifting to their sexual partners. Sexual transmission among men who have sex with men (MSM), female sex workers (FSWs), FSW clients, and clients' partners was also on the rise. According to self-reported data, two-thirds of new HIV diagnoses were among people who reported being infected through sexual contacts (IEID 2014). According to integrated biobehavioral surveillance (IBBS) data, self-reported use of clean needles during last drug injection was high (96.9 percent), and so was condom use among FSWs with clients

Table 11.1   Key National Data on Ukraine's HIV Situation and Response

Category	Data	Source
Population size estimates		
Number of FSW	79,816	2012 population size estimates
Number of MSM	175,750	2012 population size estimates
Number of PWID	310,000	2012 population size estimates
Number of PLHIV	223,000	2015 national HIV estimates (Spectrum)
Number of new HIV infections	10,000	2015 national estimates (Spectrum)
Number of people estimated to be at high risk of infection	566,000	2015 national estimates (Spectrum)
HIV prevalence (%)		
FSW	7.3	2013 IBBS
MSM	5.9	2013 IBBS
Men who inject drugs	18.8	2013 IBBS
Women who inject drugs	22.4	2013 IBBS
Key outcome data		
Number of PLHIV on ART	66,000	Program records (May 2015)
Share of all PLHIV on ART (%)	29.6	Based on program records and national estimates
Share of PWID who shared needle during last injection (%)	3.1	2013 IBBS
Number of PWID on opioid substitution therapy	8,407	2014 program records
Share of FSW using a condom with most recent client (%)	97.0	2013 IBBS
Share of MSM using a condom at last casual sex (%)	82.0	2013 IBBS

Source: As indicated in the table; Ukraine 2016 (Spectrum estimates from the Ukranian Center for Socially Dangerous Disease Control).

Note: Data presented represent the latest data available at the time that the allocative efficiency study was conducted. ART = antiretroviral therapy; FSW = female sex worker; HIV = human immunodeficiency virus; IBBS = integrated biological and biobehavioral surveillance; MSM = men who have sex with men; PLHIV = people living with HIV; PWID = people who inject drugs.

(97.0 percent). Coverage of opioid substitution therapy (OST) was limited, however, to less than 3 percent of all PWID—a low rate, even when considering that the proportion of nonopioid injectors (who do not require OST) was increasing.

Globally, the pathway for successful national HIV responses has been laid out very clearly. UNAIDS and partners have defined a global Fast Track strategy to achieve the goal of ending the AIDS epidemic by 2030 (UNAIDS 2014b). This strategy includes the ambitious target of having 90 percent of all PLHIV diagnosed and 90 percent of those diagnosed on sustained antiretroviral therapy (ART) (UNAIDS 2014a). Reaching these targets means that 81 percent of all PLHIV should receive ART by 2020. The Fast Track approach also emphasizes the need to focus on the geographical areas most affected by HIV. Another element of this global consensus is that resources should be concentrated on the programs with the greatest impact.

In Ukraine, however, less than 20 percent of PLHIV (40,000) were on ART at the end of 2013, the baseline year for the Optima allocative efficiency analysis. In early 2015, only 66,000 of Ukraine's estimated 223,000 PLHIV received ART—that is, only about 30 percent against the UNAIDS global target of 81 percent by 2020. Therefore, at the time of the analysis, although there had been successes in the response to the epidemic and HIV prevalence had stabilized in Ukraine, major efforts were still needed to achieve national targets.

Key Policy Messages of the Analysis

Optimizing the 2013 Allocation to Avert Deaths

A major component of the 2014–15 allocative efficiency analyses was an optimization analysis to determine the optimal allocation of the 2013 funding envelope for the HIV response (US$80 million).

As indicated in figure 11.2, Ukraine's 2013 funding envelope was already relatively well allocated, because it was on the whole aligned to the optimized allocations for minimizing HIV incidence and deaths. The analysis found that optimized allocations of the 2013 spending amount would cumulatively avert an additional 9 percent of deaths and 3 percent of new infections over the 2015–30 period. These results would be achieved by increasing allocations for ART and related laboratory monitoring to about 60 percent of all HIV spending, while making small savings on other programs. It should be noted that this reallocation is not because other programs are not effective but because of the critical role of ART in averting deaths. In addition, because unit costs for programs for key populations in Ukraine's national plan funded by Global Fund grants have declined as compared to 2013, coverage of prevention programs for key populations would not decline compared to 2013, despite the partial reallocation of funds to treatment. HIV testing and counseling (HTC) and ART for pregnant women—for the prevention of mother-to-child

Figure 11.2 Optimized Allocations to Minimize HIV Incidence and Deaths, Compared with 2013 Allocations of HIV Funding, Ukraine

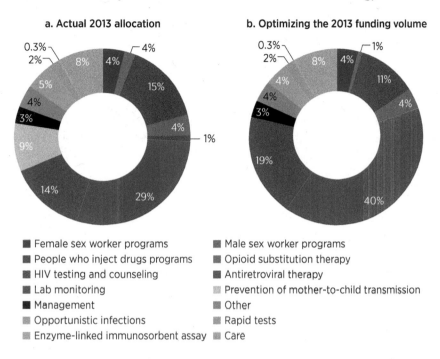

a. Actual 2013 allocation

b. Optimizing the 2013 funding volume

- Female sex worker programs
- People who inject drugs programs
- HIV testing and counseling
- Lab monitoring
- Management
- Opportunistic infections
- Enzyme-linked immunosorbent assay
- Male sex worker programs
- Opioid substitution therapy
- Antiretroviral therapy
- Prevention of mother-to-child transmission
- Other
- Rapid tests
- Care

Source: World Bank 2015.
Note: HIV = human immunodeficiency virus.

transmission (PMTCT)—as well as key populations would continue to be part of the optimized package and remain priorities for the country (unit cost assumptions are discussed later in the chapter). HTC (screening) for key populations would be part of the packages for PWID, FSWs, and MSM. HTC for pregnant women could be covered from fixed budgets for enzyme-linked immunosorbent assay (ELISA) testing and antiretroviral medicines (ARVs) for pregnant women covered from the ART budget.

Reducing New Infections

Although optimally allocating the 2013 funding envelope was estimated to avert 3 percent of new infections over the 2014–30 period compared to maintaining the 2013 allocation, reallocating would not be enough to reverse the increasing trend in new infections. There were an estimated

18,000 new infections in 2014; this number was projected to rise to 22,000 new infections per year in 2030 if the 2013 allocation were maintained, or to 20,000 new infections per year if funds were optimally allocated.[4]

The allocative efficiency study highlighted that cutting HIV budgets by half (compared to 2013 spending) in Ukraine would have had catastrophic effects. Estimated annual new infections could have risen from below 18,000 in 2014 to 31,000 in 2030—or cumulatively 440,000 new infections between 2015 to 2030. Understanding the impacts of such funding decisions, the government and partners acted and increased allocations to the HIV response.

Additional analyses were performed to estimate the effects of reduced and increased investment (figure 11.3). Reduced investment would have substantial negative effects on the HIV response and epidemic. If funding were cut by half or a quarter compared to the 2013 level, the results obtained from an unconstrained optimization analysis imply that prevention interventions for key populations would be most cost-effective. Because it was considered a condition in the model that no one on ART or OST should have to go off treatment, a constrained optimization analysis was run and found that the majority of funds would need to be allocated to ART in case of reduced funding. Reducing HIV funding by 50 percent compared to 2013 spending—a situation that could have occurred if support from the Global Fund had ended—would have meant that, under the cost conditions studied in the allocative efficiency analysis, new infections would have risen from 18,000 in 2014 to 31,000 by 2030, because with such budget cuts all funds would be absorbed by existing treatment commitments.

The analysis found that, by increasing total HIV spending from US$80 million to US$160 million (or US$113 million with additional efficiency gains), Ukraine could avert 5 out of 10 new infections and 6 out of 10 HIV deaths by 2030. Even with such increases, HIV spending would remain relatively low—between 0.9 percent and 1.5 percent of total health spending.

With increasing levels of funding, the results of the allocative efficiency analysis suggest substantial increases in funding for ART, while simultaneously sustaining funding for prevention programs for key populations. Unit costs for prevention programs were reduced in the process of developing the 2015–17 Concept Note to the Global Fund and the 2015–18 national strategic planning (see annex 11A). These reductions mean that coverage of prevention programs for key populations could moderately increase even if funding remained at 2013 levels.

The 2014–15 study found that the effects of a 50 percent increase in annual investments (to US$120 million per year) would be substantial: relative to a scenario in which the 2013 funding envelope was annually

Figure 11.3 Optimized Allocations to Minimize HIV Incidence and Deaths in Ukraine with Different Levels of Funding

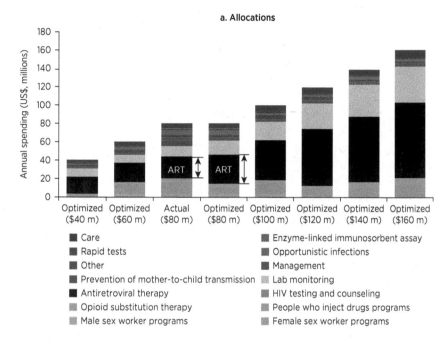

a. Allocations

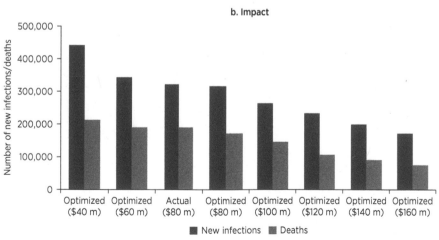

b. Impact

Source: World Bank 2015.

Note: Funding amounts are expressed in US dollars. ART = antiretroviral therapy; HIV = human immunodeficiency virus; m = million; US$ = US dollar.

available and allocated as it was in 2013, this combination of a funding increase and a reallocation could reduce cumulative new infections over the 2014–30 period by 27 percent and cumulative deaths by 43 percent (figure 11.3). This effect would be sufficient to reverse the trending increase in new infections, with the result that annual new infections in 2030 would be 17 percent lower compared to 2014 and deaths would be 46 percent lower. The analysis also found that, by doubling funding to US$160 million, the national targets of halving new infections and deaths relative to 2013 levels could be achieved for new infections and exceeded for reducing deaths. With this level of funding, new infections would decline by 39 percent by 2030 compared to 2014 and deaths by 65 percent. Relative to a scenario in which the 2013 funding envelope was annually available and allocated as it was in 2013, a doubling of annual investments combined with an optimized allocation of these investments would translate to 154,000 (48 percent) new infections and 114,000 (61 percent) deaths averted by 2030. The number of people on ART could be increased from 66,000 to over 130,000. Options for obtaining the same results but with lower levels of investment are explored further below.

If Ukraine realizes the potential for savings in procurement costs, investing US$113 million per year (US$33 million more than 2013, but less than in the costed national strategy) would avert an estimated 154,000 new infections by 2030—translating into a total saving of US$2.4 billion in lifetime costs of treatment.

The Importance of Initiating ART Early

As part of the 2014–15 allocative efficiency analysis, a scenario analysis was carried out to test the effect of implementing different eligibility criteria for ART (figure 11.4), with 2015 conditions defined as keeping 66,000 PLHIV on ART (which was the coverage level when the analysis was conducted in early 2015). In figure 11.4, ART at CD4 below 350 and 500 cells per cubic millimeter reflects a scenario in which 85 percent of PLHIV diagnosed and 90 percent of those diagnosed with the respective CD4 levels of 350 and 500 are on ART. The ART for all CD4 levels scenario assumed 85 percent of PLHIV diagnosed are on ART. In line with the relevant UNAIDS definitions, the 90–90–90 targets were defined for the scenario analysis as 90 percent of all PLHIV having been diagnosed (and knowing their status), 90 percent of those diagnosed on ART, and

90 percent of those on ART with viral suppression. The resulting analysis suggested that higher rates of HIV diagnosis followed by ART initiation for PLHIV with CD4 counts above 350 and CD4 counts above 500 would reduce deaths by approximately 50 percent by 2030 compared to 2015 levels of ART coverage. The analysis suggested that, if 81 percent of PLHIV in Ukraine were on sustained ART in line with the 90-90-90 targets (yellow line in figure 11.4), deaths would decline by more than 80 percent in 2030 relative to 2013 levels.

Figure 11.4   Effects of Different Antiretroviral Therapy Eligibility Criteria on the Number of AIDS-Related Deaths in Ukraine

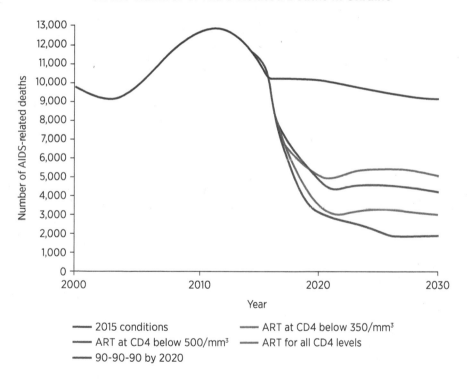

Source: World Bank 2015.

Note: AIDS = acquired immune deficiency syndrome; ART = antiretroviral therapy; 90-90-90 = Joint United Nations Programme on HIV/AIDS targets of 90 percent of people living with HIV (PLHIV) knowing their status, 90 percent of those diagnosed on ART, and 90 percent of people on ART having viral load suppression by 2020.

Figure 11.5   Estimated and Projected Numbers of Annual New Infections in Ukraine

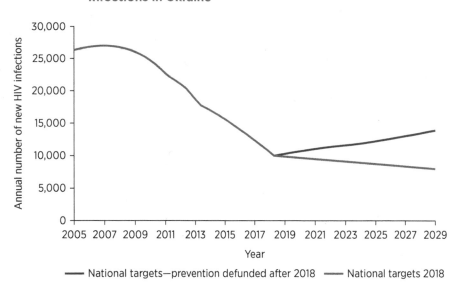

Source: World Bank 2015.
Note: HIV = human immunodeficiency virus.

The Importance of Key Population Prevention Programs

At the time that the 2014–15 allocative efficiency analysis was conducted, the understanding was that prevention programs for key populations (PWID, MSM, and FSWs) would be supported by the Global Fund until midyear in 2018. Figure 11.5 shows the impact of defunding these prevention programs for key populations after 2018, under the assumption that the government would not be able to continue financing at the same level those prevention programs that were supported by the Global Fund (FSW, MSM, needle and syringe exchange programs, and other prevention for PWID).

For both scenarios within this analysis, it was assumed that ART coverage would increase between 2015 and 2018 in order to reach the national 2018 target of 114,000 PLHIV on ART. ART coverage was then held constant out to 2030, which was done simply in order to provide a worst-case scenario baseline so that the impact of the withdrawal of prevention funding could be examined within a context where no assumptions were made about treatment scale-up beyond 2018. In the scenario "National targets 2018," it was assumed that rates of condom use and needle sharing would be sustained at the level of the 2018 targets; in the scenario with prevention defunded, it was assumed that prevention behaviors among key populations would deteriorate as Global Fund investments were withdrawn (see figure 11.5 and annex 11B). The model results illustrated that, despite the increase in coverage of ART to the level of the national 2018 target, defunding prevention programs for key populations could lead to increasing new infections. Using a life-time cost of ART of US$18,700 per person,[5] achieving national prevention targets would translate into a savings of US$670 million for the new infections averted between 2018 and 2030. Under the conditions studied in the model, by 2030, 36,000 additional HIV infections would occur, and levels of new infections would be 75 percent higher in 2030 if prevention programs were stopped rather than sustained.

The analysis therefore concluded that it is imperative that Ukraine sustains and transforms basic programs for PWID, FSWs, and MSM. In addition to achieving the 2018 national targets for condom use among FSWs and MSM, as well as use of clean needles among PWID, the analysis highlighted a need to further strengthen the capacity of prevention program implementers to enhance the effectiveness of prevention programs in identifying and referring PLHIV to ART, as well as supporting the retention of PLHIV on ART. The analysis also found that expanding OST services with non-HIV resources is critical considering the wider health and social benefits of OST.

Positive Impacts of Optimization

As part of the 2014–15 allocative efficiency study, an additional analysis was carried out to establish how much it would cost to achieve national targets with reduced costs in the program areas of ART and viral load monitoring—the areas that were projected to absorb the largest share of resources between 2015 and 2030. The analysis assumed that ART cost could be reduced by 33 percent by procuring generic drugs. It also assumed the cost of viral load monitoring could be reduced from US$55 to US$9 per test in line with the negotiated price in the Global Access Program, a global initiative to reduce the cost of viral load monitoring; that would translate into a 50 percent reduction in the total laboratory monitoring cost. Together, these two measures would reduce the total annual cost of the HIV response from US$160 million to US$113 million, while still achieving the national targets—producing an estimated reduction of half of new infections and over 60 percent of deaths between 2015 and 2030 (figure 11.6).

Comparing the optimized allocations with savings from reduced costs of services (US$113 million) to 2013 spending levels (US$80 million) highlighted a need for additional investments of US$33 million per year or about US$530 million between 2015 and 2030. This additional investment would also lead, however, to future savings in additional treatment costs.

Figure 11.6 Combined Effects of Optimized Allocations with Savings, Ukraine

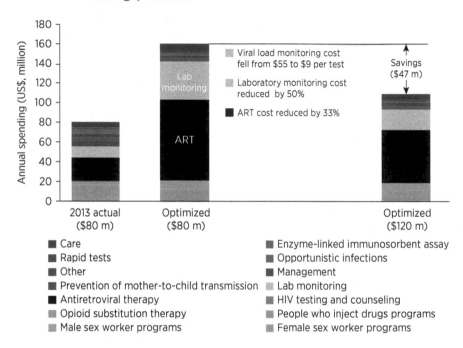

Source: World Bank 2015.

Note: The cost of antiretroviral therapy (ART) was reduced by procuring generic drugs. The cost of viral load monitoring was negotiated down by the Global Access Program. Funding amounts and costs are expressed in US dollars. HIV = human immunodeficiency virus; m = million; US$ = US dollar.

Because this allocation would avert an estimated 154,000 new infections, it would translate into reduced lifetime costs of treatment of US$2.89 billion against a cumulative cost of US$0.53 billion.

Integrating Services in Decentralized Settings

HIV/tuberculosis (TB) coinfections play an important and growing role in Ukraine. As of 2015, however, HIV and TB services were delivered by two separate national programs. The level of integration and coordination differed from region to region, but HIV and TB services were generally delivered separately. The 2015 study found that further aligning HIV and TB services would create opportunities for efficiency gains that should be exploited systematically. The study recommended that HIV patients have access to a TB test, and new TB cases should routinely receive HIV testing services. Another strategy would be to increase integration and decentralization by providing more HIV-related services at the primary health care level and doing so in an integrated manner using public funding.

The final recommendation of the 2014–15 allocative efficiency analysis was that a major transition was needed in financing for services: from funding inputs according to the line-item budgeting to a model of "per case" payment. Risk-adjusted capitation—a mechanism to optimize the allocation of resources across health facilities providing outpatient services using population data weighted by relevant risk factors and taking various health and demographic specifics into account—could be used. Adding "per case payment" elements related to specific HIV services for key populations to the capitation-based budget could motivate providers to offer more of these services.

Whereas HIV-related clinical services are mainly provided by health care facilities, nonclinical and social services for HIV prevention, as well as for care and support for PLHIV, are provided by regional nongovernmental organizations (NGOs) and community-based organizations. Close cooperation between local NGOs and health care facilities allows for the provision of effective medical and social services in the area of HIV/AIDS and increases the adherence of patients to particular services. Nevertheless, local governments face barriers to funding NGOs to provide HIV services. Promoting cooperation between NGOs and local authorities in programming and monitoring, as well as improving capacity at the regional level to define needs and manage social contracting, would enable the implementation of cost-effective intervention models.

Recommendations from the Analysis

The 2014–15 allocative efficiency analysis concluded that there were major opportunities but also major risks in relation to HIV investment decisions in Ukraine. Whereas decreasing funding would lead to a marked increase in deaths, new infections, and future health care costs, a smart approach to increasing HIV investment could avert about half of the new infections and deaths up to 2030, compared to continuing with the 2013 funding envelope and allocation. The study concluded that the keys to success would be the following:

1. Scale up ART.
2. Reform procurement to reduce unit costs for drugs and diagnostics.
3. Sustain prevention programs for key populations and further enhance coverage with strong geographical prioritization.

4. Establish domestic financing and management of community systems for prevention and treatment adherence support.
5. Strengthen integration of HIV efforts with other health, social, and drug-use treatment programs.

The analysis determined that bold, immediate investment in key programs and measures to improve efficiency were needed to avoid large increases in future health care costs and, most importantly, to prevent over 150,000 new infections and save over 110,000 lives by 2030.

Actions Taken and Next Steps

For the past several years, significant economic and political changes have affected the HIV response. On the macroeconomic front, the political turnovers and economic crisis fueled by the armed conflict in the eastern part of the country caused Ukraine's gross domestic product per capita to decline from US$4,400 in 2013 to less than US$2,100 in 2016. In 2016, economic growth resumed and gross domestic product per capita in 2017 was forecast at US$2,250.[6] The government has also started 68 reforms under an Association Agreement (2014) with the European Union, but implementation challenges and partial resistance to reform continue to slow down critical changes.

Ukraine has been able to mobilize more than US$353 million in international donor funding over the period from 2014 through 2020 to cover gaps in domestic resources for TB and HIV to achieve the 90-90-90 targets of 90 percent of PLHIV knowing their status, 90 percent of those on ART (81 percent of all PLHIV), and 90 percent of people on ART (73 percent of all PLHIV) having viral load suppression by 2020. These funds include US$100 million from PEPFAR (the US President's Emergency Plan for AIDS Relief) for 2015–17, and two tranches from the Global Fund in the amounts of US$134 million (2014–17) and US$119 million (2018–20). The Global Fund's Emergency Fund provided an additional US$3.7 million in 2016 and another US$ 4.3 million in 2017 to cover ART gaps in the non-government-controlled areas of Lugansk and Donetsk.

Using the results of the allocative efficiency study (World Bank 2015) and the earlier Ukraine HIV Program Efficiency Study (World Bank 2014), HIV prevention and care services have realized efficiency gains of 30–50 percent. Through Global Fund financing, together with PEPFAR investments and additional resources for ART scale-up, the risk of ART interruption due to failure of the state procurement was mitigated in 2014–15. The ART scale-up toward the 90-90-90 targets started with Ukraine's adoption of the Treat All guidelines of the World Health Organization (WHO 2016) and approval of the UNAIDS Fast Track targets (UNAIDS 2014b). By the end of 2016, 85,025 PLHIV were on ART, including PLHIV in non-government-controlled territories (Ukraine 2017). By late 2018, the number of people on treatment exceeded 100,000.

Ukraine has also made major progress in funding and improving the efficiency of HIV procurements as well as in improving the management structure for the public health system, including HIV/AIDS. As an anticorruption response to the stagnation of the national procurement procedures, procurement of ARV drugs and laboratory commodities was transferred to international agencies under a memorandum of understanding with the Ministry of Health for 2016–19 and considerable cost savings were realized beginning in 2016.

After intense advocacy from civil society and the newly created National Center for Public Health, the state budget for HIV procurements increased by 132 percent (in Ukrainian hryvnia). These increases resulted in government financing to cover up to 63 percent of the funding needed for ARVs, and the allocation of up to US$0.5 million to purchase methadone for all current clients in the OST program.

Advocacy from the civil society PLHIV Network on pricing and patent protection brought reductions in ARV prices, including for a generic version of Atripla and for dolutegravir. There has also been a breakthrough in the optimization of treatment schemes: all ART procurements under Global Fund and PEPFAR financing will use optimized ART regimens. This breakthrough, combined with the reductions in ARV prices, will ensure the ability of Ukraine to provide treatment for 196,000 PLHIV by 2020, thus meeting the relevant Fast Track target.

On the basis of the WHO 2016 guidelines, the Ministry of Health has worked on new comprehensive guidelines for the HIV treatment cascade with pre-exposure prophylaxis (PrEP), prevention for key populations, test and treat (a WHO-backed approach in which key populations are targeted for testing and early treatment), new effective testing and referral algorithms, decentralization of treatment, and a deemphasis of CD4 testing. The new guidelines will open the gates for innovations in service delivery and further strengthening the role of civil society in service provision by state funding.

The Global Fund and PEPFAR remain the key donors for outreach prevention programs and care and support for key populations. To address the planned transition of responsibility (including financing) for prevention and care to the government, the Ministry of Health, with support from international organizations and donors, developed the National HIV and TB Transition and Sustainability Strategy for 2017–2020, with an action plan based on the UNAIDS Fast Track Strategy and the Public Health System Reform including a reform of health care financing and primary health care. The Transition Strategy action plan will be gradually implemented though the Global Fund 2018–20 grant and with PEPFAR investments in strategic information, HIV research and surveillance, and health system strengthening.

Annex 11A: Populated Optima Spreadsheet Showing Differences in Cost per Person Reached

Program	Ukraine (average in US$)	
	2013	2015–18 plan
Prevention for female sex workers	113	52
Prevention for men who have sex with men	48	22
Needle and syringe exchange programs and prevention for people who inject drugs	67	32
Opioid substitution therapy	431	248
Treatment		
Antiretroviral therapy	668	631
Laboratory monitoring	184	304
Prevention of mother-to-child transmission	1,959	1,120

Source: World Bank based on Optima model.
Note: US$ = US dollar.

Annex 11B: Scenario Analysis Showing Assumptions Made

	Time frame	Scenario 1: Prevention sustained	Scenario 2: Prevention defunded from 2018
Number of PLHIV on ART	2018	—	114,000
	2030	—	114,000
Needle-sharing, PWID (%)	2018	—	2
	2030	2	8
Condom use, FSW (%)	2018	—	98
	2030	98	85
Condom use, MSM (%)	2018	—	75
	2030	75	60

Source: World Bank based on Optima model.
Note: ART = antiretroviral therapy; FSW = female sex worker; MSM = men who have sex with men; PLHIV = people living with HIV; PWID = people who inject drugs; — = not available.

Notes

1. Against a total estimated PLHIV number of 1.5 million according to 2014 UNAIDS estimates (UNAIDS 2015).
2. Data from the World Health Organization's National Health Accounts online resource, http://apps.who.int/nha/database/country_profile/Index/en.
3. These policies included the Ukraine–European Union Association Agreement (March 2014), the World Health Organization Treat All policy (2016), and the 2014 Fast Track Strategy and the 90-90-90 targets of the Joint United Nations Programme on HIV/AIDS (UNAIDS 2014a, 2014b).
4. The difference between optimized allocations and business as usual is estimated at about 10 percent in 2030 and about 3 percent cumulatively. The cumulative proportion of new infections averted is lower because most of the effect of optimized allocations would be incurred in the second half of the 2015–30 period.
5. Using ART cost of US$631 and laboratory monitoring cost of US$304, this would translate in US$935 per year, as life-expectancy projections extend beyond the time frame for which this allocative efficiency analysis was conducted (2015–30). An average life-expectancy on ART of 20 years was considered here as a proxy. This may appear low, but the allocative efficiency analysis team considered it realistic in this context because of the high background mortality among PWID.
6. According to data as of October 2016 from the International Monetary Fund's World Economic Outlook Database, https://www.imf.org/external/pubs/ft/weo/2016/02/weodata/index.aspx.

References

Association Agreement between the European Union and Its Member States, of the One Part, and Ukraine, of the Other Part. 2014. OJ L 161, 29.5.2014, 3–2137.

IEID (Institute of Epidemiology and Infectious Diseases of the Academy of Science of Ukraine). 2014. "Information Bulletin 40: HIV Infection in Ukraine." Kyiv.

IEID (Institute of Epidemiology and Infectious Diseases of the Academy of Science of Ukraine). 2017. "Information Bulletin 47: HIV Infection in Ukraine." Kyiv.

Ukraine. "2017 Global AIDS Monitoring Report: Ukraine 2017." Government of Ukraine, Kyiv. Available with English language summary at http://www.unaids.org/sites/default/files/country/documents/UKR_2017_countryreport.pdf.

Ukraine, UCDC (Ukrainian Center for Socially Dangerous Disease Control). 2016. Estimates produced in Spectrum model. UCDC, Kyiv.

UNAIDS (Joint United Nations Programme on HIV/AIDS). 2014a. "90-90-90: An Ambitious Treatment Target to Help End the AIDS Epidemic." UNAIDS, Geneva.

UNAIDS (Joint United Nations Programme on HIV/AIDS). 2014b. *Fast-Track: Ending the AIDS Epidemic by 2030*. Geneva: UNAIDS.

UNAIDS (Joint United Nations Programme on HIV/AIDS). 2015. "Global HIV Estimates." UNAIDS, Geneva.

United Nations. 2015. *The Millennium Development Goals Report 2015*. New York: United Nations.

World Bank. 2014. "Ukraine HIV Program Efficiency Study: Can Ukraine Improve Value for Money in HIV Service Delivery?" World Bank, Washington, DC. https://www.medbox.org/ukraine-hiv-program-efficiency-study-can-ukraine -improve-value-for-money-in-hiv-service-delivery/preview.

World Bank. 2015. "Value for Money in Ukraine's HIV Response: Strategic Investment and Improved Efficiency." World Bank, Washington, DC.

WHO (World Health Organization). 2016. *Consolidated Guidelines on the Use of Antiretroviral Drugs for Treating and Preventing HIV Infection: Recommendations for a Public Health Approach*, 2nd ed. Geneva: WHO.

12

Uzbekistan
Toward Effective Prevention and Treatment for Key Populations

Predrag Duric, Christoph Hamelmann,
and John Macauley

Briefly

- The trends of the human immunodeficiency virus (HIV) epidemic in Uzbekistan are similar to those in most of the other countries in the Commonwealth of Independent States.
- The proportion of people on antiretroviral treatment (ART) has been too small to have a significant preventive effect on HIV transmission at the population level.
- The HIV epidemic indicators, service coverage, and modeling forecast showed that overall the HIV response was underfunded to an extent that precluded meeting the effort's stated objectives and fulfilling the commitments for universal coverage of essential HIV services.
- The Ministry of Finance has been developing a plan to guide the transition from donor funding to full state funding of HIV programs. The United Nations Development Programme (UNDP) modeling report has been used to help develop this transitional plan.

Introduction

Among countries in the Commonwealth of Independent States (CIS), Uzbekistan is the second largest by population. It lies on the Silk Road, which connected East and West, and China with the Middle East and Rome. Cities like Tashkent, Samarkand, Bukhara, and others are witnesses of magnificent history, trade, and culture.

The first HIV case in Uzbekistan was recorded in 1987; but, before the 2000s, little was known about HIV in Uzbekistan. By the end of 2000, 230 people had been diagnosed with HIV and officially registered (Duric et al. 2015). At the end of 2015, it was estimated that there were more than 52,000 people living with HIV (PLHIV) in Uzbekistan, of whom 32,872 were registered.[1] The trends of the HIV epidemic in Uzbekistan are similar to those in most of the other CIS countries.

For years, the epidemic was mainly concentrated among people who inject drugs (PWID), but since 2010 sexual transmission has become the predominant mode of transmission (figure 12.1). One of the important attributes of the HIV epidemic in Uzbekistan is nosocomial HIV transmission (transmissions occurring in hospital settings), which particularly affected children. Until 2004, fewer than 10 children were diagnosed with HIV annually, but then the number of new HIV infections among children

Figure 12.1 HIV Infection in Uzbekistan, Self-Reported Modes of Transmission, 2000–15

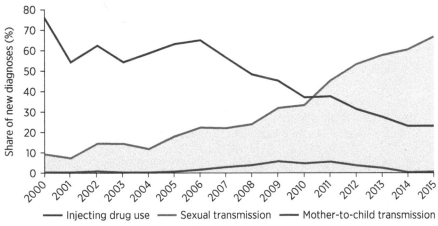

Source: World Bank based on Republican AIDS Center data for 2015 and 2017.
Note: HIV = human immunodeficiency virus.

increased substantially. It peaked in 2011 with 870 new HIV infections among children (190 as a result of mother-to-child transmission), accounting for one out of every four new HIV diagnoses that year; the rate has decreased since that peak.

Another shift in the HIV epidemic was observed between 2000 and 2014: the proportion of new HIV infections diagnosed in women increased from 16 percent of all diagnosed cases in 2000 to 45 percent in 2014. Finally, despite a high HIV prevalence among men who have sex with men (MSM) found in biobehavioral surveys, there is no HIV infection officially registered in this population. Opioid substitution therapy (OST) is not available in Uzbekistan, and less than one-third of men and women from key populations reported having an HIV test during the past 12 months (before the biobehavioral survey).

To ensure their consistency and relevance, and unless otherwise indicated, the data provided in this chapter relate to the situation in Uzbekistan at the time the analysis was conducted.

Analysis of the HIV Response

Scenarios and Objectives

In response to a clear need for data analysis to inform decision-making on how to spend the limited funds available for HIV programming, a research team was assembled to take on the project. The team developed scenarios the government of Uzbekistan could use to make the right investment decisions for its national HIV response, keeping in mind that the response had been highly dependent on international support. Using 2012 as the reference year, the team considered the following three scenarios:

- *Scenario 1*: Continue with the existing investment allocations and budget ceiling.
- *Scenario 2*: Continue with optimized investment allocations and the existing budget ceiling.
- *Scenario 3*: Continue by scaling up to universal coverage for essential HIV prevention and treatment services.

The analysis had the following objectives:

- To provide model estimates of future epidemic trajectories in the context of the development of an HIV investment case and sustainable financing strategies for the national response for Uzbekistan under the three scenarios described above.
- To estimate and compare the program costs and the impact (that is, return on investment, expressed in new HIV infections averted and

disability-adjusted life years [DALYs] averted) of the three scenarios in the medium term (2020) and the long term (2030). These estimations and comparisons kept in mind short-term objectives such as the development of a Concept Note for the Global Fund to Fight AIDS, Tuberculosis and Malaria (the Global Fund) using the new funding model (NFM), and long-term objectives such as the "Getting to Zero" goals of the Joint United Nations Programme on HIV/AIDS (UNAIDS), the "Together We Will End AIDS" campaign, and the "End of HIV/AIDS Epidemic" target by 2030 proposed for the Sustainable Development Goals (SDGs) (UNAIDS 2010, 2014; United Nations General Assembly 2015).[2]

The findings from the analysis, which used the Optima HIV model, were assembled in a modeling report published by UNDP in 2015 (Duric et al. 2015).[3]

HIV Prevalence in Key Populations

HIV prevalence among PWID declined to 5.5 percent in 2015. The prevalence has been stable among sex workers (2.1 percent) and uncertain among men who have sex with men (MSM)—3.6 percent in 2013 but ranging from 0.7 percent to 10.0 percent in previous surveys conducted between 2005 and 2011 (figure 12.2). Significant differences in prevalence exist by gender (for example, 7.1 percent among men who inject drugs and 16.5 percent among women who inject drugs) and subnationally (for example, much higher rates among PWID in Tashkent and Samarkand) (Uzbekistan 2015). The modeling indicates that HIV prevalence may also slow for intimate female partners of men who inject drugs. Prevalence estimates for the lower-risk general population, however, are highly uncertain because of the lack of prevalence data.

Many people are still diagnosed late, resulting in late initiation of ART. In turn, this leads to poorer clinical outcomes as well as longer and higher infectiousness because of uncontrolled viral load. The number of PLHIV needing ART outstrips supply; and that number is expected to increase more in the near future, including the need for second-line regimens. Although ART treatment greatly improves a person's quality of life, many PLHIV in Uzbekistan were still not receiving treatment in 2014. Furthermore, the proportion of people on treatment has been too small to have a significant preventive effect on HIV transmission at the population level. According to national estimates, there were 52,569 PLHIV in Uzbekistan in 2015 (table 12.1), of whom 32,872 (63 percent) had been diagnosed. Of these, 13,186 were on ART (25 percent of the estimated total number of PLHIV).

Figure 12.2 HIV Prevalence and Prevalence Trends in Key Populations, Uzbekistan, 2005–15

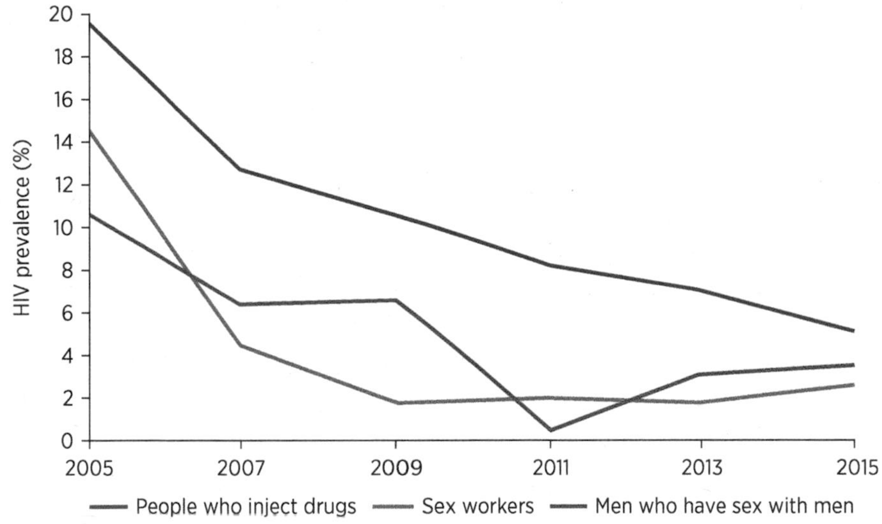

Source: Integrated biobehavioral surveys 2006–16.
Note: HIV = human immunodeficiency virus.

Maintaining Current Allocations and Budget

Assuming that the conditions as of the time of the analysis (behaviors and program coverage) remain stable, the Optima epidemic modeling analysis for Scenario 1 (maintaining 2012 investment allocations and budget level) in Uzbekistan results in six main findings (figure 12.3):

1. For the future projection, the model-estimated annual HIV incidence shows a moderate decline from approximately 3,300 in 2012 to about 2,500 in 2020.
2. The projected declining incidence is driven by both key populations at higher risk of HIV exposure and the general population; among sex workers incidence is projected to decline by 74 percent, among PWID by 22 percent, and among low-risk men and women by 39 percent and 27 percent, respectively. It is estimated that the incidence in MSM will increase by 14 percent.
3. HIV will continue to be transmitted among PWID in Uzbekistan, but the trend toward a larger share of sexual transmissions will progress.
4. The estimated number of PLHIV is projected to slightly decrease from about 37,000 in 2012 to 35,000 in 2020.

Table 12.1 Summary of Key National HIV Data, Uzbekistan, 2000–15

Cumulative HIV diagnoses	2000	2005	2010	2013	2014	2015	Source
Cumulative number of people diagnosed with HIV, total	230	7,810	24,399	36,111	40,347	44,518	Republican AIDS Center
Cumulative registered number of people diagnosed with HIV and alive, total	–	–	18,758	28,250	30,315	32,872	Republican AIDS Center
Estimated number of people living with HIV, total	37,322	47,564	40,959	36,692	–	52,569	Republican AIDS Center
New HIV diagnoses							
Number of people newly diagnosed with HIV, total	154	2,198	3,795	4,247	4,236	4,171	Republican AIDS Center
Number of people newly diagnosed with HIV (ages 15 and older)	154	2,153	2,957	4,149	–	–	Republican AIDS Center
Number of people newly diagnosed with HIV (ages 0–14)	0	45	838	98	–	–	Republican AIDS Center
Number of people newly diagnosed with HIV, women	25	478	1,697	1,968	1,889	1,860	Republican AIDS Center
Number of people newly diagnosed with HIV, men	129	1,720	2,098	2,279	2,347	2,311	Republican AIDS Center
HIV-related deaths							
Annual registered number of HIV-related deaths, total	–	–	330	–	–	–	Republican AIDS Center
Cumulative registered number of HIV-related deaths, total	–	–	828	–	–	–	Republican AIDS Center

continued next page

Table 12.1 (continued)

Cumulative HIV diagnoses	2000	2005	2010	2013	2014	2015	Source
HIV prevalence among key populations (%)							
Sex workers	–	14.7	–	2.1	–	2.8	Biobehavioral surveys 2000–2015
Men who have sex with men	–	10.8	–	3.3	–	3.6	Biobehavioral surveys 2000–2015
People who inject drugs	–	19.7	–	7.3	–	5.5	Biobehavioral surveys 2000–2015
Service coverage and utilization							
Total number of HIV testing performed	573,916	835,657	1,677,462	2,816,424	2,859,575	–	Republican AIDS Center
Number of people receiving antiretroviral therapy	–	–	2,463	8,120	10,948	13,186	Republican AIDS Center
Sexual transmission	9.0	18.0	37.5	58.4	64.7	–	Republican AIDS Center
Transmission through injecting drug use and unsafe blood or blood products	76.6	64.0	33.7	27.8	24.4	–	Republican AIDS Center
Mother-to-child transmission	0.0	0.5	6.3	2.3	0.2	–	Republican AIDS Center

Sources: Combined data from Uzbekistan 2012, 2014, 2015; personal communication with the Republican AIDS Center (RAC); and unpublished RAC data.

Note: The analysis was based on historical data available at the moment of analysis, up to 2013 data. Please note that number of people living with HIV registered and number of new infections include reported cases only and they do not necessarily reflect the HIV incidence presented in the analysis. HIV prevalence in key populations should be interpreted according to the methodology used in integrated biobehavioral studies. AIDS = acquired immune deficiency syndrome; HIV = human immunodeficiency virus; — = not available.

Figure 12.3 Estimated Numbers of PLHIV, ART-Eligible PLHIV, and PLHIV on ART under Scenario 1 in Uzbekistan

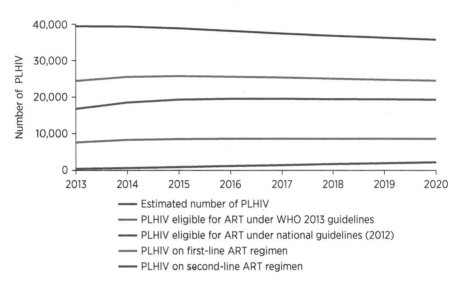

Source: Duric et al. 2015.

Note: ART = antiretroviral therapy; PLHIV = people living with HIV; WHO = World Health Organization.

5. Without increased testing rates, 14,200 PLHIV will go undiagnosed, representing about 40 percent of all PLHIV.
6. Because the total number of PLHIV on ART would slightly decrease because of budget constraints and the increasing number of second-line ART, and because the model predicts that the number of PLHIV will only slightly decrease, ART coverage in 2020 would remain low, with 31 percent of the estimated number of PLHIV receiving ART (11,000 out of 35,000).

The resource allocation at the time of analysis struck a compromise between an incidence-reduction strategy and an optimal DALY-reduction strategy. The allocation of resources across program components in Uzbekistan was considered generally well balanced and close to optimal for minimizing HIV incidence and DALYs (with the exception of the unclear situation of MSM).[4] Some potential still exists, however, for refinement toward better allocative efficiency.

Optimizing Underfunded Program Efficiency

The analysis identified that overall the 2012 budget envelope was insufficient to scale up all effective standard interventions to achieve universal coverage.

Therefore, the results for an optimized allocative efficiency for the under-funded programming required careful consideration in the context of service rationalization—keeping in mind the competing effectiveness of essential key interventions in terms of reducing infections, disease burden, and death.

With these constraints in mind, the model suggested only small changes for an optimized resource allocation under the 2012 budget constraints by shifting resources from general prevention among youth toward HIV testing and counseling (HTC) and treatment (figure 12.4).

In late 2013, the government of Uzbekistan committed to allocate US$2 million to ART and other costs. As of June 2015, US$894,697 had been spent—US$775,312 for antiretroviral (ARV) procurement and delivery and US$119,385 for CD4 and viral load tests. Considering this amount and adding it to the 2012 budget ceiling, the modeling allocative efficiency results under Scenario 2 (optimizing the investment allocations at the 2012 budget level) led to the following estimated numbers of PLHIV, ART-eligible PLHIV, and PLHIV on ART by 2020 (figure 12.5):

- An estimated 36,000 PLHIV
- An estimated 19,000 of PLHIV eligible for ART based on the 2012 national guidelines, and 24,000 based on the World Health Organization (WHO) 2013 guidelines (WHO 2013)
- 10,500 PLHIV on ART (8,300 on the first-line ART and 2,200 on the second-line ART) with an estimated ART coverage of 29 percent among the total estimated number of PLHIV (10,500 out of 36,000)

A Rights-Based Approach

The modeling results of Scenarios 1 and 2 clearly demonstrated the limitations of the 2012 budget level: too many PLHIV will remain undiagnosed and without essential services, even under optimized allocative efficiency and reduced program management and human resources costs. Moreover, the impact on HIV incidence and DALYs remained limited.

"Doing more and better with less" is an important mantra in the effort to ensure continuous quality improvement and efficiency gains. Clearly, however, a minimum spending threshold exists below which a budget simply becomes insufficient to fully meet the objectives. In Uzbekistan, the HIV epidemic indicators, service coverage, and modeling forecast showed that overall the HIV response was underfunded to an extent that precluded meeting the effort's stated objectives and fulfilling the commitments for universal coverage of essential HIV services. Starting at the estimated service coverage levels for HTC, ART, prevention of mother-to-child transmission (PMTCT), and special interventions for key populations in 2012, the model assumed an approximately linear increase

Figure 12.4 Comparison of Budget Allocations under the 2012 Budget Envelope, Uzbekistan

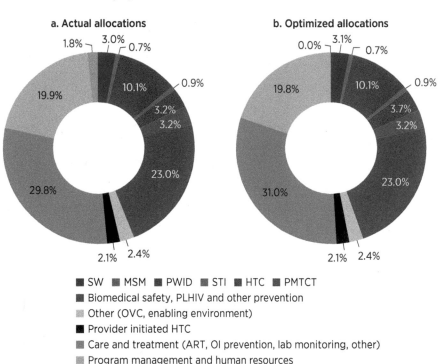

a. Actual allocations

1.8% | 3.0% | 0.7%
0.9%
10.1%
3.2%
3.2%
19.9%
23.0%
29.8%
2.1% | 2.4%

b. Optimized allocations

0.0% | 3.1% | 0.7%
0.9%
10.1%
3.7%
3.2%
19.8%
23.0%
31.0%
2.1% | 2.4%

■ SW ■ MSM ■ PWID ■ STI ■ HTC ■ PMTCT
■ Biomedical safety, PLHIV and other prevention
■ Other (OVC, enabling environment)
■ Provider initiated HTC
■ Care and treatment (ART, OI prevention, lab monitoring, other)
■ Program management and human resources
■ Youth

Source: Duric et al. 2015.

Notes: Allocations to key populations refer to interventions specific for the respective key population at higher risk of HIV infection. For example, specific funding for key populations does not include their treatment or testing costs; however, care and treatment includes care and ART for key populations. The budget breakdown data were available only for US$16.9 million out of US$18.3 million for 2011 and US$21.3 million out of US$23.9 million for 2012. ART = antiretroviral therapy; HTC = HIV testing and counseling; MSM = men who have sex with men; OI = opportunistic infections; OVC = orphans and vulnerable children; PLHIV = people living with HIV; PMTCT = prevention of mother-to-child transmission; PWID = people who inject drugs; STI = sexually transmitted infection; SW = sex worker.

over time to reach universal coverage for the key prevention and ART services by 2020.

For ART services, the model investigated alternatively the following three options to determine universal coverage under Scenario 3:

1. Option A: 95 percent of diagnosed PLHIV and those eligible for ART under the existing national ART guidelines

Figure 12.5 Estimated Numbers of PLHIV, ART-Eligible PLHIV, and PLHIV on ART under Scenario 2, Uzbekistan

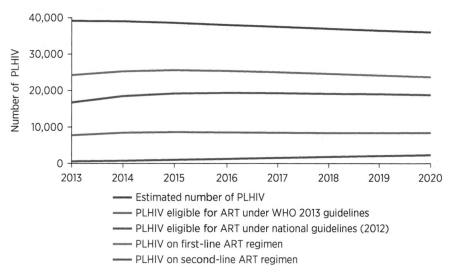

Source: Duric et al. 2015.

Note: ART = antiretroviral therapy; PLHIV = people living with HIV; WHO = World Health Organization.

2. Option B: 95 percent of diagnosed PLHIV and those eligible for ART under WHO 2013 guidelines
3. Option C: 95 percent of all diagnosed PLHIV—in accordance with the "test and treat" concept, in which individuals are offered treatment as soon as they test positive for HIV (Dodd, Garnett, and Hallett 2010)

For PMTCT, the objective of the modeling was to achieve 95 percent coverage; for harm reduction specific to PWID and special preventive service for other key populations, 80 percent coverage of estimated need was used. For HTC, the objective was that 80 percent of key populations at higher risk would know their status.

To achieve universal treatment access under Scenario 3, Option C (test and treat), the number of PLHIV on ART would need to reach about 25,800; for Option B (WHO 2013 guidelines) approximately 23,300; and for Option A (2012 national guidelines) about 20,000 by 2020. These numbers reflect a two-and-a-half- to threefold increase of 2013 ART figures. Because coverage for PMTCT services was already high, these services would see only modest scale-ups by 2020. The same applies to harm-reduction programs for PWID, with the exception of OST, which is currently not being offered. Assuming universal coverage for key preventive interventions, the epidemic impact would depend on which criteria were applied for determining ART eligibility, as shown in table 12.2.

Comparing Impacts of the Three Scenarios

Compared to the counterfactual scenario of no HIV programs at all, Scenario 1 (maintaining 2012 investment allocations and budget level) would avert about 12,500 new HIV infections and 49,000 DALYs until 2020 at a total program cost of US$167.1 million (2014–20, not counting inflation). Compared to the counterfactual scenario of no HIV programs at all, Scenario 2 (optimizing the investment allocations at the 2012 budget level) would avert approximately 13,000 new HIV infections and 74,000 DALYs until 2020 at a total program cost of US$174.1 million (2014–20). The model predictions showed the highest impact for Scenario 3 (scaling up to universal coverage) in terms of averting new HIV infections and DALYs by 2020; it is also the only scenario fulfilling international commitments made and core objectives of the Strategic Program on Fighting HIV Infection in the Republic of Uzbekistan in 2013–17 (Uzbekistan 2012). Table 12.3 summarizes the comparisons of projected impact and costs.

The long-term impact of Scenario 3 until 2030 is even more impressive. Figure 12.6 shows comparisons of all of the scenarios. Under Scenario 3, the estimated number of PLHIV would be about 35,000 using the 2012 national guidelines, approximately 33,000 using WHO 2013 treatment

Table 12.2 Projected Estimated Epidemiological Impact and Program Costs (Point Estimates) Using Three Options for Antiretroviral Therapy Eligibility Criteria in Scenario 3, Uzbekistan

By 2020	Universal ART Coverage		
	Option A	Option B	Option C
Estimated PLHIV	39,586	38,755	33,799
Estimated new HIV infections averted	20,270	21,150	26,818
Estimated DALYs averted	222,622	229,149	232,061
Total program costs, 2014–20 (US$)	210.6 million	228.1 million	248.8 million

Source: Duric et al. 2015.

Note: Program costs are for the period of 2014–20, not accounting for inflation. The options are compared to the counterfactual scenario of no HIV/AIDS programs at all. See narrative in chapter for further explanation of Options A, B, and C. ART = antiretroviral therapy; DALYs = disability-adjusted life years; HIV = human immunodeficiency virus; PLHIV = people living with HIV; US$ = US dollar.

guidelines, and about 23,000 using the test and treat approach (figure 12.6, panel a). The variations can be explained by long-term dynamics of differences in averted HIV infections and averted HIV-related deaths.

An estimated cumulative total of about 103,000 new HIV infections would be averted between 2014 and 2030 under Scenario 3 using the test and treat approach, approximately 91,000 would be averted using WHO 2013 guidelines, and 88,000 would be averted using the 2012 national guidelines. The differences arise mainly because of the higher impact in earlier years under options with more inclusive eligibility criteria for ART. Scenarios 2 and 1 achieve significantly lower numbers of averted HIV infections—approximately 70,000 and 65,000, respectively (figure 12.6, panel b).

Between 2014 and 2030 about 870,000 DALYs would be averted under Scenario 3 using the test and treat approach, 822,000 would be averted using WHO 2013 guidelines, and 796,000 would be averted using 2012 national guidelines. For new HIV infections averted, the differences arise mainly because of the higher impact during the earlier years under options with more inclusive eligibility criteria for ART. About half as many DALYs would be averted under Scenario 2 (516,000) and Scenario 1 (430,000).

Table 12.3 Point Estimates of Cumulative New HIV Infections Averted, Cumulative Disability-Adjusted Life Years Averted, and Total Program Costs under the Three Scenarios for Uzbekistan, 2014–20

	Scenario 1	Scenario 2	Scenario 3 Option A	Scenario 3 Option B	Scenario 3 Option C
New HIV infections averted	12,869	13,151	20,270	21,150	26,818
DALYs averted	49,218	74,110	222,622	229,149	232,061
Total program costs (US$)	167.1 million	174.1 million	210.6 million	228.1 million	248.8 million

Source: Duric et al. 2015.

Note: Option A = 95 percent of diagnosed and eligible PLHIV by 2020 (2012 national guidelines); Option B = 95 percent of diagnosed and eligible PLHIV by 2020 (WHO 2013 guidelines); Option C = 95 percent of all diagnosed PLHIV by 2020 ("test and treat"). DALYs = disability-adjusted life years; HIV = human immunodeficiency virus; PLHIV = people living with HIV; US$ = US dollar.

Figure 12.6 Long-Term Comparisons of the Epidemiological Impact of Scenarios 1, 2, and 3, Uzbekistan, 2015–30

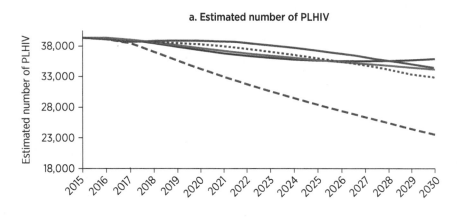

a. Estimated number of PLHIV

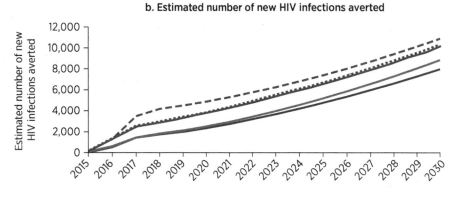

b. Estimated number of new HIV infections averted

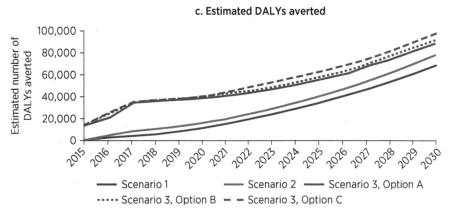

c. Estimated DALYs averted

Source: Duric et al. 2015.

Note: DALYs = disability-adjusted life years; HIV = human immunodeficiency virus; PLHIV = people living with HIV.

Conclusions

The model results suggest the following conclusions:

- The 2012 budget ceiling was too low to achieve universal coverage of essential HIV services.
- Achieving these goals and targets (Scenario 3) and universal coverage for all essential HIV services would require increasing the overall investment until 2020 by about 40 percent.
- Using the test and treat approach under Scenario 3 would avert about 103,000 new HIV infections between 2014 and 2030. Scenarios 2 and 1 avert significantly lower numbers of HIV infections—approximately 70,000 and 65,000, respectively.
- Despite the significantly higher number of HIV-related deaths averted under Scenario 3, the model predicts for this scenario the lowest number of PLHIV by 2030—ranging between 20,270 for Option A and 26,818 for the Option C).
- A transitional plan, under development by the Ministry of Finance to guide the transition to full state funding of HIV programs, is a good opportunity to address key recommendations from the UNDP modeling report.

Actions Taken and Next Steps

The Ministry of Finance has been developing a plan to guide the transition from donor funding to full state funding of HIV programs. The UNDP modeling report has been used to help develop this transitional plan.

In 2016, UNDP published a social contracting factsheet for Uzbekistan (Abdullaev et al. 2016). This document provides an overview of nongovernmental organizations for the national HIV response and emphasizes the importance of those organizations in ensuring access for key populations at higher risk of HIV exposure and ensuring access for people living with HIV to prevention, treatment, care, and support.

Notes

The mathematical model was developed and run by David Wilson and Cliff Kerr, University of New South Wales. Abdugulom Hakimov, manager of the Country Coordinating Mechanism (CCM) Secretariat in Uzbekistan, and Liya Perepada, formerly UNDP's Program Assistant for Democratic Governance and HIV/AIDS in Uzbekistan, provided information about the use of the modeling report in the national program and response planning in Uzbekistan. Rosemary Kumwenda, UNDP Team Leader for Regional HIV, Health and Development in

Europe and CIS, reviewed the chapter. The original report the chapter is based on was built on the inputs and reviews of the Uzbekistan country team working on the development of an HIV investment case for Uzbekistan: Nurmat Satiniyazovich Atabekov (RAC), Umida Islamova (Center for Economic Research), Zakir Kadirov, Liya Perepada (UNDP Uzbekistan), and Flora Sallikhova in coordination with Roman Hailevich, Jean-Elie Malkin, and Manoela Manova from the regional UNAIDS office in Moscow. Many others have participated in reviews of drafts, data verification, and translations; among them are the following individuals: Lusine Aydinyan, Victoria Froltsova, Alisher Juraev, Alexandra de Olazarra, Sophia Sul, Alexander Steven Wahn, Julia Whitman, and Karen Zhang. The study would not have been possible without the valuable comments and support from John Macauley and Boyan Konstantinov (both from the regional UNDP HIV, Health and Development Team, Regional Bureau for Europe and the CIS).

1. Republican AIDS Center data; see also UNODC 2017. Note that the information in this section draws extensively on data from the Republican AIDS Center.
2. For more information on the "Together We Will End AIDS" campaign, visit http://www.unaids.org/en/resources/campaigns/togetherwewillendaids. For more information on "Sustainable Development Goal 3: Targets and Indicators," visit https://sustainabledevelopment.un.org/sdg3.
3. Note that much of this chapter reviews the process and findings of the modeling exercise documented in Duric et al. 2015; as such, the material herein draws significantly on that report.
4. Overall program management costs accounted for 18 percent of overall funding in 2011–12. This proportion is deemed generally acceptable. A technical efficiency gain of 5 percent was considered realistic for the model.

References

Abdullaev, T., P. Duric, B. Konstantinov, and C. Hamelmann, C. 2016. "NGO Social Contracting: Factsheet Uzbekistan." Eastern Europe and Central Asia Series on Sustainable Financing of National HIV Responses, UNDP.

Dodd P. J., G. P. Garnett, and T. B. Hallett. 2010. "Examining the Promise of HIV Elimination by 'Test and Treat' in Hyperendemic Settings." *AIDS* 24 (5): 729–35.

Duric, P., C. Hamelmann, D. P. Wilson, and C. Kerr. 2015. "Modelling an Optimised Investment Approach for Uzbekistan." A joint publication of the United Nations Development Programme Regional Hub for Europe and the Commonwealth of Independent States and the Republican Center to Fight AIDS. Government of Uzbekistan, Tashkent.

UNAIDS (Joint United Nations Programme on HIV/AIDS). 2010. *Getting to Zero: 2011–2015 Strategy*. Geneva: UNAIDS.

UNAIDS (Joint United Nations Programme on HIV/AIDS). 2014. *Fast-Track: Ending the AIDS Epidemic by 2030*. Geneva: UNAIDS.

United Nations General Assembly. 2015. "Transforming Our World: The 2030 Agenda for Sustainable Development." United Nations document A/Res/70/1, October 21, United Nations, New York.

UNODC (United Nations Office on Drugs and Crime). 2017. "Republic of Uzbekistan Fact Sheet." Updated March 2017. https://www.paris-pact.net/upload/777dee 49f96d0ce4d4bef4502268d7a6.pdf.

Uzbekistan. 2012. "Strategic Program on Fighting HIV Infection in the Republic of Uzbekistan in 2013–2017." Government of Uzbekistan, Tashkent.

Uzbekestan. 2014. "Results of Epidemiological Surveillance of HIV Infection among People Who Inject Drugs in 2013." Government of Uzbekistan, Tashkent.

Uzbekestan, Ministry of Health. 2015. "Analysis of HIV Infection Triangulation Data in the Republic of Uzbekistan." Unpublished document, Ministry of Health, Tashkent.

WHO (World Health Organization). 2013. *Consolidated Guidelines on the Use of Antiretroviral Drugs for Treating and Preventing HIV Infection: Recommendations for a Public Health Approach.* Geneva: World Health Organization.

13

Optima HIV Methodology and Approach

*Cliff C. Kerr, Robyn M. Stuart, David J. Kedziora,
Amber Brown, Romesh Abeysuriya, George L. Chadderdon,
Anna Nachesa, and David P. Wilson*

Introduction

Optima HIV has grown from a simple mathematical model of human immunodeficiency virus (HIV) transmission and disease progression into a software package containing everything from epidemic indicator inferences, trend forecasting, and scenario analyses to resource need estimation, stochastic resource optimization, and user database management systems. The form of the Optima HIV software package adheres as closely as possible to its function: implementing the "Optima approach" of defining the burden of disease, identifying the programmatic responses, specifying the objectives and constraints, and applying mathematical optimization. These four components are drawn together to determine the optimal resource allocation to guide country decision-makers, funders, and their partners in order to achieve the greatest positive impact possible for the lives of people in their populations with available funding.

The aim of this chapter is to provide both a conceptual and a technical overview of the methodology underlying Optima HIV. The most comprehensive explanation of the Optima HIV methodology is the codebase itself, which has been made publicly available on GitHub with an open-source software license (github.com/optimamodel). The Optima HIV software package has been extensively documented; however, its intrinsic complexity provides a relatively high barrier of entry for people without considerable background in programming and mathematical modeling. To improve ease of use, Optima HIV also comes with a comprehensive six-volume user guide (optimamodel.com/user-guide). The guide describes in detail the layout of the interface and how to use it, and it also includes numerous worked examples.

Optima HIV has important similarities with other HIV modeling software packages, such as Spectrum/Goals (Stover et al. 2008), the AIDS Epidemic Model (AEM) (Brown and Peerapatanapokin 2014), and Thembisa (Johnson et al. 2014). For example, all are based on rate-based compartmental models, and all use similar approaches for modeling programs (for example, the use of coverage data to determine the impact of programs on the epidemiological outcomes in a defined scenario). Optima HIV, however, also has a number of unique features, including (1) how epidemiological and program data are integrated with a mathematical optimization function to determine optimal resource allocations and (2) how all components have been integrated into a friendly, web-based interface allowing analyses to be easily and flexibly performed on any modern computer (or indeed smartphone) from anywhere in the world.

The structure of this chapter recapitulates the structure of the Optima software itself, which in turn is based on the Optima approach. The chapter begins by discussing the epidemic module of HIV transmissibility and disease progression. It then describes how programs and interventions are modeled in the Optima framework. Next, it discusses objectives and constraints, and how they are used in the optimization algorithm. Finally, it describes the technical implementation of the software in terms of its Python backend and JavaScript frontend.

The Epidemic Model

Understanding the burden of disease overall and in subpopulations, as well as epidemiological trends over time, is a crucial first step in any HIV allocative efficiency analysis. The epidemic model within Optima HIV provides the necessary support for completing this step. This section describes the model in detail. It begins with a description of the model's structure, which can be described in very broad terms as a compartmental epidemic model. The classical susceptible–infected–recovered (SIR) structure is the canonical foundation example of this type of model. In more general terms, however, a compartmental epidemic model divides the entire population into compartments that (1) characterize their risk of transmitting a pathogen associated with disease or (2) characterize their chance of experiencing morbidity or mortality (or both). Movement between compartments is determined by a set of population-average rates of transition, which can be translated to probabilities of transition for individuals; details of the equations used to model these transition rates are provided in the next section. Finally, the section explains the statistical methods used to fit the model to data.

Model Structure

The risks of transmitting, acquiring, and dying from HIV depend on a host of different factors that can vary across the population, across partnerships, and over time. In the Optima HIV epidemic model, the population is stratified in three different ways in order to reflect this variation: by demographic or risk group, by health/disease state (stratified by CD4 [cluster of differentiation 4] count as an immunological marker), and by care stage. In Optima HIV, the different demographic/risk groups are defined as populations, the different disease progression stages as health states, and the different care and treatment stages as care states. For example, a given person might be a female sex worker (her population) and be living with HIV with a CD4 count of 350–499 (her health state) and currently be linked to care but not on treatment (her care state).

In the Optima HIV epidemic model, the entire population can be divided into as many subpopulations as required to capture variation in vulnerability to HIV. These subpopulations (henceforth simply referred to as populations) will be denoted by P_i, with $i = 1, \ldots, N$ for N different population groups.

Three different types of HIV transmission are modeled: transmission between sexual partners, transmission via sharing injecting equipment, and mother-to-child transmission. The input data associated with populations, sexual partnerships, injecting partnerships, and births are outlined in table 13.1. In any given application of the Optima HIV epidemic model, the populations can be chosen to capture the differences in the characteristics associated with both the populations themselves, and in the partnerships in which these populations engage.

For female populations, the analysis models seven states related to the care and treatment cascade (susceptible, undiagnosed, diagnosed and never linked to care, in care and not receiving antiretroviral therapy [ART], receiving ART and not virally suppressed, receiving ART and virally suppressed, and, finally, lost to follow-up) and eight for male populations (as for females but with the susceptible compartment divided into those who have been circumcised versus those who have not been circumcised). All infected stages are further disaggregated into six CD4-related health states (acute HIV infection, >500 cells per microliter [µL], 350–499 cells/µL, 200–349 cells/µL, 50–199 cells/µL, and <50 cells/µL). Taken together, these

Table 13.1   Input Variables Used to Characterize Population Groups in the Optima HIV Model

Sexual risk factors

$circ_{i,t}$	Prevalence of circumcision in population P_i at time t (defined for male populations only)
$sti_{i,t}$	Prevalence of ulcerative sexually transmitted infections in population P_i at time t
$prep_{i,t}$	Proportion of population P_i using pre-exposure prophylaxis at time t
$pmtct_{i,t}$	Proportion of population P_i covered by prevention of mother-to-child transmission at time t (defined for female populations only)
sex_i	The sex of population P_i (can be male, female, transgender, or unspecified)

Factors influencing mortality

$d_{i,t,dt}$	Probability of dying of non-HIV-related causes in population P_i between time t and $t+dt$
$tb_{i,t}$	Prevalence of tuberculosis in population P_i at time t

Factors influencing testing and treatment uptake

$test_{i,t,dt}$	Probability of taking and receiving the results of an HIV test between time t and $t+dt$ for population P_i
$link_{i,t}$	Average time taken for population P_i to be linked into care at time t
$loss_{i,t,dt}$	Proportion of people from population P_i who are lost from care between time t and $t+dt$

Factors specifying sexual partnerships

$c_{i,j,f,a,t}$	Probability at time t that condoms are used in partnerships of type f and act a between populations P_i and P_j (where $f \in$ {regular, casual, commercial} and $a \in$ {insertive penile-anal, receptive penile-anal, insertive penile-vaginal, receptive penile-vaginal})
$n_{i,j,f,a,t,dt}$	Number of interactions that occur between time t and $t+dt$ of type f and act a between populations P_i and P_j
$inj_{i,j,t,dt}$	Number of shared injections that occur between time t and $t+dt$ between populations P_i and P_j

Factors specifying births

$birth_{i,j,t,dt}$	Number of births between time t and $t+dt$ where population P_i gives birth into population P_j
$breast_{i,j,t}$	Proportion of population P_i that breastfeeds population P_j at time t

Source: World Bank.

Note: HIV = human immunodeficiency virus.

states give 38 care and health states (figure 13.1), one of which is empty for female populations (susceptible circumcised; not shown). The prevalence of HIV at time t among population P_i is denoted by $p_{t,i}$.

Model Transitions

During any given interval of time, people can move between population groups and health states according to a set of allowable transitions. One can use $k_t = (k_{t,i,h,c})$ to describe the distribution of people in each compartment at time t, where $k_{t,i,h,c}$ denotes the number of people in health state h, care state c, and population group P_i at time t. The general format of the transitions between all the states can be expressed by defining a function f that takes as inputs (1) the model parameters, θ; (2) a d-dimensional array of exogenous data, X_{t+dt} (such as numbers of people receiving treatment); and (3) the distribution of people at time t, k_t. This function then maps these inputs to a distribution of people at time $t+dt$:

$$k_{t+dt} = f(\theta, X_{t+dt}, k_t). \tag{13.1}$$

This section provides an overview of how each individual transition is modeled. Finally, it provides an overview of how the individual transitions are combined together to give the function f.

Adult HIV transmission is modeled by the movement of people from the susceptible compartments to the acute undiagnosed compartment. To derive this transition, one first considers the probability of sexual transmission. The set of sexual partnership types will be denoted by $F = \{$regular, casual, commercial$\}$, and the set of sexual acts will be denoted by $A = \{$insertive penile-anal, receptive penile-anal, insertive penile-vaginal, receptive penile-vaginal$\}$. The set of sexual partnerships is given by the following formula:

$$Q_{sex} = \{(i,j,a,f)|P_i \text{ and } P_j \text{ engage in sexual act } a\ (a \in A) \text{ of type } f\ (f \in F)\}. \tag{13.2}$$

The number of sexual partnerships (i,j,a,f) that occur between time t and $t+dt$ is denoted by $n_{t,dt,i,j,f,a}$. The sexual partnerships that a person from population P_i engages in are defined as $Q_{i,sex} = \{(j,a,f) \mid P_i \text{ and } P_{j'} \text{ engage in sexual acts } a\ (a \in A) \text{ of type } f\ (f \in F)\}$.

To model the effect of prevention, ω is defined as the efficacy of condoms, $c_{t,i,j,f}$ as the probability at time t that condoms are used in partnerships of type f between populations P_i and $P_{j'}$ and R as the power set of $\{PrEP, circumcision\}$. An act a that occurs at time t between a susceptible person from population P_i covered by prevention type $r \in R$ and a partner from population P_j who is in health state h is associated with the per-act transmission probability $\beta_{t,i,j,a,h,c,r}$.

Figure 13.1 Disease- and Care-Related Transitions in Optima

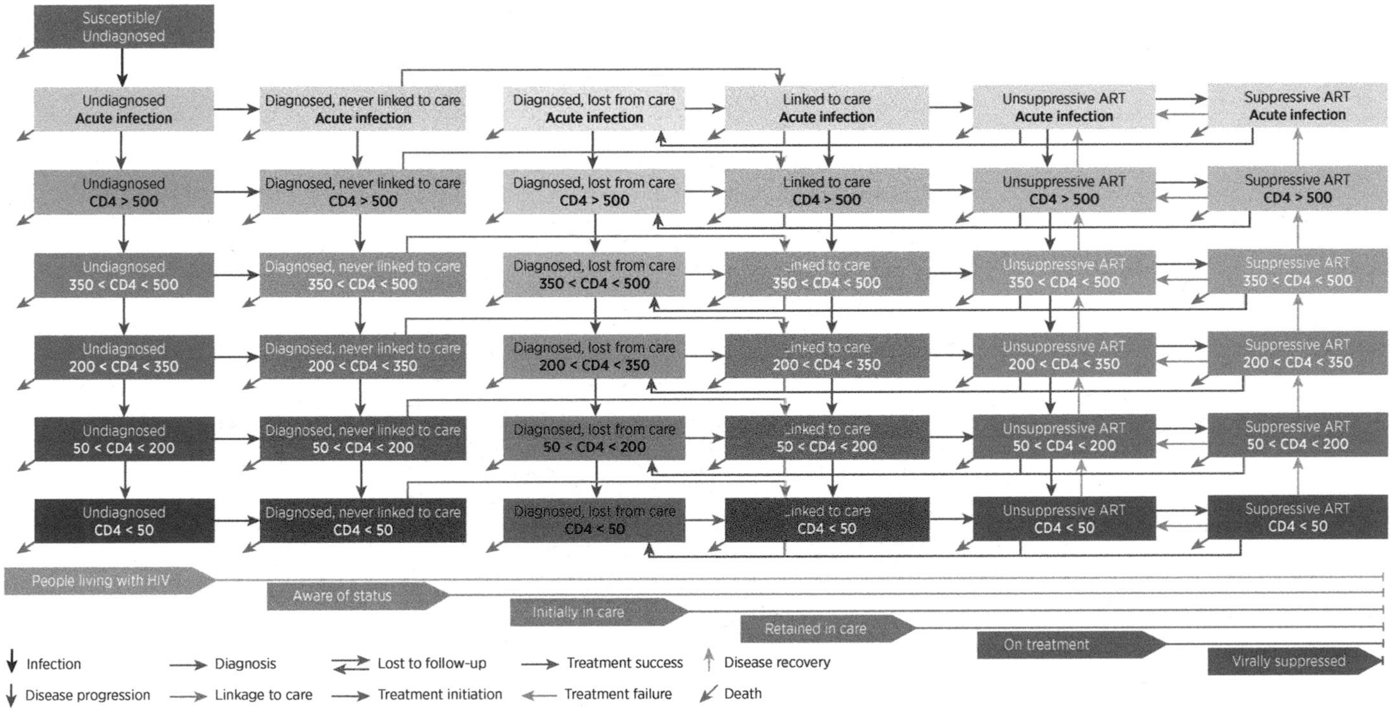

Source: World Bank based on Optima model.

Note: Horizontal movements represent movements between care states, while vertical movements represent movements between health states. ART = antiretroviral therapy; CD4 = cluster of differentiation 4; HIV = human immunodeficiency virus.

For example, the per-act transmission probability associated with condomless receptive penile-vaginal intercourse between a susceptible female and an undiagnosed HIV-positive male with CD4 count of 200–349 cells/µL is estimated as approximately 0.0008 (Padian et al. 1997). If one takes this as the base case, and for illustrative purposes takes point estimates of relevant metrics, then

1. Use of pre-exposure prophylaxis (PrEP) by the female lowers the per-act transmission probability (relative to the base case) by 73 percent (Baeten et al. 2015) to 0.000216;
2. If the male is receiving viral-suppressive treatment, it lowers the per-act transmission probability (relative to the base case) by 92 percent (Cohen et al. 2011) to 0.000064; and
3. If the male is in the acute/primary infection stage, it increases the per-act transmission probability (relative to the base case) by 560 percent (Pilcher et al. 2004) to 0.00448.

One can then define an expression for the probability that a susceptible person from population P_i who is covered by prevention type $r \in R$ acquires HIV between time t and $t+dt$ from a sexual partnership (i,j,a,f) where the partner from population P_j is in health state h and care state c:

$$
\begin{aligned}
1-\lambda^{sex}_{i,j,t,dt,a,f,r,h,c} \\
= (1-p_{t,j,h}\beta_{i,j,t,a,h,c,r}\ \omega c_{i,j,f,t}\ (n_{t,dt,i,j,f,a}-\lfloor n_{t,dt,i,j,f,a}\rfloor))(1-p_{t,j,h}\beta_{i,j,t,a,h,c,r}\ \omega c_{i,j,f,t})^{\lfloor n_{t,dt,i,j,f,a}\rfloor} \\
\times (1-p_{t,j,h}\beta_{i,j,t,a,h,c,r}(1-c_{i,j,f,t})(n_{t,dt,i,j,f,a}-\lfloor n_{t,dt,i,j,f,a}\rfloor)) \\
\times (1-p_{t,j,h}\beta_{i,j,t,a,h,c,r}(1-c_{i,j,f,t}))^{\lfloor n_{t,dt,i,j,f,a}\rfloor}.
\end{aligned}
\tag{13.3}
$$

Finally, one can define the probability that a susceptible person from population P_i would become infected via sexual transmission between time t and $t+dt$ as

$$
\Lambda^{sex}_{i,t,dt} = 1 - \prod_{h \in H, (j,a,f) \in Q_{i,sex}, r \in R}\left(1 - \lambda^{sex}_{i,j,t,dt,a,f,r,h,c}\right).
\tag{13.4}
$$

In a similar fashion, one can derive an expression for the probability that a susceptible person from population P_i would become infected via sharing injecting equipment between time t and $t+dt$:

$$
\Lambda^{inj}_{i,t,dt} = 1 - \prod_{h \in H, j \in Q_{i,inj}}\left(1 - \lambda^{inj}_{i,j,t,dt,h}\right),
\tag{13.5}
$$

where $Q_{i,inj}$ is the set of injecting partnerships that a person from population P_i engages in with population(s) P_j, and $1-\lambda^{inj}_{i,j,t,dt,h}$ is the probability that a susceptible person from population P_i acquires HIV between time t and $t+dt$ from an injecting partnership with someone from population P_j in health state h, defined as

$$1-\lambda^{inj}_{i,j,t,dt,h}=(1-p_{t,j,h}\beta_{i,j,t,h,inj}(n_{t,dt,i,j,inj}-\lfloor n_{t,dt,i,j,inj}\rfloor))\ (1-p_{t,j,h}\beta_{i,j,t,h,inj})^{\lfloor n_{t,dt,i,j,inj}\rfloor}, \qquad (13.6)$$

where $\beta_{i,j,t,h,inj}$ is the per-act transmission probability associated with a shared injection that occurs at time t between a susceptible person from population P_i and a partner from population P_j who is in health state h, and $n_{t,dt,i,j,inj}$ is the number of injecting interactions between populations P_i and P_j between time t and $t+dt$.

Putting the sexual and injecting transmission probabilities together, one can derive the final expression for the probability that a susceptible person from population P_i acquires HIV between time t and $t+dt$ as

$$\Lambda_{i,t,dt} = \theta_i \left(1- \prod_{h\in H(j,a,f)\in Q_{i,sex},r\in R,j\in Q_{i,inj}} \left(1-\lambda^{sex}_{i,j,t,dt,a,f,r,h,c}\right)\left(1-\lambda^{inj}_{i,j,t,dt,h}\right) \right). \qquad (13.7)$$

To evaluate this expression, one collates data on sexual and injecting behavior and uses estimates from trials and other empirical estimates to inform the per-act transmission probabilities. (For a full list of input data, see the online user guide at optimamodel.com/user-guide.) The parameter θ_i is an element of the p-dimensional parameter vector θ; details of how these parameters are estimated are provided later in the chapter.

When the probability $\Lambda_{i,t,dt}$ is multiplied by the number of susceptible people in population P_i, it corresponds to the estimated number of people who become infected between time t and $t+dt$. In compartmental models this can be translated to an average time for people in population P_i to become infected. This translation from individual-level probability to population rate is an important element for all transitions in Optima HIV, as in all compartmental models.

The probability that a person from population P_i will be diagnosed between time t and $t+dt$ is

$$diag_{t,dt,i,h} = p_{t,i}test_{t,dt,i,h}, \qquad (13.8)$$

where $test_{t,dt,i,h}$ is the probability that a person from population P_i in health state h will get tested between time t and $t+dt$.

The probability that a person from population P_i in health state h is linked to care between time t and $t+dt$ is

$$link_{t,dt,i,h} = \left(1-e^{-\frac{dt}{linktime_{i,t,h}}} \right), \qquad (13.9)$$

where $linktime_{t,i,h}$ is the average time that it takes for a person from population P_i in health state h to be linked into care at time t.

The probability of treatment initiation is determined by the number of treatment spots available. These spots are first filled by those with lower CD4 counts.

The probability that a person in health state h achieves viral suppression between time t and $t+dt$ is

$$vs_{t,dt,h} = \left(1 - e^{-\frac{dt}{timetovs}} + treatfail_{dt} propvlmon_{t,dt} \right), \qquad (13.10)$$

where $timetovs$ is the time after initiating ART to achieve viral suppression, $treatfail^{dt}$ is the probability over dt units of time of having treatment failure, and $propvlmon_{t,dt}$ is the proportion of people on treatment who receive a viral load test between time t and $t+dt$.

The probability that a person receiving virally-suppressive treatment experiences treatment failure between time t and $t+dt$ is $treatfail_{dt}$ $(1-propvlmon_{t,dt})$.

The probability that someone transitions from a health state h to a health state with a lower CD4 count in dt units of time is given by

$$cd4progress_{dt} = \left(1 - e^{-\frac{dt}{progresstime_h}} \right). \qquad (13.11)$$

For someone on suppressive ART, the probability of transitioning from a health state h to a health state with a higher CD4 count in dt units of time is given by

$$cd4recover_{dt} = \left(1 - e^{-\frac{dt}{recovertime_h}} \right). \qquad (13.12)$$

The probabilities of transitioning from any given compartment to a compartment with either a higher or a lower CD4 count are updated from the best available clinical data—such as from the CASCADE study (Huang et al. 2012; Lodi et al. 2011).

The probability that a person from population P_i transitions to population P_j in dt units of time is given by

$$risktrans_{i,dt} = \left(1 - e^{-\frac{dt}{time_i}}\right).$$ (13.13)

Age transitions $agetrans_{i,dt}$ are defined by the reciprocal of the width of the age bin. For example, if a population is defined to be aged 25–34 inclusive, then the rate of transition will be 0.1.

The probability of someone in health state h and care state c dying from HIV-related causes in dt units of time is $d_{dt,h,c}$ and the probability of someone in population P_i dying of non-HIV-related causes between time t and $t+dt$ is $d_{t,dt,i}$.

From each compartment within the model structure, a person may transition to multiple other compartments. The following example illustrates how these probabilities are combined. For example, a diagnosed HIV-positive female aged 15–24 years with a CD4 count between 200 µl⁻¹ and 349 µl⁻¹ who is diagnosed but not yet linked to care may

1. Transition to the female sex worker (FSW) population *(poptrans_{i,dt})*,
2. Age into the female 25–34-year-old population *(agetrans_{i,dt})*,
3. Have her CD4 count decline to below 200 µl⁻¹ *(cd4progress_{dt})*,
4. Be linked to care *(link_{t,dt,i})*,
5. Die of HIV-related causes *(d_{t,dt,i})*, or
6. Die of non-HIV-related causes *(d_{dt,h})*.

Excluding the death transitions, she may move to 24 possible compartments: *{female 15–24, female 25–34, FSW}×{200<CD4<350, 50<CD4<200} ×{diagnosed, linked to care}*.

Model Calibration

As equation (13.1) demonstrates, it is possible to calculate k_{t+dt} (the distribution of people across all model compartments at any point in time) given (1) the functional form of f, which determines how the individual transition probabilities are modeled and were described for each transition; (2) the exogenous data X_{t+dt}, which consists of all the variables described in table 13.1; (3) the distribution of people at the previous time, k_{t+dt}; and (4) the parameter vector θ. In fact, because the equations are dynamic, k_{t+dt} can be calculated using X_{t+dt}, f, θ, and k_0, where k_0 is the initial distribution of people at time 0. The process of ensuring that the model produces estimates that resemble reality is called model calibration. This section describes first how the goodness-of-fit of the model is measured and then how the goodness-of-fit is optimized.

Like any system of differential equations, the model requires initial conditions to be specified. Doing so corresponds to defining the distribution $k_{t,i,h,c}$ for $t = 0$.

If the input parameters were known precisely and the model was a perfect representation of reality, then no parameter fitting would be required and the epidemic would be accurately represented by a single parameter set. In practice, however, large uncertainties in input parameters exist. Furthermore, the structure of Optima HIV does not necessarily capture all relevant aspects of the real-world epidemic; thus, even with perfect information on parameters, one would expect some discrepancy between model estimates and measured values. Exacerbating the problem, the data used for calibration are also typically not exact, because there is some uncertainty even in HIV prevalence data from population-based surveys, which may be subject to selection bias.

These data correspond to various indicators of the epidemic state. The indicators vary depending on context, but they may include time series of HIV prevalence, the number of acquired immune deficiency syndrome (AIDS)-related deaths, and the number of new HIV diagnoses, HIV incidence among (sub-)populations, and (if available) country-endorsed estimates of trends in the number of people living with HIV (PLHIV) and total annual number of new HIV infections. One can denote the observed epidemic state indicators by $y_{t,obs}$. Each epidemic state indicator for which data or estimates are collated equates to an epidemic state indicator for which the Optima HIV model produces estimates. Because the Optima HIV model's estimates depend on the model parameters θ, one denotes the model's estimates of the epidemic state indicators by $y_{t,est}(\theta)$. (Note that the variables in y_t, model$[\theta]$ can all be derived from k_t and k_{t-dt}. For example, the number of new infections that occurred between time t and dt is calculated by taking the difference in the number of people in all the infected compartments between the two times. Thus, equation [13.1] is sufficient to determine any of the model outputs.) The goodness-of-fit of the model is measured by comparing the model's estimates of the epidemic state indicators to the observed epidemic state indicators.

If the goal is to minimize the difference between the model's estimates of the epidemic state indicators and the observed epidemic state indicators, a natural approach would be to set $\theta = \theta^*$, and minimize a distance metric such that

$$\theta^* = \arg \min_{\theta} \sum_{t \in T} \frac{\left| y_{t,est}\left(\theta, k_0\right) - y_{t,obs} \right|}{y_{t,obs}}, \qquad (13.14)$$

where T is the set of times at which one observes some epidemic state indicator. Mean absolute percentage errors are used in the distance metric because the data are measured on different scales. (Note that this estimator minimizes the median error, whereas using mean squared percentage errors would minimize the mean error.) There is no closed-form solution to this equation, so instead one proceeds by choosing an initial θ_0 and refining iteratively. This is an instance of a nonlinear, data-fitting problem, for which many numerical algorithms exist. By default, Optima uses the adaptive stochastic descent (ASD) algorithm described later in the chapter.

Minimizing the distance metric defined in equation (13.14) corresponds to finding the best possible match between the model and the data. It thus approximates the maximum likelihood estimate of the model parameter values. To quantify uncertainty in the parameters, one can use a modified Bayesian framework, beginning with Bayes' theorem:

$$p(\theta \mid y_{obs}) = \frac{p(y_{obs} \mid \theta)p(\theta)}{p(y_{obs})},\qquad(13.15)$$

where $p(\theta \mid y_{obs})$ is the posterior distribution of the model parameters given the data (the quantity to be estimated), $p(y_{obs} \mid \theta)$ is the likelihood (the probability of the data given the parameters), $p(\theta)$ is the prior (the initial degree of belief in the parameter values), and $p(y_{obs})$ is the evidence (how likely one is to have observed the data one observed). Because the only interest is the dependence of the posterior probability on the parameters, one can set $p(y_{obs}) = 1$. Because the prior range on the model parameters is also typically unconstrained (although assumptions can be made), implying $p(\theta)=const.$, Bayes' theorem can be rewritten as

$$p(\theta \mid y_{obs}) \propto p(y_{obs} \mid \theta).\qquad(13.16)$$

This equation implies that the density of the posterior is proportional to the density of the likelihood. The likelihood is impossible to derive precisely, given that the Optima HIV model is not formulated in a way that allows its probability density function to be estimated. The likelihood can be approximated, however, by a distance metric that is assumed to be proportional to it. An appropriate distance metric is provided by equation (13.14), which approaches zero as the model estimates and the data converge, as intuitively expected. Replacing the likelihood with a distance metric then allows for the estimation of the posterior using approximate Bayesian computation Markov chain Monte Carlo (ABC-MCMC; Marjoram et al. 2003). Using the Metropolis-Hastings sampling approach (Hastings 1970), the algorithm proceeds as follows:

1. Begin with an initial parameter set, θ, and a corresponding approximate likelihood estimated from the prior distribution and the inverse of the distance metric above:

$$E = p(\theta) = \left(\sum_{t \in T} \frac{\left| y_{t,est}(\theta, k_0) - y_{t,obs} \right|}{y_{t,obs}} \right)^{-1}.$$

2. Draw a candidate parameter set, θ', by sampling from a proposal density centered on θ (that is, for each parameter i, a Gaussian distribution with mean θ_i and standard deviation $\alpha\theta_i$, where α is the step size, e.g., 10 percent).
3. Compute the approximate likelihood, E', corresponding to this candidate parameter set, using the formula shown in step 1.
4. Calculate the acceptance ratio $\alpha = \dfrac{E'}{E'}$; accept the new parameter set (that is, $\theta \leftarrow \theta'$) with probability α.
5. Store θ as a sample from the posterior distribution (regardless of whether or not the candidate parameter set was accepted).
6. Repeat steps 2–5 until sufficient parameter samples have been drawn to estimate the posterior to the desired level of precision (typically 100–10,000 samples).

From the posterior distribution of the parameters obtained using the algorithm above, one can generate posterior predictive distributions of $y_{t,model}$. Furthermore, the empirical posterior distribution can be bootstrapped (that is, Monte Carlo sampling with replacement) to generate parameter sets for use in further analyses (for example, scenarios and optimizations). Note that, rather than beginning with a single set of parameters, θ, it is possible to begin with a Monte Carlo initialization of θ, leading to multiple (noninteracting) chains.

Understanding Responses

Programs that provide HIV care, treatment, and prevention are the direct means by which national governments, donors, and partners aim to have an impact on the HIV epidemic. Enabling a successful HIV response of course requires other essential components, including community engagement and empowerment, removing legal barriers, and so on. In its current form, however, the Optima HIV model can include interventions only if they impact directly on one of the proximal determinants of HIV. This section describes how direct programmatic interventions are defined within Optima HIV. Strictly speaking, programs do not have to be defined for Optima HIV analyses to be run; however, most of the key functionality of Optima HIV—namely running optimization analyses or coverage and budget scenarios—requires such programs; thus, in practice, they are required for all but the simplest of forward projection analyses.

Defining Programs

Optima HIV includes a list of predefined default programs, which are intended to cover the key aspects of most national HIV responses (see table 13.2). These default programs are based on the key National AIDS Spending Assessment (NASA) categories. Programs are divided into four broad categories: prevention, care and treatment, management and administration, and other. Because programs that provide HIV care, treatment, and prevention are what national governments, donors, and

Table 13.2   Default Programs Included in Optima HIV

Program name	Category	Target population(s)	Target outcome(s)
Condom programs	Prevention	All	Casual condom use
Social behavior change communication	Prevention	All	Casual condom use
Sexually transmitted infection (STI) programs	Prevention	All	STI prevalence
Voluntary medical male circumcision	Prevention	Male populations	Circumcision prevalence
Programs for female sex workers	Prevention	Female sex workers	Commercial condom use, HIV testing rates
Programs for men who have sex with men	Prevention	Men who have sex with men	Casual condom use, HIV testing rates
Programs for people who inject drugs	Prevention	People who inject drugs	Needle-syringe sharing rate
Opioid substitution therapy	Prevention	People who inject drugs	Number of injections

continued next page

Table 13.2 *(continued)*

Program name	Category	Target population(s)	Target outcome(s)
Cash transfers	Prevention	Female populations	Number of casual sexual acts
Pre-exposure prophylaxis (PrEP)	Prevention	All	PrEP prevalence
Post-exposure prophylaxis (PEP)	Care and treatment	All	PEP prevalence
HIV testing and counseling	Care and treatment	All	HIV testing rates
Antiretroviral therapy (ART)	Care and treatment	People living with HIV (PLHIV)	Number of people on ART
Lab monitoring	Care and treatment	PLHIV on ART	Number of viral load tests
Adherence support	Care and treatment	PLHIV on ART	Rate at which people leave care
Pre-ART tracing	Care and treatment	PLHIV on ART	Rate at which people are linked to care
Prevention of mother-to-child transmission (PMTCT)	Care and treatment	Pregnant and breastfeeding women	Number of pregnant or breastfeeding women receiving PMTCT
Orphans and vulnerable children	Care and treatment	n.a.	n.a.
Other care	Care and treatment	n.a.	n.a.
Management	Management/ administration	n.a.	n.a.
Human resources and training	Management/ administration	n.a.	n.a.
Enabling environment	Management/ administration	n.a.	n.a.
Social protection	Other	n.a.	n.a.
Monitoring, evaluation, surveillance, and research	Other	n.a.	n.a.
Health infrastructure	Other	n.a.	n.a.
Other	Other	n.a.	n.a.

Source: World Bank.

Note: HIV = human immunodeficiency virus; n.a. = not applicable.

partners use to address the HIV epidemic, allocative efficiency analyses typically include only prevention and care and treatment programs, although other programs can also be included in technical efficiency analyses, with cost savings redirected toward "direct-impact" (also called targeted) programs.

Each program has a defined list of target populations and target outcomes, which define the possible impacts of that program. Programs can be quantified in terms of their total spending, total coverage, and unit costs. Only two of these three quantities are required for all three to be calculated; countries most typically have information on total spending (from NASA reports) and total coverage (from monitoring and evaluation units), from which unit costs can be calculated. In some contexts, however, coverage values are calculated from total spending and unit costs (which are often calculated using an ingredients-based method). One issue for consideration when performing an Optima analysis is whether management costs should be included within other programs or as a distinct program. Because management often accounts for 30–40 percent of the total HIV budget, its inclusion can make a significant difference to the unit costs and thus the cost of covering additional people with a given program. Depending on the context, either approach can be justified; however, it is critical that a consistent choice be made across all programs. The historical approach taken in Optima HIV analyses is to take the NASA-reported total programmatic cost to wash over all of the nominated programmatic factors that contribute toward achieving the reported programmatic coverage in the target population. This is admittedly a crude measure of cost, but it is typically likely to be more inclusive than if a bottom-up costing study was done of commodities, labor costs of primary staff, and basic overheads. The Global Health Costing Consortium is currently developing a costing reference case, framework, and database for HIV unit costs. As this becomes available, it will be used to provide additional inputs for Optima HIV.

Cost Functions

Optima HIV links program spending to the underlying epidemic model and thus to possible epidemic impact via cost functions. There are two complementary types of cost functions. The primary type is the cost-coverage function, which relates the amount of spending on a given program to the number of people covered by that program. The second type is the coverage-outcome function, which relates the number of people covered to the change in the values of one or more model inputs.

Data available to inform cost functions are typically very limited. Thus, it is often necessary to make assumptions regarding the parameters of the cost functions. One such assumption is that, with zero spending, the coverage of a given program is zero. This assumption does not, however, imply that the affected parameters are also zero. For example, if spending for a condom program is zero, then zero people will be covered by that program; but condom usage rates will be above zero because of private spending. Furthermore, because of the strict upper limit on the number of people reached by a given program (that is, the target population size), and because it becomes increasingly difficult to reach new people as program coverage scales up (and because some people are likely to be entirely unreachable no matter how much funding is allocated toward a given program), the cost-coverage function must asymptote toward a saturation value that is somewhat less than the total target population size. The simplest equation that meets these requirements is a modified logistic function:

$$c = \frac{2c_{max}}{1+e^{-2s/(c\,max^u)}} - c_{max},$$ (13.17)

where c is the coverage, c_{max} is the saturation coverage value (for example, 90 percent of the target population size), s is the spending, and u is the unit cost at zero coverage (or, equivalently in this case, marginal cost). Note that this equation does not include start-up costs. Although these costs can be included within Optima HIV, by default they are not, because (1) few or no data typically exist to constrain the shape of this part of the curve, and (2) programs considered in allocative efficiency analyses are typically already implemented at scale, and thus start-up costs do not necessarily apply.

Note that the nonlinearity of this curve is one of the primary drivers of the difference between the Optima approach and a simple cost-effectiveness league table. With a nonlinear cost-coverage function, programs saturate slowly as they scale up toward optimal coverage. In contrast, with linear cost functions, the most cost-effective program would be scaled up to maximum coverage, followed by the next most cost-effective program, and so on (ignoring the contributions of nonlinearities in the epidemic model including interactions between programs on epidemic outcomes).

Compared to the cost-coverage function, the coverage-outcome function is relatively simple. It is assumed that (1) a given person is either covered by a program or not (if a person is partially covered by a program, or provided with a different quality of service, then this service can be defined as a separate program), and (2) the impact of a program on a given person is independent of the impact of that program on any other person. These two assumptions imply a simple linear relationship between coverage and outcome:

$$o = o_{min} + c\,(o_{max} - o_{min})$$ (13.18)

where o is the outcome (that is, the value of the given outcome), o_{min} is the minimum value this outcome would have with no interventions, o_{max} is the value this outcome could have under maximum coverage of this program, and c is the coverage as determined by equation (13.17) (except here expressed as a fraction of the target population rather than as an absolute number). Together, the cost-coverage and coverage-outcome functions specify the impact a program will have on the model inputs, as shown in figure 13.2.

Panel a of figure 13.2 shows the cost-coverage function for an example of 10,000 FSWs, with a saturation coverage of 90 percent and a unit cost of

Figure 13.2 Schematic Illustration of Cost Functions in Optima HIV

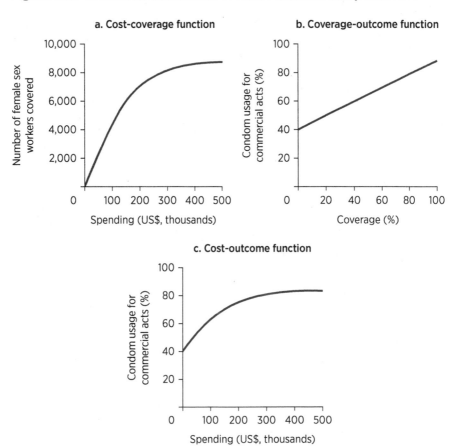

Source: World Bank based on Optima data.

Note: HIV = human immunodeficiency virus; US$ - US dollar.

US\$20 per person covered. Panel b shows the coverage-outcome function, where condom usage for commercial sexual acts is 40 percent in the absence of any interventions, and 90 percent given full coverage of this particular program. Panel c shows the cost-outcome function, which is the result of multiplying these two functions.

Combining Modalities

Further complications arise when different service modalities exist for a given program. For example, consider multiple interventions that each aim to increase the HIV testing rate (a community-based advertising campaign, workplace- and school-based programs, and a program targeting FSWs). Three possible coverage assumptions are available in Optima HIV.

The random assumption is that any given person has a finite probability of being covered by a given program, which is independent of whether or not that person is covered by any other program. For example, if community-based programs have coverage of 60 percent and workplace-based programs cover 20 percent, then 12 percent (=60%×20%) of people will be covered by both programs, 8 percent by the workplace program only (=20%×40%), 48 percent (=60%×80%) by the community program only, and 32 percent (=40%×80%) by no program.

The nested assumption is that a person is covered only by a lower-coverage program if that person is also covered by a higher-coverage program; for example, it could be assumed that all people who are in the workplace are also exposed to community advertisements. In this case, 20 percent of people would be covered by both programs, 40 percent by the community program only, and the remaining 40 percent by no program (no one is covered by only the workplace program).

Finally, the additive assumption is that the overlap between target populations is minimized. For example, it is unlikely that someone exposed to the school-based program would also be exposed to the workplace program. Assuming coverage of the school-based program is 50 percent, then 50 percent of people would be covered by the school program only, 20 percent would be covered by the workplace program only, and the remaining 30 percent would be covered by no program (no one is covered by both programs).

Although the examples above illustrate only two modalities, they can be extended to any number of interacting programs. In addition to the afore-mentioned choices regarding how coverage across programs combines, various assumptions can be made about how programs interact within a given individual: in some cases, the outcome for that individual may simply be equal to the outcome of being covered by the single most effective program; in other cases, programs may have synergistic effects within that

annual increases or decreases in program funding are not to exceed 30 percent).

Using Optimization to Achieve Strategic Goals

For complex epidemiological systems, it is difficult to determine which programs have the greatest marginal impact. This challenge is especially true when interventions do not target the same populations, do not have the same type of effects, or do not have simple linear cost functions. In most cases, the net epidemiological impact of a resource allocation will not be known before a full model run. Moreover, when a large number of interventions is involved, the combinatorial explosion of possible budgets makes it computationally infeasible to explore different possible funding combinations in using an undirected approach.

Mathematical Optimization Algorithm

Optima HIV circumvents this obstacle by anchoring all optimization analyses on an algorithm called adaptive stochastic descent (ASD) (Kerr et al. under review). This algorithm consists of five steps:

1. Select an initial distribution of funding across programs, typically drawn from the most recent available spending data.
2. Run the model using the given resource allocation, and calculate the epidemiological outcome.
3. Increase or decrease funding to one program chosen stochastically (but based on probability distributions learned from previous iterations), redistribute funding evenly across remaining programs so that the total budget stays the same, and rerun the model to compute the new epidemiological outcome.
4. If the outcome improved, accept the new funding distribution; otherwise, keep the current spending distribution.
5. Repeat steps 2–4 until the solution converges.

By using this algorithm, Optima HIV is able to greatly reduce the number of model runs it requires when calculating an optimal resource allocation. Of course, solution space for the objective function is large and nonlinear, meaning that ASD can occasionally be caught in local extrema. For this reason, Optima HIV typically repeats the chain of iterations several times for different initial funding distributions; this Monte Carlo (MC) process increases the probability of finding a true optimum. By using MC-ASD, Optima HIV is thus able to determine an optimal resource allocation and epidemiological outcome with high computational efficiency. An example outcome of such an optimization is shown in figure 13.3.

The standard form of optimization consists of redistributing a fixed sum of funds among a set of programs, aiming to maximally improve an epidemiological outcome—for example, to minimize the number of cumulative AIDS-related deaths between 2015 and 2030.

Through the use of MC-ASD, Optima HIV explores varying resource distributions and aims to find the global minimum of the objective function. Aside from context-specific constraints, every iteration of the algorithm ensures that the sum of funds across all programs is kept constant. The result is that the original and optimal budgets are always equal in net size,

Figure 13.3 Example Optimization Result, Showing the Current Budget Allocation, the Optimal Budget Allocation, and the Change in the Allocation

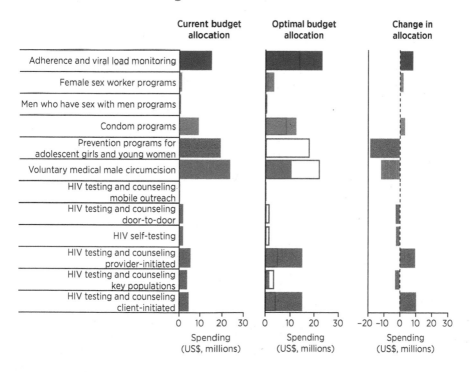

Source: World Bank based on Optima data.

Note: Transparent columns show initial allocation. HIV = human immunodeficiency virus; US$ = US dollar.

but the optimal distribution of the budget among possible programs can be markedly different from the status quo. Programs with high impact will be prioritized, whereas less cost-effective interventions will be defunded.

Minimizing Funding Required to Meet Objectives

Although boosting allocative efficiency is desirable (subject to caveats regarding equity, ethical, and other considerations), available funds may not be sufficient to achieve aspirational epidemiological targets. Optima HIV thus provides an alternative optimization procedure that seeks to estimate the minimum funding required to achieve or maintain a given epidemiological impact. In one sense, this procedure is a reversal of a standard optimization: resources are variable and outcomes are fixed; however, it is typically not possible to identify an exact allocation that produces a desired outcome. The algorithm employed is thus more complicated:

1. Run the model for an initial allocation, typically for the most recent available budget allocation.
2. If a desired epidemiological impact is achieved, scale the allocation down proportionally by a predetermined factor; otherwise, scale it up by that same factor.
3. Repeat step 2 until an upper and lower bound on total funding size are established, for which the desired outcome is and is not achieved, respectively.
4. Select a total budget amount within this range, then optimize and determine whether an allocation exists for which the impact is attained.
5. Depending on whether the solution exists or does not, set the budget amount as the new upper or lower bound, respectively.
6. Repeat steps 4–5 until satisfied with solution accuracy.

In this way, Optima HIV estimates the optimal resource allocation with the smallest net funding that still achieves a desired epidemiological outcome.

The process of cost optimization implicitly investigates optimal resource allocations for a number of total budget sizes. It can often be instructive for policy makers to make this exploration explicit; when done for a regular array of budget sizes, the result is referred to as an "investment staircase" (Stuart et al. 2017). Figure 13.4 depicts such a visualization, with the bar chart on the right of the diagram indicating how best to apportion funds between interventions, given a linearly increasing total funding amount. Corresponding bars on the left of the diagram indicate epidemiological impact associated with each optimal allocation. Accordingly, the value of each bar shows the best outcome that can be achieved for each budget—for example, the minimum number of DALYs.

Figure 13.4 The "Investment Staircase": The Optimal Budget Allocation at Each Different Funding Level, from 0 Percent of Current Budget through 200 Percent of Current Budget, Showing an Exponential Saturation of Outcome

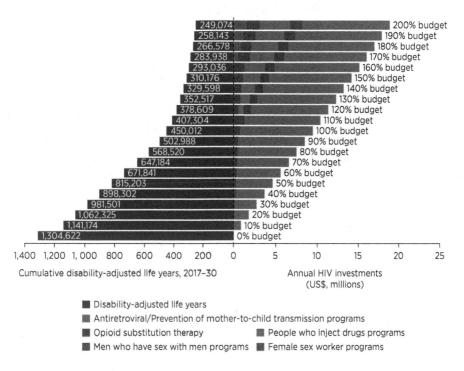

Source: World Bank based on Optima data.

Note: HIV = human immunodeficiency virus; US$ = US dollar.

Geospatial Optimization

This series of optimal impact values is referred to as a budget-outcome curve (BOC) within the Optima HIV framework and notably tends to be concave (that is, it shows diminishing returns). It reflects the typical asymptotic cost-coverage functions of programs; any initial spending can often have a large impact on controlling an epidemic, but these effects are eroded by smaller benefits for increased spending.

Optimizing a national, regional, or global response to an epidemic can often involve distributing funding not just between interventions but between geographic localizations as well. Standard Optima HIV projects can already handle this situation by cloning populations and programs for geospatial components, which can be sufficient for simple urban–rural or other bilateral splits. The number of different population groups and programs in an aggregate model can quickly become computationally intractable.

If an assumption is made that epidemics are localized and populations do not interact between boundaries, which is reasonable for large scales, it is much simpler to advise on resource allocations. In Optima HIV, this process is called geospatial analysis (GA). It requires every atomic component of the aggregate model to be a standalone project, enabling all standard epidemic and optimization analyses. These analyses are then grouped together as a collection of projects, referred to as a portfolio.

Conceptually the GA algorithm is as follows:

1. Calculate a BOC for each constituent project in the portfolio, estimating the optimal impact attainable within its localized epidemic context for a range of budget values.
2. For a fixed aggregate budget, apply ASD to the BOCs, so as to optimize resource distribution between projects and minimize the sum of outcomes across all of the components.

The theoretical simplicity of the algorithm belies the numerical complexity involved, with GA existing as the most computationally strenuous feature within the Optima toolkit. Given that many BOCs need to be generated, depending on the number of projects within a portfolio, the BOCs themselves are typically interpolated across a small number of budget sizes, each point requiring a standard optimization to identify. Because the interpolations are estimates in the form of analytic curves, ASD is extremely quick in determining the estimated optimal funding distribution across a portfolio, but reoptimizations are still required to check the validity of the estimates. In practice, multiprocessing is required to produce results in any timely manner.

Map 13.1 shows an example result of applying GA. Not only are resources locally redistributed for greatest effect, Optima can also advise how to move funds between districts, countries, or regions in order to balance marginal impact and best influence epidemics across geographical expanses.

Software Implementation

This section describes the way the Optima HIV model is implemented in practice. Optima HIV uses a wide range of modern software technologies, ranging from scientific modeling packages to web frameworks. These technologies provide the means by which users from a wide variety of backgrounds—from programmers and mathematical modelers to epidemiologists and staff in

Map 13.1   Example of Geospatial Optimization Analysis Applied to Malawi

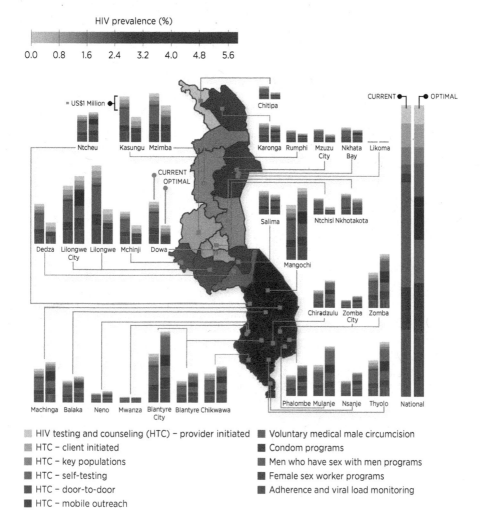

HIV prevalence (%)

0.0   0.8   1.6   2.4   3.2   4.0   4.8   5.6

= US$1 Million

CURRENT ● ● OPTIMAL

Chitipa

Ntcheu   Kasungu   Mzimba

Karonga   Rumphi   Mzuzu City   Nkhata Bay   Likoma

CURRENT ● ● OPTIMAL

Salima   Ntchisi   Nkhotakota

Dedza   Lilongwe City   Lilongwe   Mchinji   Dowa

Mangochi

Chiradzulu   Zomba City   Zomba

Machinga   Balaka   Neno   Mwanza   Blantyre City   Blantyre   Chikwawa

Phalombe   Mulanje   Nsanje   Thyolo   National

▨ HIV testing and counseling (HTC) – provider initiated
▨ HTC – client initiated
■ HTC – key populations
■ HTC – self-testing
■ HTC – door-to-door
■ HTC – mobile outreach

■ Voluntary medical male circumcision
■ Condom programs
■ Men who have sex with men programs
■ Female sex worker programs
■ Adherence and viral load monitoring

Source: World Bank 2018.

ministries of health and monitoring and evaluation units—are able to access Optima HIV's functionality.

Optima HIV comprises (1) a fully self-contained Python software package, including epidemic, programmatic, optimization, graphics, and other components; and (2) a web application (web app) that forms a wrapper around the Python module.

Structure of the Python Module

Optima HIV is written as a "module" that can be imported using the Python programming language. The structure of the code largely reflects the structure of the framework described above. The Optima HIV module can be thought of roughly as consisting of three major workflows: a project workflow, the simulation workflow, and the geospatial workflow, as shown in figure 13.5. The "project workflow" includes the key components of an Optima HIV analysis—beginning with the creation of a project, which is a Python class containing all other components (that is, attributes and methods) required for an Optima HIV analysis. It includes epidemiological data, model inputs, definitions of programs and cost functions, and specifications of scenarios and optimizations. Within the project workflow is the "simulation workflow," which consists of the steps required to

Figure 13.5   Structure of the Optima HIV Workflow Implemented in the Python Programming Language

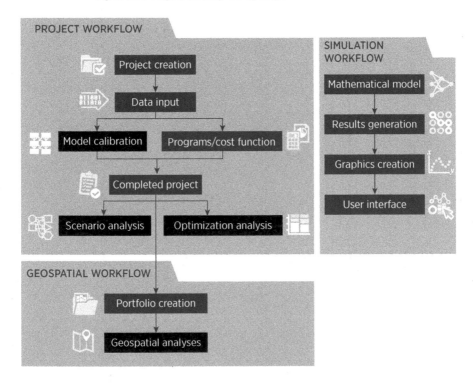

Source: World Bank.

Note: Boxes in black show the stages of the workflow that require the mathematical model to be run.

generate results—including the mathematical model that is the core of Optima HIV. Finally, multiple projects can be gathered into a "portfolio" that allows GAs to be performed. In addition to the custom classes and functions described here, Optima HIV relies on a number of other Python modules, including "NumPy" (for all numerical computations), "Matplotlib" (for graphics), "multiprocessing" (for parallel processing), and several other specific modules. All required modules are freely available and come bundled with standard scientific Python distributions (for example, Anaconda Python).

The creation of a project begins with the specification of the population groups included in the analysis. These groups typically include several low-risk or general population groups (for example, females aged 25–29 years) and several key or high-risk populations (for example, people who inject drugs). Optima HIV is completely flexible in terms of which populations are defined; it theoretically has no limit to the number of different population groups that can be defined, although in practice projects become difficult to calibrate and optimize with more than approximately 30 populations.

Once the populations are defined, Optima HIV creates a (mostly) empty Excel spreadsheet template for the user to enter data into. (This step occurs after the creation of the project and the definition of the populations, because most data are entered by population.) The input data include demographics, namely the size of each population (which, for key populations lacking good time trend data, are interpolated over time on the basis of the trends in the size of the low-risk population from the United Nations Population Division); HIV prevalence (which, together with the population sizes, defines the burden of disease for each population group); other epidemiological indicators (including sexually transmitted infection [STI] prevalence, tuberculosis prevalence, and background mortality rates for each population); testing and treatment (including the numbers of people on ART and prevention of mother-to-child transmission, HIV testing rates, and rates of PrEP, plus information on birth rates and breastfeeding required to calculate prevention of mother-to-child transmission impacts); optional indicators (including estimates of PLHIV, HIV prevalence, deaths, new infections, and other quantities, typically drawn from the Spectrum model); cascade indicators (including the proportion of people with HIV who are aware of their status, on ART, have viral suppression, or are lost to follow-up, and the average number of viral load tests for people in care on ART); sexual behavior (including average numbers of regular, casual, and commercial acts for each population, as well as corresponding condom usage rates, plus circumcision prevalence); injecting behavior (including the average number of injections per year, needle-syringe sharing rates, and the number of people on opioid substitution therapy); partnerships (matrixes specifying the weights with which populations have sexual or injection-related acts with which other populations); transitions (including the average number of years a person spends in each risk-related population group, as well as aging between population groups); and constants (including act- and CD4-related HIV transmissibilities, rates of CD4 progression [when untreated] and recovery [when successfully treated], mortality rates, intervention efficacies, and CD4-related disutilities). Note that these data requirements map onto the inputs of the model, as listed in table 13.1.

Once all input data are defined, they are loaded into the project to create a *parameter* set. The parameter set stores all the information required to run the mathematical model. Each parameter set contains the following (see the list in table 13.1):

- 33 types of time-varying input data—referred to as X_t in equation (13.1) (for example, condom usage rates)
- 59 types of time-constant input data (for example, condom efficacy)
- 2 fitted parameters—referred to as θ in equation (13.1)
- 20 other inputs—including population names and characteristics

In total, there are 109 different model inputs stored in a parameter set. These are stored in a custom Python object called an "odict" (short for "ordered dictionary"), which was created to support as fully as possible all the functionality of both a Python list and a dictionary; for example, in contrast to Python's built-in ordered dictionary class, the odict class supports retrieval by index as well as by key. Each individual quantity in the parameter set (with the exception of the "other inputs") is also a custom Python class, including attributes defining its limits (for example, [0,1] for a probability, or $[0,10^{10}]$ for a population size), the populations it targets, its prior distribution, and (for time-varying inputs) one or more control points. The control points are pairs, each consisting of a data point (or estimate) and the time at which this data point was observed; for example, the casual condom usage among FSWs might be specified as [(2000, 0.33), (2008, 0.63), (2012, 0.61)], indicating that condom use rose from 33 percent in 2000 to 61 percent in 2012. These data points are then interpolated—typically, using linear interpolation between data points and otherwise employing nearest-neighbor interpolation. These control points are defined using a custom dataframe class, similar to that provided by the "pandas" Python library, but with additional flexibility in terms of adding, removing, or sorting rows and columns.

Programs and cost functions are also specified using custom classes, using the same data structures as model inputs (that is, odicts and dataframes). Each program object stores information on its target populations, the model inputs it affects (for example, condom usage rates), and the cost function—that is, the unit cost and program coverage over time (although, in contrast to the model inputs, only the most recent data point for each is typically used in forward-looking analyses). Coverage-outcome functions are stored separately from programs, because they are defined for outcomes, rather than programs. For example, "HIV testing rate among FSWs" would be an example of an outcome that might be affected by a combination of FSW programs, social and behavior change communication (SBCC) programs, and HIV testing and counseling (HTC) programs. They are specified in terms of the intercept (that is, the value the model input would have in the absence of any interventions), saturation (that is, the maximum attainable value of the model input given full coverage of all programs), and the impact of each program (that is, the value of the model input given full coverage of that program and zero coverage of all other programs). The parameters of the cost functions can be specified as distributions (typically uniform), allowing sensitivity and uncertainty analyses to be conducted.

Scenarios are implemented as a relatively lightweight structure: they simply store the modifications to the model inputs, coverages, or budget as specified by the user (for example, scaling from 60 percent ART coverage in 2015 to 90 percent coverage in 2020). So-called parameter scenarios are used to directly modify items in the model inputs, which can then be used to run the model and thus calculate counterfactuals. Coverage scenarios are run by converting them into parameter scenarios via the coverage-outcome functions; similarly, budget scenarios are converted to coverage scenarios via the cost functions. Thus, all three types of scenarios operate by modifying the values of the inputs that are used to run the model—either directly in the case of parameter scenarios, with one conversion step for coverage scenarios, or with two conversion steps for budget scenarios.

Optimization objects store information on user-specified objectives and constraints. The objectives include the start and end years for the optimization, and which quantity is being optimized (new HIV infections, AIDS-related deaths, or HIV-related DALYs). Unlike running scenarios, however, running optimizations is a nontrivial task. Because an optimization requires the model to be run many times, it is highly computationally intensive. For this reason, optimizations are typically run in parallel. Although the ASD algorithm described above is iterative and thus cannot be parallelized, multiple ASD runs can be run in parallel. Many parallelization packages for Python exist, but most have strict requirements on the types of functions that can be parallelized. In contrast, the Optima HIV module includes a custom parallelization workflow that allows any function within scope to be parallelized, with arguments passed as standard keyword arguments (in contrast to the comparatively inflexible "pickled tuples" that most other Python parallelization methods require).

Like other Optima HIV objects, results sets are also specified using a custom class. This class stores all key outputs of the model (including HIV prevalence and incidence; numbers of PLHIV, new infections acquired and caused by population group, deaths, and DALYs; percentages of people in each stage of the care cascade; number of cases of mother-to-child transmission; and so on), both overall and for each population in the model. Once generated, custom class methods allow results sets to be easily added (for example, to aggregate different regions) or subtracted (for example, to compare the difference between a business-as-usual and a counterfactual scenario). Results sets can be exported to Excel for further analysis or plotted using the built-in Python graphical user interface (GUI). This Python interface, although designed primarily for internal use, also forms the basis of the online interface. Significant attention has been paid to provide an optimal user experience, including, for example, choosing colors that are optimal for distinguishing different population groups. For 13 or fewer populations, Optima HIV uses ColorBrewer (Harrower and Brewer 2003), which is based on psychometric studies regarding optimal color distinguishability. ColorBrewer is not available, however, for larger numbers of categories. Because some Optima HIV projects use up to 30 populations, a custom method was created for choosing optimally distinguishable colors. This method corresponds to choosing points that are uniformly spaced in the red–green–blue color cube.

Given the considerable complexity of the project, model input, program, scenario, optimization, and results data structures, saving and loading projects is a highly nontrivial task. In addition, because Optima HIV continually evolves to include new functionality, the data structures are not necessarily static. To sidestep the need to specify custom load and save functionality for each custom object, projects are saved as Python "pickles," which include not just the data but also information on the Python object containing the data. Currently, no flexible alternative exists that allows objects to be comprehensively saved and loaded. For example, the popular JSON (JavaScript Object Notation) format does not support mathematical objects like infinity or not-a-number, which can lead to data corruption when saved and reloaded. To handle the situation where Optima HIV versions may differ, every time a Python object specification is modified in the codebase (for example, if attributes are added or removed), a *migration* is created. The migration function compares the version number of the saved project to the current Optima version number and performs any operations necessary to bring the old structure in line with the latest version.

Finally, although Optima HIV features both online and Python graphical interfaces, it has also been designed to be as easy to use as possible via command-line or scripting usage, because this is the most powerful and

Figure 13.6 Example Code Listing for a Simple Optima Analysis

```
1 import optima as op          # Import the Optima module
2 P = op.Project(spreadsheet='Example.xlsx')   # Create the project and load the spreadsheet
3 R = op.defaultprogset()      # Create a default set of programs and cost functions
4 P.addprogset(R)              # Add the program set into the project
5 P.autofit(maxtime=120)       # Automatically calibrate the model
6 P.optimize()                 # Perform the default optimization
7 op.plotresults(P)            # Plot the results of the optimization
```

Source: Optima Consortium for Decision Science.

flexible way of accessing the underlying functionality of the Python code. An example of a simple Optima HIV workflow—creating a project from a data spreadsheet (that has previously been created and populated with data), using default programs, performing an automatic calibration to the data, and running a default optimization—is shown in figure 13.6. In practice, an Optima analysis will require many additional custom steps, but this example illustrates the design principle that "common tasks should be easy tasks."

Structure of the Online Interface

Optima HIV's web application is structured in (roughly) an MVC (model-view-controller) architecture, as shown in figure 13.7. The web interface, which runs in users' web browsers, is the view component and is presently implemented as a JavaScript (AngularJS/Node.js) client. At the other end, the model component is implemented as a Python module as described in the previous section and that can operate completely independently of the web interface. The controller component, which allows communication between the web interface and the backend Python model, is the web session manager, which consists of a Twisted/Flask server and a Celery task manager (both written in Python), along with a database implemented using Postgres and Redis.

The client software that allows the user to run the application from most web browsers (including Firefox, Chrome, Internet Explorer, and Safari) is implemented as a JavaScript single-page application using a blend of Angular (Version 1.2) and Require JS. This application communicates with the Twisted/Flask server through remote procedure calls (RPCs) that pass arguments for the Python functions via HTTP POST request packets, and which in turn receive JSON encodings of returned Python objects in the response packets. These response packets include Matplotlib graphics objects, which are converted to JSON via the MPLD3 Python/JavaScript library, which bridges the gap between Matplotlib graphs generated on the backend and interactive D3.js graphs that are available to the user on the

Figure 13.7 Overview of the Structure of the Optima HIV Online Interface, Web Application

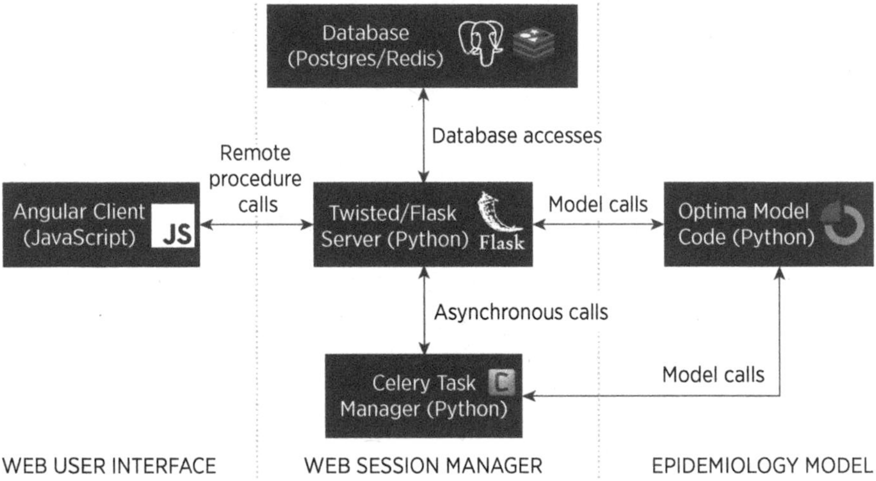

Source: World Bank.

Note: HIV = human immunodeficiency virus.

frontend. An example screenshot of the JavaScript web interface is shown in figure 13.8.

The server software is written in Python and manages web application sessions for users through an application programming interface (API) of RPCs that trigger accesses to the database and calls to the backend code. The Twisted Python framework is used to set up a pool of server threads to allow multiple users to simultaneously log in and use the site. The Flask web application microframework is used to route the requests made by the JavaScript client to targeted backend code calls and database accesses. Currently, this server code (as well as the database and task manager) is hosted on a Dell PowerEdge high-performance computer running Ubuntu Linux; however, Optima HIV is efficient enough to run effectively on most laptops and is compatible with Linux, Windows, and Mac operating systems.

A two-tiered database structure is used to store information about Optima HIV's users, their projects, and the results collected and cached by the web application during user sessions. The first tier is implemented in the PostgreSQL 9.5 relational database management system and includes information on users, projects, and results tables, each of which is associated with a unique identifier (UID) for ease of retrieval. The UIDs for the projects and results tables are used as keys to access the Python object instances in the second-tier storage, which is implemented using a

Figure 13.8 Screenshot of the Optima HIV Web-Based User Interface

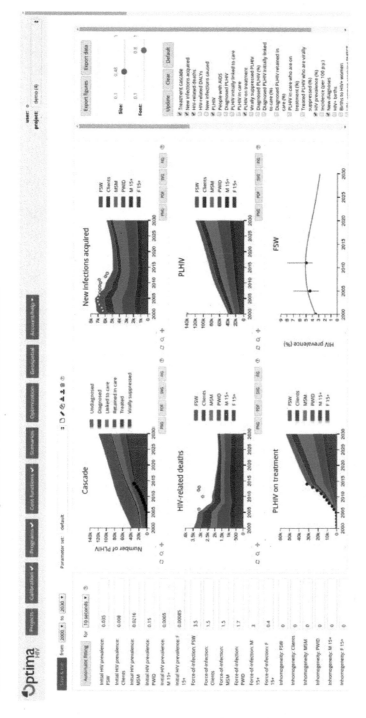

Source: World Bank based on Optima model.

Note: DALY = disability-adjusted life year; F = female; FSW = female sex worker; HIV = human immunodeficiency virus; k = thousand; M = male; MSM = men who have sex with men; PLHIV = people living with HIV; PWID = people who inject drugs.

Redis database. Redis is primarily an in-memory data-storage system, but Optima uses the default regular backup of the database to allow data persistence across user sessions, which offers the advantage of typically faster reading and writing of the Python objects because Redis fetches from and writes to memory, not disk as does a database like Postgres.

To allow some tasks to be executed in parallel via Optima's web application (for example, GAs), another Python server process running in parallel to the main server code processes asynchronous task requests passed in by the Twisted/Flask server using Celery, an open-source distributed task queue system that spawns potentially multiple "worker" processes. The Redis in-memory store is used to mediate the data transfer between the two server and task manager processes.

Summary

Thanks to its adaptability and easy-to-use interface, Optima HIV has been rapidly adopted as an analytical tool by policy makers, international funders, and other stakeholders on a global level across many countries. In turn, the adoption of Optima HIV has spurred further development, because no two countries have exactly the same requirements. For example, applying Optima HIV to Eswatini's generalized epidemic led to the extension of Optima from a simple risk-population-focused model to one that includes a comprehensive demographic model, and applying Optima to Malawi's geographically heterogeneous epidemic was the impetus for the development of geospatial optimization analysis.

Like all models, Optima HIV has several major limitations. First, as discussed previously (Kerr et al. 2015), Optima HIV's main limitation is that the results it produces can only be as good as the data provided (also known as "garbage in, garbage out"). Unfortunately, in many contexts, data—especially on cost functions—are severely limited. Second, Optima's flexibility and adaptability result in an undesirable consequence: irreducible complexity. Put another way, every time the users are given a choice, they will possibly make a poor choice. Optima HIV's ability to flexibly define population groups, for example, allows for the possibility that users will choose population groups that are not sufficiently constrained by the data, leading to poor robustness of the analysis. To balance the competing needs of flexibility and ease of use, Optima HIV comes preloaded with large numbers of defaults (for population groups, programs, and model input values), and it is then up to the user to overwrite them; however, the use of defaults has its own drawback in terms of making the software appear "black-box" to the user. There is no solution to these problems; rather, they should be thought of as competing priorities that need to be balanced, and the precise balance achieved for a given context will depend on both the user's skills and expertise and the complexity of the problem needing to be addressed. For these reasons, although wherever possible the user interface has been made transparent and easy to use, users may still require training in order to take full advantage of Optima HIV's features.

The flexibility of the Optima HIV tool as described in this chapter allows it to be extended to other areas. Critically, the framework for the budget-objective curves described can be flexibly implemented for any context in which DALYs (or another metric of interest) can be defined. This thus leads to the prospect of efficiently performing optimal allocations across diseases (for example, HIV, malaria, and tuberculosis). Our hope is that such a tool will be able to leverage our experiences and software technology into an increasingly beneficial global public good.

References

Baeten J., R. Heffron, L. Kidoguchi, N. Mugo, E. Katabira, E. Bukusi, S. Asiimwe, J. Haberer, D. Donnell, and C. Celum. 2015. "Near Elimination of HIV Transmission in a Demonstration Project of PrEP and ART." Paper presented at the Conference on Retroviruses and Opportunistic Infections (CROI), Seattle, Washington, February 23–26. Abstract number 24.

Brown T., and W. Peerapatanapokin. 2004. "The Asian Epidemic Model: A Process Model for Exploring HIV Policy and Programme Alternatives in Asia." *Sexually Transmitted Infections* 80 (Suppl. 1): i19–i24.

Cohen M. S., Y. Q. Chen, M. McCauley, T. Gamble, M. C. Hosseinipour, N. Kumarasamy, J. G. Hakim, J. Kumwenda, B. Grinsztejn, J. H. S. Pilotto, S. V. Godbole, S. Mehendale, S. Chariyalertsak, B. R. Santos, K. H. Mayer, I. F. Hoffman, S. H. Eshleman, E. Piwowar-Manning, L. Wang, J. Makhema, L. A. Mills, G. de Bruyn, I. Sanne, J. Eron, J. Gallant, D. Havlir, M.D., S. Swindells, H. Ribaudo, Vanessa Elharrar, D. Burns, T. E. Taha, K. Nielsen-Saines, D. Celentano, M. Essex, and T. R. Fleming, for the HPTN 052 Study Team. 2011. "Prevention of HIV-1 Infection with Early Antiretroviral Therapy." *The New England Journal of Medicine* 365 (6): 493–505.

Harrower, M., and C. A. Brewer. 2003. "ColorBrewer.org: An Online Tool for Selecting Colour Schemes for Maps." *The Cartographic Journal* 40 (1): 27–37.

Hastings, W. K. 1970. "Monte Carlo Sampling Methods Using Markov Chains and Their Applications." *Biometrika* 57 (1): 97–109.

Huang X., S. Lodi, Z. Fox, W. Li, A. Phillips, K. Porter, A. Kellher, N. Li, X. Xu, H. Wu, A. M. Johnson, Beijing PRIMO Cohort Study, and CASCADE Collaboration in EuroCoord. 2012. "Rate of CD4 Decline and HIV-RNA Change Following HIV Seroconversion in Men Who Have Sex with Men: A Comparison between the Beijing PRIMO and CASCADE Cohorts." *JAIDS Journal of Acquired Immune Deficiency Syndromes* 62 (4): 441–46.

Hume, D. 1740. *A Treatise of Human Nature.* Oxford: Oxford University Press.

Johnson L., R. Dorrington, T. Rehle, S. Jooste, L. G. Bekker, M. Wallace, L. Meyer, and A. Boulle. 2014. "THEMBISA Version 1.0: A Model for Evaluating the Impact of HIV/AIDS in South Africa." Working Paper, Centre for Infectious Disease Epidemiology and Research, University of Cape Town.

Kerr, C. C., T. Smolinski, S. Dura-Bernal, and D. P. Wilson. Under review. "Optimization by Bayesian Adaptive Locally Linear Stochastic Descent." *PLoS One*. http://scholar.google.com/citations?view_op=view_citation&hl=en&user =TFy7ncUAAAAJ&citation_for_view=TFy7ncUAAAAJ:Ug5p-4gJ2f0C.

Kerr, C. C., R. M. Stuart, R. T. Gray, A. J. Shattock, N. Fraser, C. Benedikt, M. Haacker, M. Berdnikov, A. M. Mahmood, S. A. Jaber, M. Görgens, and D. P. Wilson. 2015. "Optima: A Model for HIV Epidemic Analysis, Program Prioritization, and Resource Optimization." *JAIDS Journal of Acquired Immune Deficiency Syndromes* 69 (3): 365–75.

Lodi S., A. Phillips, G. Touloumi, R. Geskus, L. Meyer, R. Thiébaut, N. Pantazis, J. del Amo, A. M. Johnson, A. Babiker, and K. Porter on behalf of the CASCADE Collaboration in EuroCoord. 2011. "Time from Human Immunodeficiency Virus Seroconversion to Reaching CD4+ Cell Count Thresholds <200, <350, and <500 Cells/mm(3): Assessment of Need Following Changes in Treatment Guidelines." *Clinical Infectious Diseases* 53 (8): 817–25.

Marjoram P., J. Molitor, V. Plagnol, and S. Tavare. 2003. "Markov Chain Monte Carlo without Likelihoods." *Proceedings of the National Academy of Sciences* 100 (26): 15324–28.

Padian, N. S., S. C. Shiboski, S. O. Glass, and E. Vittinghoff. 1997. "Heterosexual Transmission of Human Immunodeficiency Virus (HIV) in Northern California: Results from a Ten-Year Study." *American Journal of Epidemiology* 146 (4): 350–57.

Pilcher, C. D., H.-C. Tien, J. J. Eron, Jr., P. L. Vernazza, S. Y. Leu, P. W. Stewart, L. E. Goh, and M. S. Cohen. 2004. "Brief but Efficient: Acute HIV Infection and the Sexual Transmission of HIV." *Journal of Infectious Diseases* 189 (10): 1785–92.

Schroeder, S. A. 2012. "Incidence, Prevalence, and Hybrid Approaches to Calculating DALYs." *Population Health Metrics* 10 (19).

Stover J., P. Johnson, B. Zaba, M. Zwahlen, F. Dabis, and R. E. Ekpini. 2008. "The Spectrum Projection Package: Improvements in Estimating Mortality, ART Needs, PMTCT Impact and Uncertainty Bounds." *Sexually Transmitted Infections* 84 (Suppl. 1): i24–i30.

Stuart, R. M., C. C. Kerr, H. Haghparast-Bidgoli, J. Estill, L. Grobicki, Z. Baranczuk, L. Prieto, V. Montañez, I. Reporter, R. T. Gray, J. Skordis-Worrall, O. Keiser, N. Cheikh, K. Boonto, S. Osornprasop, F. Lavadenz, C. Benedikt, R. Martin-Hughes, S. A. Hussain, S. L. Kelly, D. J. Kedziora, and D. P. Wilson. 2017. "Getting It Right When Budgets Are Tight: Using Optimal Expansion Pathways to Prioritize Responses to Concentrated and Mixed HIV Epidemics." *PLoS One* 12 (10): e0185077.

UNAIDS (United Nations Joint Programme on HIV/AIDS). 2014. "90-90-90: An Ambitious Treatment Target to Help End the AIDS Epidemic." UNAIDS, Geneva.

World Bank. 2018. "Improving the Allocative Efficiency of Malawi's HIV Response: Findings from a Mathematical Modelling Analysis." World Bank, Washington DC.

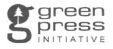